Acute Emergencies and Critical Care of the Geriatric Patient

Acute Emergencies and Critical Care of the Geriatric Patient

edited by

Thomas T. Yoshikawa

Charles R. Drew University of Medicine and Science
Martin Luther King, Jr.–Charles R. Drew Medical Center
Los Angeles, California

Dean C. Norman

VA Greater Los Angeles Healthcare System
Los Angeles, California

MARCEL DEKKER

MARCEL DEKKER, INC. NEW YORK • BASEL

ISBN: 0-8247-0345-6

This book is printed on acid-free paper.

Headquarters
Marcel Dekker, Inc.
270 Madison Avenue, New York, NY 10016
tel: 212-696-9000; fax: 212-685-4540

Eastern Hemisphere Distribution
Marcel Dekker AG
Hutgasse 4, Postfach 812, CH-4001 Basel, Switzerland
tel: 41-61-261-8482; fax: 41-61-261-8896

World Wide Web
http://www.dekker.com

The publisher offers discounts on this book when ordered in bulk quantities. For more information, write to Special Sales/Professional Marketing at the headquarters address above.

Current printing (last digit):
10 9 8 7 6 5 4 3 2 1

PRINTED IN THE UNITED STATES OF AMERICA

To our wives, Catherine Yoshikawa and Jane Norman, and our families, whose patience and support made this book possible.

Preface

The demographic shift toward an aging population is occurring now and will extend over the next 40 years in the United States and the rest of the world. Health care problems of older adults will require the primary attention of most physicians. Certainly, among those health problems of aging persons will be diseases, disorders, and injuries that require acute emergency management and critical care in an inpatient setting. This book focuses on the approach to the diagnosis and treatment of the most commonly encountered medical and surgical acute emergencies and life-threatening conditions in elderly persons. In addition, topics such as drug prescribing in critically ill patients and adverse life-threatening drug reactions, elder abuse, ethics, and nursing care of the critically ill elderly are discussed. The chapters were written by clinicians and researchers nationally recognized in their field of expertise.

There are four major sections. Part I emphasizes the principles of geriatric critical care: the geriatric patient in the emergency department, ethical issues in emergency care, drug dosing and life-threatening drug reactions, and nursing care issues of the critically ill elderly. Part II is devoted to surgical emergencies: emergency preoperative evaluation, emergency anesthesia, traumatic injuries, hip fracture, acute abdomen, and acute vascular emergencies. Part III reviews the major medical emergencies: shock, cardiac emergencies, hypertensive crises, acute respiratory failure, acute renal failure, acid-base and electrolyte imbalance, diabetic ketoacidosis and hyperosmolar hyperglycemia, infectious diseases emergencies, gastrointestinal hemorrhage, neurological emergencies, and psychiatric emergencies. Part IV completes the book with special issues related to aging: acute vision impairment or loss, thermoregulatory disorders (hypothermia, hyperthermia), diagnosis and treatment of elder abuse and neglect, and future direction of acute hospital care of the elderly.

Each chapter presents the latest and most up-to-date approach to diagnosing and treating the acutely and critically ill elderly patient. To provide quick access to information, chapters are concisely written and formatted in a consistent style.

Current and other relevant references are provided so that the reader may pursue additional information or refer to the original data or study.

This book is essential reading for health care providers who manage elderly patients, i.e., primary care physicians, geriatricians, emergency physicians, intensivists/hospitalists, surgeons, anesthesiologists, and critical care and emergency nursing staff, as well as pharmacists. The information contained in these chapters will increase the awareness of clinicians and their capacity to more rapidly diagnose acute emergencies and life-threatening conditions, as well as institute lifesaving interventions and/or seek appropriate specialty consultations. Ultimately, our goals are to reduce pain and suffering and improve the quality of life of all older people. We hope that this book will contribute to these goals.

We thank Patricia Thompson for typing the manuscripts. We are also grateful to the authors for their willingness to contribute to this book and to Russell Dekker for his belief in and support of this project.

Thomas T. Yoshikawa
Dean C. Norman

Contents

Contributors

Adebenga Adetola, M.D. Department of Internal Medicine, Charles R. Drew University of Medicine and Science, and Martin Luther King, Jr.–Charles R. Drew Medical Center, Los Angeles, California

Abbasi J. Akhtar, M.D., M.R.C.P. Department of Internal Medicine, Charles R. Drew University of Medicine and Science, and Martin Luther King, Jr.–Charles R. Drew Medical Center, Los Angeles, California

Sharon Anita Ashley, M.D. Department of Anesthesiology, Charles R. Drew University of Medicine and Science, and Martin Luther King, Jr.–Charles R. Drew Medical Center, Los Angeles, California

Merlyn M. Asuncion, M.D. Department of Internal Medicine, Charles R. Drew University of Medicine and Science, and Martin Luther King, Jr.–Charles R. Drew Medical Center, Los Angeles, California

J. Dennis Baker, M.D. Department of Surgery, UCLA School of Medicine, Los Angeles, California

Melissa M. Bottrell, M.P.H. Division of Nursing, New York University, New York, New York

Earl Warren Brien, M.D. Department of Orthopaedic Surgery, Orthopaedic Hospital, Los Angeles, California

Elizabeth L. Cobbs, M.D. Departments of Health Care Sciences and Medicine, The George Washington University Medical Center, Washington, D.C.

L. Jaime Fitten, M.D. Department of Psychiatry and Biobehavioral Sciences, UCLA School of Medicine, Los Angeles, and Department of Veterans Affairs Medical Center, Sepulveda, California

Ellen Flaherty, R.N., G.N.P. Gitt Resource Center, Yorktown Heights, New York

Arthur W. Fleming, M.D., F.A.C.S. Department of Surgery, Charles R. Drew University of Medicine and Science, and Martin Luther King, Jr.–Charles R. Drew Medical Center, Los Angeles, California

Kathy Fletcher, R.N., C.S., M.S.N., G.N.P. University of Virginia Health Sciences Center, Charlottesville, Virginia

Charles Wesley Flowers, Jr., M.D., F.A.C.S. Department of Ophthalmology, Charles R. Drew University of Medicine and Science, Martin Luther King, Jr.–Charles R. Drew Medical Center, and Jules Stein Eye Institute, UCLA School of Medicine, Los Angeles, California

Ronald L. Fong, M.D. Department of Medicine, Charles R. Drew University of Medicine and Science, and Martin Luther King, Jr.–Charles R. Drew Medical Center, Los Angeles, California

Terry Fulmer, Ph.D., R.N., F.A.A.N. Division of Nursing, New York University, New York, New York

Jeffrey B. Halter, M.D. Geriatrics Center, University of Michigan, Ann Arbor, Michigan

Robert V. Hogikyan, M.D., M.P.H. Department of Internal Medicine, University of Michigan, Ann Arbor, Michigan

Arnel M. Joaquin, M.D. Department of Internal Medicine, Charles R. Drew University of Medicine and Science, and Martin Luther King, Jr.–Charles R. Drew Medical Center, Los Angeles, California

Calvin Johnson, M.D. Department of Anesthesiology, Charles R. Drew University of Medicine and Science, and Martin Luther King, Jr.–Charles R. Drew Medical Center, Los Angeles, California

Vidya S. Kaushik, M.D., D.M., F.A.C.C. Department of Internal Medicine, Charles R. Drew University of Medicine and Science, and Martin Luther King, Jr.–Charles R. Drew Medical Center, Los Angeles, California

Anthony Kingsley, M.D. Department of Internal Medicine, Charles R. Drew University of Medicine and Science, and Martin Luther King, Jr.–Charles R. Drew Medical Center, Los Angeles, California

Jo E. Linder, M.D. Department of Emergency Medicine, Charles R. Drew University of Medicine and Science, and Martin Luther King, Jr.–Charles R. Drew Medical Center, Los Angeles, California

Edward H. Livingston, M.D., F.A.C.S. Department of Surgery, VA Greater Los Angeles Healthcare System, and Department of Surgery, UCLA School of Medicine, Los Angeles, California

William T. Long, M.D. Department of Surgery, Charles R. Drew University of Medicine and Science, and Martin Luther King, Jr.–Charles R. Drew Medical Center, Los Angeles, California

Joanne Lynn, M.D., M.S., M.A. Center to Improve Care of the Dying, The George Washington University Medical Center, Washington, D.C.

Michael E. Mahler, M.D. Department of Neurology, UCLA School of Medicine, Los Angeles, California

Glenville A. March, Jr., M.D. Department of Ophthalmology, Charles R. Drew University of Medicine and Science, Martin Luther King, Jr.–Charles R. Drew Medical Center, and Jules Stein Eye Institute, UCLA School of Medicine, Los Angeles, California

Mathy Mezey, Ed.D., R.N., F.A.A.N. Division of Nursing, New York University, New York, New York

Deborah Moran, M.D. Medical Service, Department of Veterans Affairs Medical Center, Brooklyn, New York

Keith C. Norris, M.D. Department of Medicine, Charles R. Drew University of Medicine and Science, Martin Luther King, Jr.–Charles R. Drew Medical Center, and UCLA School of Medicine, Los Angeles, California

Robert M. Palmer, M.D., M.P.H. General Internal Medicine, The Cleveland Clinic Foundation, Cleveland, Ohio

Indu Poornima, M.D. Department of Cardiology, Medical College of Wisconsin, Milwaukee, Wisconsin

Indumathi Raghavan, M.D. Department of Psychiatry and Biobehavioral Sciences, UCLA School of Medicine, Los Angeles, and Department of Veterans Affairs Medical Center, Sepulveda, California

Shobita Rajagopalan, M.D., F.A.C.P. Department of Internal Medicine, Charles R. Drew University of Medicine and Science, and Martin Luther King, Jr.–Charles R. Drew Medical Center, Los Angeles, California

Jay P. Rho, Pharm.D. Department of Clinical Pharmacy, University of Southern California School of Pharmacy, Los Angeles, California

Stephen N. Steen, Sc.D., M.D. Department of Anesthesiology, Charles R. Drew University of Medicine and Science, and Martin Luther King, Jr.–Charles R. Drew Medical Center, Los Angeles, California

Darryl Y. Sue, M.D. Department of Medicine, Harbor–UCLA Medical Center, and UCLA School of Medicine, Torrance, California

Donald D. Tresch, M.D., F.A.C.C. Departments of Cardiology and Geriatrics, Medical College of Wisconsin, Milwaukee, Wisconsin

David Vo, M.D. Department of Surgery, UCI Medical Center, Orange, California

Samuel Eric Wilson, M.D., F.A.C.S. Department of Surgery, UCI Medical Center, Orange, California

Frances S. Wong, Pharm.D. Department of Clinical Pharmacy, University of Southern California School of Pharmacy, Los Angeles, California

Cheryl E. Woodson, M.D. Ingalls Health System, Harvey, Illinois

Dean T. Yamaguchi, M.D., Ph.D. Geriatric Research, Education, and Clinical Center, VA Greater Los Angeles Healthcare System, and UCLA School of Medicine, Los Angeles, California

1

Relevance of Aging Issues in the Emergency Department

Anthony Kingsley
Charles R. Drew University of Medicine and Science, and Martin Luther King, Jr.–Charles R. Drew Medical Center, Los Angeles, California

I. CLINICAL RELEVANCE

A. Epidemiology

1. Demographics

Emergency departments (EDs) throughout the country will be receiving and managing enormous numbers of older patients over the next 30 years. The older adult population is rapidly increasing throughout the world. It is anticipated that the population of people 60 years and older will increase by 60% in developed countries and by almost 160% in less developed regions over the next 30 years (1). In the United States, the current elderly population of 33 million (13%) will nearly double to 65 million (25%) by 2020 (2). More importantly, the most vulnerable elderly population (i.e., those who are 80 years and older) will be disproportionately increasing more rapidly than younger elderly persons.

The increase in life expectancy for both males and females has contributed largely to the expanding elderly population. At the turn of the twentieth century, the average life expectancies for a male and female child at birth were approximately 46 and 48 years, respectively. Within approximately 100 years, the life expectancies at birth have increased nearly 30 years for both genders (72 and 79 years for males and females, respectively) (3). Life expectancy at age 65 years has also improved modestly during this past century—the average male and female at age 65 can expect to live another 15 and 19 years, respectively (3). Women continue to outnumber men in all older age categories. Elderly women are more likely to be widowed than elderly men, which may have an impact on the use of the ED for health care. Studies have suggested that those who live alone without adequate social support and an immediate source of help (i.e., the single, widowed, or divorced) are more likely to visit the ED (4).

B. Mortality and Morbidity

With a rising number and proportion of the total population being 65 years of age and older, it is not surprising that the elderly account for most deaths in the United States. Table 1 summarizes the total number of deaths in the United States in 1993 by age categories; nearly three-quarters of all deaths occurred in the elderly (5). In contrast, in 1900 only one-quarter of deaths occurred in persons aged 65 and older (6). Many of these deaths will occur outside a health care system; however, a substantial proportion of deaths or near deaths of older patients will occur in the ED.

On the basis of data of causes of death by age groups (Table 2), it is anticipated that the type of emergency services (excluding ED care for routine medical problems) sought by younger patients versus the elderly would be different. Whereas younger adults requiring emergency services are primarily for trauma and surgery, the elderly come to the ED seeking care for medical illnesses that most often require admission to the hospital (7). The most common causes of death in persons 65 and older are found in Table 3 (5). Thus, it is expected that the most serious and life-threatening problems encountered by older patients are often related to cardiac disorders, cancer and its complications, stroke and delirium, pulmonary diseases, infectious diseases, trauma and injuries (e.g., falls), kidney failure and its complications, and diabetic and vascular-related disorders.

Table 1 Number of Deaths By Age Categories in the United States, 1993

Age category (yr)	Total deaths (% of total)	
Under 1	33,466	(1.5)
1–4	7066	(0.3)
5–14	8658	(0.4)
15–24	35,483	(1.6)
25–44	155,683	(6.9)
45–64	373,393	(16.5)
65 and older	1,664,294	(72.8)
TOTAL	2,368,045	(100)

Source: Ref. 5.

Table 2 Top Three Causes of Death by Age Categories in the United States, 1993

Age category (yr)	Causes of death in rank order
1–4	Unintentional injuries
	Congenital anomalies
	Malignant neoplasms
5–14	Unintentional injuries
	Malignant neoplasms
	Homicide and legal intervention
15–24	Unintentional injuries
	Homicide and legal intervention
	Suicide
25–44	Unintentional injuries
	Human immunodeficiency virus infection
	Malignant neoplasms
45–64	Malignant neoplasms
	Diseases of heart
	Cerebrovascular diseases
65 and older	Diseases of heart
	Malignant neoplasms
	Cerebrovascular diseases

Source: Ref. 5.

Table 3 Most Common Causes of Death in Persons Aged 65 and Older in the United States, 1993

Causes	No. of deaths (% of total)	
Diseases of heart	619,755	(37.5)
Malignant neoplasms	371,549	(22.5)
Cerebrovascular diseases	131,551	(7.9)
Chronic obstructive pulmonary disease	86,425	(5.2)
Pneumonia and influenza	73,853	(4.5)
Diabetes mellitus	40,502	(2.4)
Unintentional injuries	27,784	(1.7)
Nephritis, nephrotic syndrome, and nephrosis	19,743	(1.2)
Septicemia	16,846	(1.0)
Atherosclerosis	16,460	(1.0)
Others	249,826	(15.1)
TOTAL	1,654,294	(100)

Source: Ref. 5.

Table 4 Most Common Chronic Conditions in Persons Aged 65 Years and Older by Race in the United States, 1993

Condition	White (%)	Black (%)
Arthritis	48.3	61.4
Hypertension	34.2	40.1
Hearing impairment	32.9	19.0
Heart disease	31.5	21.7
Orthopedic impairment	17.6	23.2
Chronic sinusitis	15.2	20.0
Cataracts	15.2	16.2
Diabetes mellitus	9.8	16.2
Visual impairment	9.7	9.5

Source: Ref. 2.

These are the predominant health problems in elderly patients seen in the ED. (Major discussions of these and other emergency medical problems are reviewed in the remaining sections of this book.)

In addition to diseases leading to death, elderly patients have numerous chronic diseases or disorders that either are exacerbated as acute diseases—many of which can be life threatening—or manifest with secondary complications (e.g., osteoarthritis complicated by septic joint infection or ischemic heart disease seen with pulmonary edema). Thus, older patients may enter the ED with an acute illness or life-threatening condition, which may be related to a more chronic underlying condition. It is imperative that ED physicians be aware of these common chronic conditions (Table 4) because the selection of diagnostic procedures and therapeutic interventions will be greatly influenced by the presence of such underlying problems (2).

II. FACTORS THAT HAVE AN IMPACT ON DIAGNOSIS AND TREATMENT

A. Aging Versus Clinical Disease

With aging, a variety of physiological and anatomical changes occur. It is beyond the scope of this chapter to describe the myriad of age-related changes. However, all clinicians who provide care for the elderly must be aware and knowledgeable of these changes to determine what is disease versus a normal process of aging. Too often, symptoms and signs of a serious disorder are overlooked by both the elderly patient and physician because these complaints are attributed to "old age" (e.g., low hemoglobin is not due to aging and requires investigation). Conversely, diagnostic and therapeutic interventions may be avoided in circumstances in which clinical findings are consistent with physiological aging rather than active disease (e.g., mild decline in creatinine clearance). Moreover, a clear understanding of the important physiological changes of aging will allow the ED physician to determine drug doses more appropriately (e.g., age-related decline in renal function); avoid drugs that might worsen aging changes (e.g., aminoglycosides affecting renal function and hearing); and limit prescribing medications that have an adverse impact on cognitive function, balance, bowel habits, urination, sleep, taste, vision, and hearing—all of which can be adversely affected by aging.

B. Polypharmacy

With the numerous medical problems associated with aging, it is not surprising that elderly patients are prescribed an inordinate number of drugs. The elderly population receive nearly one-third of all prescription drugs in the United States (8). It is critical that the initial evaluation of an elderly patient in the ED include a complete and thorough inventory of all medications—prescription and over the counter. Not infrequently an initial complaint may be caused by an adverse drug reaction (e.g., delirium or acute confusion) rather than by a pathological disease process. Thus, a drug reaction or side effect should always be considered in the differential diagnosis of an acute change in an older adult. In addition, before drug therapy is initiated, a careful assessment of current medications will minimize unnecessary duplication of drugs with similar actions, avoid drug-drug interactions, and reduce potential adverse drug reactions. (See also Chapter 3.)

C. Presentation of Illness in Elderly Persons

The clinical presentation of illness in elderly persons may be influenced by several factors. Older patients not infrequently underreport symptoms associated with serious illnesses. As stated earlier, many times older persons will attribute certain symptoms to "old age" or believe that morbidity and functional incapacities are part of "growing old" (9). Consequently, diseases may be in the advanced stage when the patient appears in the ED. In addition, the ED physician may have to be vigilant in eliciting symptoms from the elderly patient to reach a proper differential diagnosis.

Manifestations of serious illnesses may be atypical, attenuated, or absent in elderly patients (9). As examples, fever may be absent in older patients with sepsis (10), acute myocardial infarction may have minimal to no chest pain (see Chapter 12), or hyperthyroidism may not demonstrate typical hyperadrenergic symptoms ("apathetic" thyrotoxicosis) (11). Thus, it is important for the ED staff not to ignore a seriously ill older patient or dismiss a particular diagnosis because of the absence of typical symptoms. When subtle or other clinical clues suggest a serious illness despite lack of specific findings, the ED physician must be prepared to perform further diagnostic studies to ensure that a major illness has been excluded.

The presence or accumulation of multiple coexisting chronic disorders may mask or confound the clinical presentation of another acute disorder. As examples, chronic obstructive lung disease may mask an underlying bronchogenic carcinoma; degenerative osteoarthritis of the spine may confound the symptoms of a compression fracture related to multiple myeloma; or a chronic depression may cause a physician to overlook a developing dementia.

D. Functional Status

It is important to realize that for most older persons functional independence is the most important goal in their everyday life. Although the traditional approach of medicine (i.e., making a specific diagnosis to allow specific therapeutic intervention(s) to relieve symptoms and improve health) is appropriate in managing older patients, it is the impact of these diseases on functional capacity that is the critical determinant of the health and well-being of the elderly patient. Even though a disease may have been eliminated or adequately treated, if the older patient's functional capacity continues to remain unimproved, the management of the patient is deemed unsuccessful. Thus, not only should specific symptoms and signs be determined in the evaluation of the elderly sick patient, *but how the functional capacity of the patient has been disturbed by the illness* should be assessed. Often the patient's functional capacity may have deteriorated from a disease long before the illness progresses to an acute emergency. The ultimate therapeutic goal is to restore the older patient's functional status to the premorbid level.

If the patient or family is able to provide an accurate assessment of the patient's function before the acute event, this information should be recorded in the chart. The basic activities of daily living (BADLs) are skills that allow a person to perform functions for self-care: eating, dressing, bathing, toileting, continence, and transferring (some also include ambulation). Disturbances or deterioration of BADLs generally indicate the presence of a major underlying disorder. However, normal or unchanged BADLs do not exclude an active acute problem—BADLs are more specific than sensitive as parameters of function. Intermediate or instrumental activities of daily living (IADLs) assess the persons capacity to maintain an independent household (shopping, driving or using public transportation, using the telephone, meal preparation, housework, laundry, handling finances, and taking medications). Changes in the older person's IADLs may be seen earlier in the course of an acute or subacute illness compared with BADLs. Advanced activities of daily living (AADLs) assess the person's ability to fulfill roles in the occupation, as a family person, or in the community or society in general (12). AADLs will vary for each person and assessment will have to be individualized.

A screening evaluation of the older patient's cognitive status is also important and can be done by checking for orientation (time, place, person), recall of three items in 1 minute (e.g., select three items, have the patient name these, and then ask the patient to recall all items 1 minute later), serial seven test (subtracting 7 from 100 five times), and attention span (''A'' test: a random calling out of the alphabet is performed interspersed with the letter ''A,'' and the patient is asked to acknowledge whenever the letter ''A'' is noted) (12).

III. THE ACUTELY ILL OR SEVERELY INJURED ELDERLY PATIENT

Elderly patients who arrive in the ED with a severe injury, in a comatose state, in cardiovascular or respiratory compromise, or with other life-threatening conditions should be immediately managed as described in the appropriate chapters in this book. It is beyond the scope of this chapter (and it would be redundant) for the author to review the various diagnostic and therapeutic interventions for the major emergencies involving the elderly. However, it would be useful to highlight and repeat some key points described in this chapter and others throughout this book.

Age alone is not a contraindication for diagnostic and therapeutic interventions. Age is generally one of several factors in determining risks and benefits for a given diagnostic procedure or treatment. Thus, initial evaluation and therapy in the ED should not be determined solely on the basis of a patient's age.

However, if an elderly patient has an advance directive, this document should be reviewed by the ED physician after stabilization of the patient and before further interventions are pursued. In some instances, an advance directive may indicate the withholding of cardiopulmonary resuscitation, intubation, ventilators, or other ''heroic'' measures.

An assessment of the functional status of the patient before the current presenting acute event is important. This will serve as a reference point for the impact of the acute event on the patient, as well as the short-term or chronic success of therapy. If the elderly patient required a support system, it is essential to identify who provided this support and where the patient resides (home, residential care, long-term care facility). Successful discharge planning from the ED (or hospital) will be facilitated by a clear knowledge of the patient's premorbid functional capacity and existing support system.

A careful survey of all medications taken by the patient should be performed on all elderly patients. Issues of compliance, over-the-counter drugs, and potential adverse drug reactions should be reviewed. If a new drug regimen is to be initiated in the ED, the clinician should avoid drug redundancy (prescribing drugs of similar class and actions), excessive doses, and prolonged administration without monitoring. Be aware that any clinical symptom can be caused by a drug or be due to an adverse drug reaction. Reducing the number of drugs taken by an elderly patient without compromising their care and health on discharge from the ED is a highly desirable outcome and should be a goal of all physicians.

Many elderly patients will be transferred from a long-term care facility to the ED because of an acute change in their status or development of clinical findings of an acute process. The most common reasons nursing home residents are transferred to an ED are fever and infections, congestive heart failure, respiratory distress, injuries, delirium and altered consciousness, and gastrointestinal problems (13,14). Conversely, elderly patients may be brought to the ED by a family member or significant other who can no longer provide care at home and wishes to have the patient admitted to the hospital or long-term care facility.

Psychiatric problems or abnormal behavior in the elderly will often prompt the family or significant other to bring the elder to the ED. It is important that in the initial assessment of the patient potential medical conditions or medications be excluded as cause of the behavior pattern (e.g., acute delirium or confusion caused by pneumonia or by a medication). (See also Chapter 21.)

A multidisciplinary approach to an acutely ill elderly patient will facilitate optimal care and rapid and appropriate disposition. Availability or access to a geriatric nurse specialist, geriatrician, geropsychiatrist, or social worker with skills in gerontology will add immensely to the ED staff's capacity and ability to provide the highest and most appropriate levels of care to elderly patients.

IV. CONCLUSION

The ED physician will most often be the first health provider to encounter the elderly patient who seeks medical care or who needs immediate atteniton to a life-threatening condition or injury. An in-depth understanding and knowledge of the principles of aging, diseases of the elderly, unique features of disease presentation and manifestations in the older patient, and special precautions of diagnosis and treatment will greatly ensure that elderly patients will receive quality care, as well as services, with dignity and compassion.

REFERENCES

1. U.S. Department of Commerce, Economics and Statistics Administration, Bureau of Census. Global Aging—Comparative Indicators and Future Trends. September 1991.
2. Jackson S. The epidemiology of aging. In: Hazzard WR, Blass JP, Ettinger Jr W, Halter JB, Ouslander JG, eds. Principles of Geriatric Medicine and Gerontology, 4th ed. New York: McGraw-Hill, 1999, pp. 203–225.
3. National Center for Health Statistics. Life expectancy at birth, at age 65 and at 75 years of age, according to race and sex: United States, selected years 1900–1994. Health United States 1995, DHHS Pub. No. (PHS) 96-1232, Hyattsville, Maryland, 1996, p. 109.
4. Dove AF, Dave SA. Elderly patients in the accident department and their problems. BMJ 292:807–809, 1986.
5. National Center for Health Statistics. Leading causes of death and number of deaths according to age: United States, 1980 and 1993. Health United States 1995, DHHS Pub. No. (PHS) 96-1232, Hyattsville, Maryland, 1996, p. 117.
6. Castillo PA, Pousada L. Emergency services use by elderly individuals. Clin Geriatr Med 9:491–497, 1993.
7. Ettinger WH, Casani JA, Coon PJ. Patterns of use of the emergency department by elderly patients. J Gerontol 42:638–642, 1987.
8. Health Care Financing Administration Office of National Cost Estimates. National health expenditures, 1988. Health Care Financing Rev 11:1–6, 1990.
9. Williams ME. Approach to managing the elderly patient. In: Hazzard WR, Blass JP, Ettinger Jr W, Halter JB, Ouslander JG, eds. Principles of Geriatric Medicine and Gerontology, 4th ed. New York: McGraw-Hill, 1999, pp. 249–253.
10. Yoshikawa TT, Norman DC. Fever in the elderly. Infect Med 15:704–708, 1998.
11. Cohen JL. Thyroid disorders. In: Yoshikawa TT, Cobbs EL, Brummel-Smith K, eds. Practical Ambulatory Geriatrics, 2nd ed. St. Louis: Mosby–Year Book, 1998, pp. 384–395.
12. Reuben DB. Comprehensive assessment in the office. In: Yoshikawa TT, Cobbs EL, Brummel-Smith K, eds. Practical Ambulatory Geriatrics, 2nd ed. St. Louis: Mosby–Year Book, 1998, pp. 85–105.
13. Gordon WZ, Kane RL, Rothenberg R. Acute hospitalization in a home for the aged. J Am Geriatr Soc 33:519–523, 1985.
14. Tresch DD, Simpson Jr WM, Burton JR. Relationship of long-term and acute-care facilities. The problem of patient transfer and continuity of care. J Am Geriatr Soc 33:819–826, 1985.

2

Ethics in Emergency Care of Critically Ill Patients

Elizabeth L. Cobbs and Joanne Lynn
The George Washington University Medical Center, Washington, D.C.

"The ethics of care, then, both elevates care to a central value in human life and recognizes that care requires a complicated process of judgment. People need to make moral judgments, political judgments, technical judgments, and psychological judgments in their everyday caring activities. Caring, then, is neither simple nor banal; it requires know-how and judgments, and to make such judgments as well as possible becomes the moral task of engaging in care. In general, care judgments require that those involved understand the complexity of the process in which they are enmeshed" (1).

Ethical issues are pervasive in geriatric medicine, but perhaps nowhere are they seen in such intensity as in the emergency setting, where information and time are often in short supply and the outcomes are potentially dramatic. Ethical standards are useful to physicians as principles to guide decision making for individual patients but also to foster ongoing efforts that enrich systems of care that improve health outcomes for elderly persons.

I. CLINICAL RELEVANCE AND CLINICAL SITUATIONS

A. Goals of Care

Over the past 15 years, a Presidential Commission (2), a series of court rulings, and multiple other writings have contended that decisions about medical treatment should reflect the informed preferences of individual patients and the expected outcomes of alternative treatments. When an ill older patient seeks medical attention and the happy discovery is that cure can be easily achieved with little risk or burden to the patient, the goal of care is usually simply to cure the patient. What is more frequently the case, however, is that the ill older patient has more than one medical problem, challenging diagnostic dilemmas and treatment choices with significant risks and burdens.

Older patients who seek emergency care do so for a variety of reasons. Like other age groups, older persons seek emergency services when they are acutely ill or injured. In addition to acute illness, older adults may also be brought to the emergency department by caregivers or family members because of functional decline and other complications of chronic progressive illness. A functional decline sometimes signals a major new medical problem, but usually it just heralds the expected progression of chronic disability.

Emergency physicians cannot find time to address problems and concerns beyond the urgent reason for the visit. Admitting these patients to the hospital might allow problems to be identified and addressed comprehensively. Patients who go home from the emergency department, however, are likely to have no comprehensive evaluation and care plan (3). Repeatedly patching up acute problems without having a comprehensive plan of care is virtually certain to yield inadequate and incoherent treatment, marked by vague and conflicting goals of care.

The identification of goals of care is key to the practice of geriatric medicine, but no one can discuss prospects and values when urgent action is needed to stabilize a critically ill elderly patient. Seriously ill elderly patients frequently cannot provide accurate information about medical history or personal values. Despite shortages of information and direction, emergency care providers are expected to make important and immediate decisions about the treatment and disposition of these patients. Under these circumstances, it is certain that errors will occur, and that most will be errors of having tried to restore physiology or to rescue from imminent death. One important question, therefore, is whether care systems can reduce the rate and seriousness of such errors.

Emergency physicians must quickly gather all possible information about the patient's past medical history, current illness, and preferences for care to make the best possible short-term plan for caring for the patient. The irreversibility of forgoing treatment makes it obviously justifiable to treat to stabilize the patient's medical condition while awaiting important information about the patient's past condition and advance directives. Later on, treatment plans can be implemented in accord with better defined goals of care. For example, endotracheal intubation and ventilator support may be used early on to stabilize the medical condition of an acutely ill patient. Later, as the full scope of diagnosis and prognosis becomes clear, the family or surrogate may decide with the health care team that further life-sustaining treatment is not in keeping with the overall goals of the patient. Ventilator support would then be discontinued, and other treatments would be developed in accord with a recognition that goals of care are properly focused on achieving comfort.

Thus, one strategy for managing the problem of ambiguous information and a shortage of time is to do all one can to rescue the sick person long enough to allow more well-informed decisions. To use this course, the emergency personnel must work in a care system in which they can rely on others (e.g., in the intensive care unit) to be willing to stop life-supporting treatment that proves to be useless or harmful (from the patient's perspective).

A second strategy is to reduce the rate of inadequate information available in the emergency setting. Most elderly persons who are seen for emergency care have been sick. Plans could be made for exacerbations, complications, and life-threatening situations. Those plans could be immediately available to emergency care providers. In La Crosse, Wisconsin, more than eight patients in every 10 who die have written advance directives, usually rather specific and established, on average, a year before death (4). As a result, 98% of decedents had a deliberate forgoing of a life-extending treatment. Emergency care personnel cannot accomplish this on their own, but they should know that having a clear and available plan for an emergency situation is an effective strategy for avoiding having to treat just because the goals of care are ambiguous.

Physicians desire to do what is best for the patient, but defining what is ''best'' requires time, information, and communication with the patient and significant others—elements that may not readily be available in the emergency setting. When the patient is quite elderly or quite ill, the usual landmarks of patient welfare are in doubt. No substitute exists for knowing what the patient and family value and for having plans that reflect those judgments.

B. Provider-Patient Relationship

The ''moral heart'' of medicine is the concern for the welfare of the patient (5). Ill patients depend on their physicians and must perceive them to be trustworthy. Patients usually seek improvements in their health through relationships with physicians; however, for emergency cases, the patient (and family) must trust a health care system. Emergency department physicians must seek to ensure a climate of trust and to quickly engender a collaborative and understanding relationship with their patients. No expectation exists that this relationship will endure into the future, yet it can be quite intense and satisfying.

One threat to perceived trustworthiness is the physician's inability to promise to focus on the specific patient's concerns and challenges. The ability of the physician to devote time and energy to individual patients is influenced by the sum of events occurring in the department. Critically injured persons with as yet unknown diagnoses and prognoses arrive without warning, interrupting the process of delivering care to patients who are already present. Often patients and families must have some of this explained and be reassured that delays and multiple providers being involved will eventually be in the best interest of each patient. Obviously, a climate of trust is ordinarily essential if decisions about life-sustaining treatment must be made quickly. In addition, strategies of engaging primary care providers and quickly moving sick patients to other more predictable settings are also helpful.

C. Confidentiality

Americans value privacy highly, and health care professionals must always treat patient information as private and confidential. To share patient information, the practitioner must explicitly seek permission from the patient. In an emergency situation, the concern for confidentiality often competes with other important concerns of the patient (e.g., preservation of life, alleviation of suffering) or the welfare of someone else. Providers may set aside the commitment to confidentiality to promote a higher good, such as saving the patient's life. Telephone communications between physicians to share information about critically ill patients in the emergency room are often carried out. In addition, hospitals may release critically important information to emergency care providers who are seeking to learn more about the patient's condition for purposes of making key decisions. For critically ill older adults, past medical history is likely to be complex and vitally important to make the best possible diagnostic and treatment decisions.

However, practitioners must guard against any unnecessary transmission of patient information that breaches confidentiality. For example, when a critically ill patient is transported by emergency medical personnel, patient information may be transmitted over a radio or portable phone that is easily heard by unauthorized listeners. Providers should transmit only that information vital to the patient's well-being during transport, while reserving additional, but nonessential information for communication in private on arrival in the emergency department. In addition, one must not release information to bystanders or the press.

D. Prognosis

Uncertainty is at the very core of clinical medicine. The heterogeneity and multiplicity of medical problems in older adults make prognostication exceedingly difficult. Age in itself is not a reliable prognostic indicator. As an example, even patients older than 100 can enjoy good outcomes from surgery and anesthesia (6). Patients and families quickly lose trust in the physician who forecasts too definite a prognosis. Under emergency conditions, the physician may communicate with the patient and family effectively by sketching potential futures for the patient. Describing the best and worst likely outcomes serves to construct boundaries as to what can be expected in terms of a recovery. The physician seeks to paint a reasonable picture of what the future may hold, without destroying all hope or falsely inflating the chances for recovery.

By acknowledging and defining the uncertainties that exist, physicians contribute to the dialogue with patients and surrogates to develop patient-centered plans of care. In this context, patients or surrogates share information about the potential outcomes and the relative desirability (to the patient) of the accompanying risks, burdens, and benefits of different treatment options. Sometimes patients and families will flatly decline treatment options when the burdens and risks are too great. Others may agree to a time-limited trial of an intervention, with the condition that the intervention be withdrawn after a period of time if certain benefit is not achieved. In either event, it is more useful to patients and families to be aware of the magnitude of the uncertainty in the prognosis rather than to rely on information that is inaccurate.

Uncertainty is quite uncomfortable for all concerned, even when they all know that it is the best that can be done. Often, it is helpful to patients and family to know the likely time course of the situation coming clear. Families structure their lives around statements like "the next 24 hours will tell us whether he will pull through," or "we are doing some critical tests and should have much more information to talk over with you by midnight." Another clinical strategy to help patients and families with situations of great uncertainty is to help them talk through the "worst case." Often, it helps just to ask "if things don't go well and he seems likely to die, what would be important to do?" Follow-up inquiries as to who else might need to be present and whether any particular religious practices are to be followed are useful for care providers to know and help the patient and family manage the situation in constructive ways.

E. Truth Telling

Truth telling is essential to a sustainable patient-physician relationship, perhaps especially when this entails the acknowledgment of uncertainty. Patients are entitled to honest disclosure about the nature of their condition, treatment options, and prognosis. In the past, physicians at times made decisions not to tell patients that they had cancer (7). One of the most significant bioethical advances in practice today is the emphasis on clinical honesty between patients and physicians (8). Truth telling has a profound consequence for the nature of the physician-patient relationship. With a foundation of trust and honesty, the physician-patient relationship transforms from a paternalistic one toward a true partnership. In this partnership, physicians function as consultants, advocates, and purveyors of knowledge and skill. In the event that a mistake is made, the commitment to truth telling offers the best hope for a patient to understand how the physician could make an error and still be worthy of continued confidence and trust.

F. Informed Consent

Every adult person of sound mind has the right to determine what will be done to his or her body. This right is protected by the process of obtaining informed consent before diagnostic procedures or treatments are administered. Although one might assume that by virtue of the patient's arrival in the emergency department, an inclination toward consenting to treatment has been demonstrated, this is not always the case. Elderly patients may be brought to the emergency department without their consent or against their wishes by families, friends, landlords, or others. In such cases, consent to evaluation and treatment cannot necessarily be assumed.

Informed consent is accomplished when patients who are capable of making decisions receive sufficient information and therapeutic options concerning their condition to allow them to reach a decision in concert with their physicians. The ideal of informed consent cannot often be achieved. At times, for example, informed consent cannot be obtained because a patient arrives in the emergency department critically ill, lacking the ability to communicate about health decisions and having no advance directives or surrogate. In this event, the physician must make the best judgment about tests and treatments given the information available, seeking to err on the side of preserving life until more information becomes available and recognizing that treatments can be withdrawn at some later time. However, reasonable attempts should be made to accomplish informed consent with the patient or surrogate. If the patient lacks the capacity to make health care decisions, the physician should document this carefully and seek to identify a surrogate as soon as possible.

G. Surrogate Decision-Makers

When a patient lacks the capacity to make health care decisions, the physician must turn to a surrogate who tries to decide as the patient would. Surrogate decision makers may be named through a variety of mechanisms. A durable power of attorney names an individual to make health care decisions for the patient in the event that the patient loses the capacity to make health care decisions. The designation of the durable power of attorney is made through the execution of a document by the patient in the presence of two witnesses who are not members of the health care team. The person named as a durable power of attorney is authorized to make health care decisions on behalf of the patient in the event that the patient loses the capacity to make personal health care decisions. The durable power of attorney endures through the time when the patient lacks decisional capacity. This form of surrogate decision-maker designation is often executed by patients who lack close family or choose an individual outside the family to serve as surrogate decision maker. A guardian is a surrogate decision maker who is appointed by a judge when a patient has been deemed incompetent by a court. For example, a guardian of the person is appointed when a patient is judged to lack the capacity to make decisions about personal care. Or, a guardian of finance is a person the court has named to make decisions about the management of the patient's personal finances. The court makes such determinations after reviewing evidence and testimony that show the facts and reasons for the patient's inability to manage vital affairs adequately.

In most states, the patient who is decisionally incapacitated is represented by a surrogate from the following prioritized list: a court-named guardian of the person, a person named by the patient as a durable power of attorney for health care, a spouse, other first-order relatives, and more distant relatives or friends. The attending physician should document his or her decision as to who is appropriately speaking as surrogate and why, especially if it is a controversial choice or is a choice that is not in accord with the usual priorities.

H. Assessing Decision-Making Capacity

In the course of providing emergency care to critically ill patients, physicians must often evaluate patients' capacity to make and communicate health care decisions. The assessment of such capacity is multidimensional but focused on the particular questions at hand.

Certification of decision-making capacity is issue specific. Patients may possess the capacity to make some decisions but not others. For example, a patient may lack the capacity to execute a will or to make detailed arrangements for home care services but retain the capacity to make decisions about personal health care choices. Critically ill geriatric patients commonly manifest changes in sensorium and other aspects of mental status. Delirium is a common finding in ill elderly patients and is likely to affect decision-making capacity. Cognitive abilities of elderly patients may fluctuate considerably when they are acutely ill, dehydrated, malnourished, or in pain. Serial determinations of capacity over time often show improvement as the patient's overall condition is stabilized.

A lack of decision-making capacity should not be inferred from a single incident in which a decision or statement appears irrational. A patient who is frightened, angry, confused, or otherwise distressed is at risk for appearing irrational in a single episode of evaluation. It is the responsibility of the physician to re-evaluate decisional capacity over time, especially once acute stresses have been alleviated for the patient. Consistency of preferences and beliefs over time may be useful to shed light on the patient's capacity to understand the implications of treatment decisions. For example, when an individual has persistently avoided doctors and hospitals and declined medical interventions in the past, refusal of services in the emergency department appears consistent with past patterns of behavior, which supports a decision that the patient has the capacity to make health care decisions.

Assessment tools such as mental status examination and attention testing may be helpful in evaluating decisional capacity, but none of these tools is an adequate substitute for a patient-specific capacity evaluation that is directed at ascertaining the patient's ability to rationally negotiate a particular decision. Under these circumstances, a provider must determine whether the critically ill patient has the capacity to make a decision about the question at hand. (See Table 1.)

Decisional capacity should be addressed in its most specific context. For example, if the question at hand is whether the patient has the capacity to make decisions about emergency surgery, the assessment of capacity should include whether the patient understands the options (surgery, medical therapy), the possible consequences of the various options (cure, death, stroke, bleeding, infection, heart attack), and the risks and burdens of the options and is able to communicate a decision. In the absence of any of these components, the patient is deemed to lack the capacity to make a decision, and a surrogate decision maker should be identified when there is time to do so (9).

I. Advance Directives

Advance care planning by older adults has been increasingly recognized as a highly desirable practice and morally good. Advance directives have been encouraged by health care institutions, professional societies, consumers, policy makers, and the courts as a means to communicate patients' wishes about care near the end of life. The Patient Self Determination Act is a federal mandate that went into effect in December of 1991 and was designed to promote the use of advance directives. (See Table 2.)

Advance directives are documents in which an individual states preferences for health care or names another individual who may make health care decisions

Table 1 Elements of Determining Decisional Capacity

1. Can the patient receive information about the circumstances surrounding the dilemma?
2. Does the patient understand the treatment choices?
3. Does the patient understand the consequences of the various treatment (or nontreatment) alternatives?
4. Can the patient make and communicate a choice?

Source: Mishkin B. Determining the capacity for making health care decisions. In: Billig N, Rabins PV, eds. Issues in Geriatric Psychiatry. Adv Psychosom Med Bawl: Karger, 1989; 19:151–166.

Table 2 Requirements of the Patient Self-Determination Act

1. Participating institutions must provide written information to patients admitted regarding their right to make medical care decisions, including the right to accept or refuse medical or surgical treatment and the right to formulate advance directives according to state law.
2. Written information must be provided at the time of admission about the institution's policies regarding advance directives.
3. Health care providers must document, in each patient's medical record, whether the patient has executed an advance directive.

Source: Cox DM, Sachs GA. Advance directives and the patient self-determination act. In: Sachs GA, Cassel CK, eds. Clinics in Geriatric Medicine, Philadelphia: Saunders, 1994; 10:431–443.

if the individual becomes incapacitated. A living will is an advance directive document in which an individual makes statements about providing or withholding certain medical interventions in the event of terminal illness and incapacity to make health care decisions.

In recent years significant efforts have been undertaken to develop and implement mechanisms that ensure that patients' wishes to have or forego life-sustaining treatments will be observed. In Oregon the ''Physician Orders for Life-Sustaining Treatment'' (POLST) are printed on bright pink paper and have been tested and retested across multiple settings (e.g., the nursing home, the ambulance, and the hospital) (10). It is broadly recognized that a need exists for improved mechanisms to recognize and to communicate patients' wishes regarding limits on life-sustaining treatments. Several states have developed policies that enable emergency medical personnel to accept ''Do Not Resuscitate'' orders for patients who are being transported to the hospital (11).

Because most people who are seriously ill are also chronically ill, most people would benefit from advance care planning, which aims to avert having to make decisions with inadequate information. Persons with heart failure or severe bronchitis, for example, should have plans in place as to how to manage the next exacerbation. Persons who are severely frail and demented should have explicit plans about use of the emergency medical systems (12). Emergency care providers can be powerful advocates for systemwide attention to these issues in primary care, hospital, and long-term care settings.

J. Recommending Treatment

The physician is responsible for articulating the differential diagnosis and treatment options. Emergency physicians must be alert to the presence of other conditions that may affect the patient's situation and outcomes (13). In the development of appropriate treatment recommendations, the importance of unrelated chronic disorders may be of significance because it greatly influences the risks and burdens of treatment options. Practitioners should guard against any tendency to undertreat patients on the basis of age (14).

Treatment recommendation is not difficult when a treatment exists that promises much benefit and little burden or risk to the patient. Such is the case when a recently healthy elderly patient comes to the emergency department ill with a high fever, cough, hypoxemia, and a pulmonic infiltrate on chest x-ray examination. Prompt treatment with intravenous antibiotics and supplemental oxygen would be recommended to the patient as a treatment of great value, little risk, and little burden. Treatment recommendations become more problematic when the benefit of treatment is uncertain, the potential risks of treatment are high, and the burdens associated with treatment are significant. For example, a chronically ill older adult with chronic obstructive pulmonary disease and severe dementia comes to the emergency department because of a sudden decline in sensorium, which is revealed to be due to a large hemorrhagic stroke. Should the patient be intubated? Should surgery be considered for decompression of the intracranial hemorrhage? The risks and burdens to the patient are significant, and the chance of significant recovery is slim. In such a case, the physician should communicate openly with the surrogate decision maker to describe the possible outcomes of aggressive and comfort-focused treatment plans, emphasizing that the patient would continue to have treatments for comfort and for complications if no surgery is to be done. Physicians should avoid describing a less aggressive course of treatment as ''doing nothing'' because this implies abandonment of the patient.

K. Creating Options

The physician bears the important responsibility of identifying options for each patient. When the most aggressive or conventional treatment plan is not acceptable to the patient or surrogate, physicians can often construct a modified treatment plan, which blends elements of the more aggressive treatment with other modalities, perhaps those focused on comfort and symptom control for the patient. For example, cancer patients may reject the most aggressive and toxic chemotherapy treatment because of fear of the debilitation, risk, and general misery associated with the treatment. Instead, patients may agree to a palliative course of radiation therapy, delivered over several weeks, in combination with some less toxic chemotherapy. Such a regimen might be less effective at diminishing the tumor burden but more consistent with living the remaining life meaningfully. Patients have values and personal goals that influence their willingness to choose treatment options, and physicians can construct the best fit between patient and treatment by negotiating and adjusting treatment options as needed. This ''mixed management'' approach, in which elements of aggressive care are blended with palliative care, is often appealing to frail older adults and their surrogates, who desire to continue with some treatment but do not want to assume the risks and burdens associated with the most aggressive forms of treatment.

L. Cardiopulmonary Resuscitation and Futility

During the process of clinical decision making, physicians are constantly formulating predictions about outcomes from various treatment interventions for their patients. Those treatments that have absolutely no hope of achieving a desired objective can be labeled ''futile.'' Physicians are under no obligation to provide treatments they believe to be futile (15). Dilemmas often arise, however, because in many cases of patients who are critically ill, uncertainty exists about the expected outcomes of various treatments, and criteria for futility are only rarely met.

Outcomes of cardiopulmonary resuscitation (CPR) have been shown to be very poor in some patient populations (See Table 3.) However, the group of patients for whom CPR would be absolutely futile is unclear. In essence, the label is not of much use because it applies to virtually no actual cases and invites overuse by physicians.

Table 3 Factors Associated with Poor Outcomes of Cardiopulmonary Resuscitation

Hypotension
Oliguria/azotemia
Pneumonia
Asystole/electromechanical dissociation
Unwitnessed arrest
Anemia
More than two acute diseases
$Po_2 < 60$ mm Hg
Underlying malignancy
Sepsis
No history of angina
Homebound condition

Source: Clark DE, Goldstein MK, Raffin TA. Ethical dilemmas in the critically ill elderly. In: Sachs GA, Cassel CK, eds. Clinics in Geriatric Medicine, Philadelphia: Saunders 1994; 10:91–101.

M. Working with Patients who Refuse Treatment

Critically ill patients who can make decisions for themselves may decline aggressive medical treatment despite the fact that they have permitted evaluation in an emergency department. Every competent adult has the right to self-determination and thus the right to refuse medical treatment, even if doing so is potentially life threatening. This right is supported by other rights such as the right to privacy, the right to determine what shall be done with one's body, and the right to religious freedom. As in many other areas of clinical medicine, negotiation is a useful tool to develop alternatives of care with the goal of achieving a treatment plan that is acceptable to the patient, the provider, and, if appropriate, significant others.

When a patient refuses a treatment, the patient has not refused all care. Refusal of a treatment certainly signals that the patient's preferences need to be re-examined and goals of care need to be redefined. When a patient refuses a treatment, the physician is not authorized to abandon the care of the patient. Instead, the physician should talk with the patient or surrogate to identify reasons for refusal. It is useful to reassess the available data and understand the patient's overall situation, with the potential treatments, risks, burdens, and benefits for each. The physician seeks to achieve as much accord as possible with the patient around goals of care, which should be made on the basis of patient preferences. When conflicts cannot be resolved around goals of care (e.g., the patient and physician disagree), the physician should consider seeking outside help to gain a different perspective on the patient's situation, to develop more alternatives for care, and to negotiate with the patient or surrogate.

N. Withholding or Withdrawing Treatments

Withholding treatment is entirely permissible on both ethical and legal grounds if the patient wishes it. If the patient has undergone a trial of therapy and goals of care cannot be achieved, withdrawing therapy is also permissible. Patients may articulate in advance that they do not wish certain treatments to be initiated, such as CPR in the event of cardiopulmonary failure, endotracheal and ventilator support in the event of respiratory failure, or feeding tube placement in the event of inability to take sufficient nutrition by mouth. Additional interventions that patients and surrogates may choose to forgo include hemodialysis, intravenous fluids and antibiotics, and hospitalization. These are all interventions that can also be stopped after a therapeutic trial of their use fails to achieve the desired goals of treatment. If the patient has articulated preferences, they should be documented clearly in an advance directive kept on the chart. This is especially important for chronically ill persons residing in long-term care settings, who are at high risk for acute illnesses that may warrant consideration of such interventions.

O. Interdisciplinary Team Communication

Emergency department providers are members of an interdisciplinary team who work closely together, often under extreme pressure, to achieve the best health outcomes for their acutely ill patients. Teams function best when accountability is shared by all members. When difficult decisions need to be made in the treatment of critically ill patients, the physician can support this shared accountability and ownership of the outcomes of the team's work by soliciting opinions and recommendations from the team members. Often a difficult decision is made easier by the suggestions of a team member, and mistakes may be avoided. At the very least, consulting with other team members about a potentially sensitive decision is helpful to build team solidarity and to prevent dissonance within the team. It is worth remembering that the care team around any one patient often includes long-term care providers and family caregivers. Their views and information are often helpful.

P. Assuring Comfort

Palliation is a morally important medical goal at all times, but especially for patients who are dying. Seriously ill elderly patients who come to the emergency department may be in various stages of dying. Furthering outcomes of comfort and dignity requires a holistic approach that addresses the multiple dimensions contributing to the experience of each patient. Whenever possible, the patient should be positioned comfortably and safely, which may require extra pillows, side rails, and frequent observation. Precautions must be taken to prevent injury, such as a fall or a pressure ulcer. Keeping the patient warm, clean, and dry is often of great importance to overall comfort. Extra blankets and attentive nursing care may achieve the better part of the foundation of symptom management for the seriously ill older person. Conversely, a pressure ulcer from a hard stretcher or a fracture while in the emergency department are very troubling calamities.

Careful physical assessment provides the basis for good symptom management. Pain may manifest in a variety of ways. If the patient is not able to verbally report pain, the clinician should note behaviors such as agitation or aggression that may reflect pain. Opioids should be used if needed. To begin, small doses of morphine can be used, and the dose and frequency can be increased as needed to achieve comfort. Opioid drugs that are titrated to effect are rarely a contributing cause of death. If anything, they are likely to extend life by preserving energy and allowing more movement. Even when they might accelerate dying, they still should be used. Patients near death deserve relief from suffering, and slight risks on survival are considered justified. Sometimes, law and ethics rely on a justification known as the principle of double effect. In short, this requires that the physician must be prudently balancing risks and benefits and cannot ever aim to cause death (16).

Q. Communicating with Family and Significant Others

If the patient is able to consent, permission should be sought before communicating with family or others. If the patient is not able to consent, the surrogate should be contacted and permission sought before communicating with others. Frail older persons living in the community are typically tended by an extended network of family and friends, who coordinate support and surveillance to enable the older adult to continue to live independently. Family caregivers are frequently knowledgeable about the patient's various conditions. Detailed information about the events leading up to the acute illness is often available from the caregivers. This information may be unobtainable from any other source because the critically ill patient is often a very poor historian. Timely and appropriate communication about the condition of the patient is of significant comfort to the family. Family members should be updated frequently on the condition of the patient and the upcoming plans for tests or treatment.

Emergency departments should have thoughtful and effective arrangements for supporting family and other loved ones. Some emergency providers have found that families do want to stay with patients, especially at the time of death. Even in a failed attempt at CPR, the time of death is often spiritually important, and family often want to have "seen him breathe his last." Certainly family need to be able to see and be with the body of a recently deceased patient, and they need some private setting in which to hear bad news and begin to cope.

R. Restraints

The use of physical restraints in long-term care settings has received a tremendous amount of attention in recent years, and health care institutions have been reexamining the benefit and burdens of restraints. In the absence of evidence that restraint use improved the health of residents, long-term care institutions have taken steps to reduce and usually to eliminate the use of physical restraints in patient care. More recently, acute care institutions have been examining their opportunities for maintaining safety for their patients while providing the least restrictive care environment. Justification of physical restraint use has included prevention of falls and other injury and the guarding against dislodging catheters and tubes. Like long-term care settings, hospitals and other acute care institutions have been developing alternatives to restraints that can markedly reduce the need for their use. In addition to the risk of harm engendered by the use of a restraint, loss of dignity occurs whenever a patient is placed in physical restraints. Dying in restraints is particularly repugnant. Recent writings emphasize that all individuals have the right to be free of unreasonable restraint.

S. Managing Death

Although the emergency department is designed to be a high-technology setting prepared to efficiently and effectively diagnose and treat acute traumatic or medical problems, often the emergency team is faced with the task of managing the care of the dying patient. Under such circumstances, the emergency team must create the opportunity for a dying patient to die a ''good death,'' with adverse symptoms relieved and surrounded by family and friends. Emergency departments must find ways to treat the ''whole person,'' including the spiritual and psychological dimensions that are often paramount for dying patients and their families. Providing information and explanation to the patient and family is essential. Close attention should be paid to continuous monitoring of the patient's comfort, with treatment of pain, shortness of breath, tachypnea, and other uncomfortable symptoms as needed until they are relieved. Even when the patient is not awake, the appearance of tachypnea raises concern that the patient is experiencing distress and warrants treatment. Securing a measure of privacy shows respect for the patient and family and is appreciated. The presence of a spiritual counselor such as the hospital chaplain may be welcomed.

The responsibility for determining death and for notifying the next of kin falls to the physician, and yet other members of the interdisciplinary team are inevitably involved in the care of the patient and communication with the family or significant others. Although in the aftermath of an intense though ultimately unsuccessful resuscitation effort, the process of notification may seem anticlimactic, this is an extremely important communication. Family members may be shocked by the turn of events, even when the patient had been seriously ill for some time. The physician who pronounced the fact of death is in the best position to tell the family, to provide an explanation for why death occurred, and to answer questions. The personal involvement of the physician in the care of the patient brings meaning and comfort to the family. If the family or significant other is not present in the emergency department, efforts should be made to quickly locate the family and convey information with tact and sensitivity. Special arrangements such as a home visit or a police escort to the emergency department might be considered to ease the burden for the bereaved family. Adequate space should be secured so that family members may grieve privately. The physician should provide information for the death certificate, offer autopsy, notify the medical examiner, and attend to the other tasks that arise on the death of a patient in the emergency department.

II. FOSTERING SYSTEMS OF CARE TO ACHIEVE SUSTAINED EXCELLENCE

In addition to the application of ethical standards in daily activities of caring for individual patients through the emergency medical systsem, physicians have significant opportunities to achieve ethical goals by fostering excellence throughout the systems that make up the care network for patients.

A. Measuring Outcomes

Individuals and organizations concerned with improving health and health care have become increasingly attentive to identifying and measuring outcomes as a means of improving care. Outcomes research has evolved significantly over recent years. The measurement of biomedical outcomes (incidence of postoperative complication, infection, mortality, etc.) has been used for years and has been extremely helpful. Recognition that iatrogenic illness is not uncommon in hospitalized patients has spurred quality improvement activities to identify these occurrences and develop mechanisms to prevent them. Falls, institutionally acquired pressure ulcers, and adverse drug reactions have been of particular interest in older adults.

More recently, attempts have been made to identify other outcomes that reflect patient and family experience of the care process, such as the occurrence of pain and other adverse symptoms. Scales for measuring pain and other symptoms have been developed and are increasingly used to aid assessment and treatment. Quality improvement efforts to optimize symptom relief for critically ill patients in the emergency department are highly appropriate, just as they are in other aspects of the health care system. Proactive approaches to quality improvement activities for functionally frail older persons are likely to be required because they comprise a patient population whose satisfaction with care is not easy to measure. Frail older persons are unlikely to complete a written evaluation without help, thus completion often depends on a motivated scribe or interviewer. Similarly, telephone surveys are not likely to reach frail older patients who may be cognitively impaired, unable to talk on the phone, or unreachable because they have moved to a nursing home. Patient and family satisfaction should be a very important avenue of pursuit for quality improvement. Telephone calls to patients or surrogates to ask about the emergency room experience should be considered as a potentially valuable aspect of quality improvement activities.

B. Fostering Respect and Compassion

The patient's overall perception of the experience in the emergency department is shaped by the total of encounters that occurs. Every encounter that the patient has with a care provider should be characterized by an attitude of patient-centered concern, respect, and compassion. Patients should be addressed by their surnames (e.g., Mr. Jones) not by diminutive nicknames or terms of endearment. Adequate draping and privacy should be provided at all times. Patients should be offered an explanation for any delay in care. When the stay is extended, periodic offerings of water, food, and an opportunity to empty bladder and bowels with adequate privacy and comfort are also necessary.

When mistakes occur, they should be identified and corrected as quickly as possible. Prompt and honest acknowledgment of mistakes should be made, and apologies should be rapidly forthcoming. If such amends are not made in a timely fashion, patient and family trust in the health care team is likely to be severely damaged and can result in a prolonged and unhappy episode of care for all concerned.

Inappropriate handling of ill, older patients may complicate medical outcomes and diminish dignity and comfort. For example, sudden, rough handling can render a demented, ill person frightened and agitated. The patient may manifest distress through increased motion and striking out at providers, who are then tempted to use psychotropic and physical restraints. Some patients may become withdrawn and noncommunicative in response to such treatment. A frail patient may be humiliated by an episode of incontinence, when cleanup is not conducted promptly and delicately, with attention to the need to restore dignity and comfort to the person. Such a patient might subsequently refuse all manner of care in the hospital setting for fear of further degradation. Any intervention should always be preceded by an explanation to the patient, the opportunity to ask questions, and seeking permission before beginning the procedure.

C. Enabling Appropriate Transfer

Critically ill patients who are evaluated in the emergency department are often admitted to the hospital, but they may also be transferred to other settings, depending on the goals of care. Transfers from the emergency department to non-hospital settings may become increasingly frequent as prospective systems of financing care involving more than one setting become more common. For example, an elderly woman who was brought to the emergency department in a stupor was discovered to have suffered a large stroke. Although the patient lacked the capacity to make health care decisions because of her impaired sensorium, her advance directive clearly stated that she did not want aggressive medical care under such circumstances but wanted the goals of her care to be focused on comfort and dignity. The emergency department staff, the primary care physician, and her family agreed that hospice care would be most appropriate. She was transferred from the emergency department to the inpatient hospice facility in the community.

Emergency department staff will need to be familiar with available community resources and settings where care can be delivered in the event that patients or families decide against hospitalization. Many communities are seeking to increase home care resources to provide alternatives to institutionalization. The emergency medical system is part of a loosely interwoven set of services. Practitioners in the emergency department must know a substantial amount about the functioning of the rest of the system. Can you promise an emergency department patient that the nursing home will be effective at managing his cancer pain? Can you promise a person with a recent heart attack that the cardiac surgeons are good? Emergency department personnel who understand and seek to improve the rest of the care system are invaluable to patients and families.

D. Fostering Systems of Follow-up

Follow-up of hospitalized patients is useful to ascertain diagnosis and identify any complications of care from the emergency department. When a pressure ulcer develops during the hospitalization, it may have originated during the time the patient was in the emergency department, where the sacrum and heels are particularly vulnerable to prolonged pressure from lying on a thinly padded stretcher. Simple interventions might include the use of inexpensive low-pressure mattresses for frail patients at high risk for pressure injury in the emergency department. These mattresses could be transferred with the patient to the bed in the hospital when the patient is admitted. However, the need for this innovation would not be known without a routine of follow-up. When an unexpected death occurs, the medical examiner may decide to perform an autopsy. Autopsy results should be vigorously sought by the emergency department physicians because autopsies not infrequently reveal causes of death and comorbidities that were not suspected during life.

E. Networking with Long-Term Care

The patient's experience in an emergency department is but one episode of a series of events of care, occurring across the spectrum of settings in which health care is provided, including the home, nursing home, ambulatory practice, hospital, rehabilitation hospital, and others. When caring for patients from long-term care settings, the emergency department physician and staff should seek information about the patients' advance directives and encourage means to routinely communicate this information reliably. The POLST model from Oregon has proved effective in providing reliable information that can be transferred across settings.

F. Resource Utilization Management

Over recent years the growth of the aged population has been remarkable in the United States, and with this growth has come a rise in associated costs for health care. Many questions have been raised about how best to manage resource utilization in the health care of older persons. The fee-for-service structure of Medicare has gradually been joined by alternative payment mechanisms that provide incentives to ''manage'' the care episodes more efficiently. Although some argue that managed care intrudes on the trusting relationship between physician and patient because of the incentives to curb costs in patient care, various forms of managed care approaches to financing health care continue to appear. Diagnostic related groups for acute hospital stays for Medicare beneficiaries were introduced in the early 1980s as a mechanism for paying hospitals for episodes of care. Increasingly prospective payment systems are being implemented to provide incentives for different segments of the health care system to work together to manage the health service delivery for elderly patients. As this financial integration evolves, emergency departments will be sharing reimbursement with other elements of the system, such as skilled nursing facilities. This integration will provide an opportunity to provide appropriate care for individual patients, but to accomplish this, information about past medical history and goals of care will be very important to the emergency department team. Similarly, when a patient is discharged from the emergency department to the skilled nursing facility, information about diagnostic test results and treatment rationale should be sent with the patient to guide further evaluation and treatment. Certainly, financial concerns loom large for families caring for older adults with serious illness (17). The emergency department often finds itself monitoring the crossroads of families and patients' decisions about whether home care can be continued or whether institutionalization is necessary. Significant innovation and reform in health care financing are likely to occur over the next few years.

REFERENCES

1. Tronto JC. An ethic of care. Ethics and aging: Bringing the issues home. Generations 3:15–20, 1998.
2. President's Commission for the Study of Ethical Problems in Medicine and Biomedical and Behavioral Research. Deciding to Forgo Life-Sustaining Treatment: A Report on the Ethical, Medical, and Legal Issues in Treatment Decisions, Washington, DC: Government Printing Office, 1983.
3. Miller DK, Lewis LM, Nork MJ, Morely JE. Controlled trial of a geriatric case-finding and liaison service in an emergency department. J Am Geriatr Soc 44:513–520, 1996.

4. Hammes BJ, Rooney BL. Death and end of life planning in one midwestern community. Arch Intern Med 158:383–390, 1998.
5. Pelligrino ED. Doctors and ethics, morals and manuals. Ann Intern Med 128:569–571, 1998.
6. Warner MA, Saletel RA, Schroeder DR, Warner DO, Offord KP, Gray DT. Outcomes of anesthesia and surgery in people 100 years of age and older. J Am Geriatr Soc 46:988–993, 1998.
7. Novack DH, Plummer R, Smith RL, Ochitill H, Morrow GR, Bennett JM. Changes in physicians' attitudes toward telling the cancer patient. JAMA 241:897–900, 1979.
8. Sulmasy DP. Ethics, outcomes, and end-of-life care. J Clin Outcomes Mgmnt 5:36–42, 1998.
9. High DM. Surrogate decision making. In: Fein AM, Adelman RD, eds. Clin Geriatr Med Philadelphia: Saunders, 10:445–462, 1994.
10. Tolle SW, Tilden VP, Nelson CA, Dunn PM. A prospective study of the efficacy of the physician order form for life-sustaining treatment. J Am Geriatr Soc 46:1097–1102, 1998.
11. Sachs GA, Miles SH, Levin RA. Limiting resuscitation: emerging policy in the emergency medical system. Ann Intern Med 114:151–154, 1991.
12. Teno JM, Lynn J. Putting advance-care planning into action. J Clin Ethics 7:205–213, 1996.
13. Redelmeier MD, Tan SH, Booth MD. The treatment of unrelated disorders in patients with chronic medical diseases. N Engl J Med 338:1516–1520, 1998.
14. Gurwitz JH, Fore JM, Goldberg RJ, Rubinson M, Chandra N, Rogers WJ. Elderly patients received thrombolytic agents less often. Recent age-related trends in the use of thrombolytic therapy in patients who have had acute myocardial infarction. National Registry of Myocardial Infarction. Ann Intern Med 124:283–291, 1996.
15. Waisel DB, Truog RD. The cardiopulmonary resuscitation-not-indicated order: futility revisited. Ann Intern Med 122:304–308, 1995.
16. Sulmasy DP. The use and abuse of the principle of double effect. Clin Pulm Med 3:86–90, 1996.
17. Covinsky KE, Goldman L, Cook EF, Oye R, Desbiens N, Reding D, Fulkerson W, Connors AF, Lynn J, Phillips RS. The impact of serious illness on patients' families. JAMA 272:1839–1844, 1994.

3

Drug Dosing and Life-Threatening Drug Reactions in the Critically Ill Patient

Frances S. Wong and Jay P. Rho
University of Southern California School of Pharmacy, Los Angeles, California

I. CLINICAL RELEVANCE

A. Adverse Drug Reactions and Events

The purpose of this chapter will be to examine the pharmacological approach to the critically ill geriatric patient. Particular consideration will be given to the recognition and prevention of adverse drug reactions (ADRs) and adverse drug events (ADEs) in critically ill geriatric patients. Although these two terms may appear synonymous and are often used interchangeably in the literature, an ADE is generally considered a broader definition, which can include injuries caused by errors in administration or noncompliance. An ADR, on the other hand, is regarded as ''any response to a drug which is noxious and unintended and which occurs at doses normally used in man for prophylaxis, diagnosis, or therapy of disease for the modification of physiological function'' (1). For reporting purposes, the U.S. Food and Drug Administration categorizes a serious adverse reaction (events relating to drugs or devices) as one in which ''the patient outcome is death, life threatening (real risk of dying), hospitalization (initial or prolonged), disability (significant, persistent, or permanent), congenital anomaly, or required intervention to prevent permanent impairment or damage.''

It is recognized that ADRs occur frequently in the critical care setting and that the harm associated with drug-related morbidity and mortality is exceedingly high. It has been estimated that fatalities directly attributable to ADRs place

ADRs as the fourth to sixth leading cause of death in U.S. hospitals, exceeding deaths caused by pneumonia and diabetes mellitus. A meta-analysis of 39 prospective studies from U.S. hospitals found the incidence of serious and fatal ADRs to be extremely high, ranking fatalities attributable to drugs just behind heart disease, cancer, stroke, pulmonary disease, and accidents (2). The overall incidence of serious ADRs for 1994 was 6.7% (95% confidence interval, 5.2%–8.2%) and of fatal ADRs was 0.32% (95% confidence interval, 0.23%–0.41%) of hospitalized patients (2). Although most ADRs are mild in nature and generally self-limiting, many can result in serious illness or death. In a study reviewing admissions to a public hospital, 35 of 45 (78%) iatrogenic admissions were considered drug related (3). Among the drug-related causes, 19 (54%) were attributed to side effects, 8 (23%) were related to therapeutic overdose, 7 (20%) were immunological in nature, and 1 (2%) was considered a drug-disease interaction.

Despite the enormity of serious and fatal injuries resulting from ADRs, the risk to patients from drugs is considerably greater if one includes the injuries resulting from inadvertent errors in medication administration or through noncompliance (ADEs). What is particularly disconcerting regarding these statistics is that many ADEs are potentially avoidable. In fact, results from the Adverse Drug Event (ADE) Prevention Study suggest as many as 28% of ADEs could be prevented (4). Although nearly all drugs are capable of producing an injury, certain drugs are more likely than others to be toxic. Prevention of drug-related morbidity and mortality has become an increasingly important requirement for reducing health care expenditures. For example, routine adjustment of drug dosages for a patient's age, weight, and renal function could greatly reduce ADEs.

The economic burden associated with drug-related morbidity and mortality has been shown to be extremely costly to both the patient and society. In one cost-of-illness model developed by Johnson and Bootman, drug-related morbidity and mortality was estimated to cost $76.6 billion in the ambulatory setting in the United States (5). The largest component of this total cost was associated with drug-related hospitalization. In a worst-case scenario, estimated costs were reported as high as $136.8 billion. As stated earlier, many ADEs are considered preventable. Greater attention to monitoring drugs with predictable toxicity and avoidance of drugs considered to be problem-prone can result in fewer ADEs and considerable cost reductions. Increased efforts should be made toward a better understanding of drug pharmacokinetics and dynamics of drugs with narrow therapeutic indices. Programs should also be implemented that improve medication use practices among health care providers.

B. Elderly

It has been well documented that the elderly experience a higher number of ADRs. Risk factors for ADRs associated with the aged include increased medica-

Table 1 Steps to Reduce the Occurrence of an Adverse Drug Reaction

Take a careful medication history; this may prevent repetition of a previous untoward experience.
Prescribe a minimum number of drugs.
Start at conservative dosage levels and gradually increase to achieve optimal therapeutic benefit.
Monitor patients carefully for symptoms or signs of adverse drug reactions, bearing in mind the similarity with disease progression.
Monitor appropriate laboratory tests for therapeutic levels and evidence of toxicity.
Discontinue a drug as soon as possible.

tion use, the type of medications prescribed, altered pharmacological response, the number of illnesses, the severity of illness, the length of hospitalization, and lower compliance. In a large multicenter study examining the cause of reported ADRs, risk factors such as age, gender, and cigarette smoking were excluded as significant predictors of ADRs. Rather, the use of four or more drugs, hospital stays lasting more than 14 days, having more than four active medical problems, hospitalization in a medical ward instead of a geriatric ward, and the consumption of alcohol were positively correlated with the occurrence of adverse reactions (6). Thus, no clear agreement is found in the literature about a possible age-related increase in the incidence of ADEs. The ambiguity remains whether the increased reports of ADEs in elderly patients are caused by chronological age per se or with other factors frequently associated with aging, such as polypharmacy and chronic disease states.

As the number of medications given increases, the risk of an ADR developing increases exponentially. This effect may be due in part to the increasing number of possible drug interaction combinations created when additional drugs are added. Other risk factors include the type and dose of the drug taken. Certain physiological conditions, such as impaired renal function, may also increase the risk for having an ADR. Although it may be difficult to prevent an ADR altogether, certain interventions or actions may help to minimize a potential occurrence (Table 1).

II. ALTERED PHARMACOKINETICS AND PHARMACODYNAMICS IN THE CRITICALLY ILL ELDERLY

The relationship between drug dose and response can be influenced by a variety of pharmacokinetic and pharmacodynamic effects that exist in the critically ill geriatric patient.

Pharmacokinetics refers to how the body handles the drug over time, that is, how it is absorbed into the body, distributed into the tissues and organs, and eventually eliminated. In the critical care setting the most important pharmacokinetic parameters associated with a drug are the bioavailability, volume of distribution, clearance, and half-life. Bioavailability refers to the amount of drug that reaches the systemic circulation. The degree of bioavailability is based on the percentage of drug absorption and degree of metabolism before the drug enters the systemic circulation. The volume of distribution (Vd) refers to the space in which the drug enters the body. It relates to the amount of drug administered and the concentration of the drug measured in the blood or serum (Vd = dose/drug concentration in plasma). For example if a 500-mg dose of vancomycin is administered intravenously and a peak serum concentration is measured as 40 mg/L, the estimated volume of distribution would be 500 mg/40 mg/L or 12.5 liters. It is important to note that the volume of distribution does not necessarily correlate with the physiological size of a patient. Half-life ($t^{1/2}$) is defined as the time required for the concentration of the drug to decrease by 50%. Changes in both clearance and volume of distribution will affect half-life. Thus, a drug in a patient will have a long half-life if the patient's renal clearance is decreased or the volume of distribution is large. This may result in a prolonged effect of the drug. Pharmacodynamics refers to the relationship between drug concentration and effect at the receptor site, that is, what the drug does to the body.

A. Absorption

The aging gastrointestinal tract normally undergoes physiological changes that include decreased gastric acidity, delayed gastric emptying, and decreased splanchnic blood flow (7). A reduction in the number of mucosal cells lining the gastrointestinal tract reduces the surface area available for absorption. The extent of drug absorption is not significantly altered with aging; however, the rate of absorption may be decreased. Critically ill patients, however, often have gastrointestinal mucosal damage, decreased gut motility, and decreased splanchnic circulation. Therefore, absorption of drugs following oral administration may be unreliable in these ill patients, requiring that drugs be administered intravenously to ensure therapeutic drug concentrations are achieved.

B. Distribution

Drug disposition is affected by changes in body composition and various disease states. With aging, the percentage of fat relative to lean body mass is higher, total body water is decreased, and the plasma albumin concentration is decreased (8). Therefore, lipophilic drugs, such as diazepam, barbiturates, and antidepressants, will have a larger volume of distribution and will be more widely distributed throughout the body with aging. The effect of a drug may be prolonged as a result of the slow release of drug from the fatty tissue site. Drugs that are water-soluble may produce an exaggerated initial effect because of higher blood concentrations. However, in the critically ill patient, the drug volume of distribution increases as a result of expanded fluid volume or a hypermetabolic state. These changes in volume of distribution are necessary to understand because volume of distribution is often used to predict the loading dose required to achieve a given plasma concentration of a drug. For example, larger doses of an aminoglycoside may be required to achieve a therapeutic concentration. Distribution may also be affected by changes in protein concentration and affinity of the protein to bind the drug molecule. Albumin concentrations are decreased in the elderly because of poor nutrition and chronic disease states. Critically ill patients may also have decreased serum albumin concentration as a result of increased capillary permeability and decreased hepatic synthesis. This combination of factors leads to more active unbound drug being available. This would result in a larger volume of distribution because a higher free drug concentration is available to distribute throughout the body. Proper interpretation of drug serum levels is necessary because serum drug levels are usually measured in total concentrations (bound + unbound). For example, a subtherapeutic serum phenytoin concentration (<10 μg/ml) obtained in a patient with a low serum albumin concentration may actually be therapeutic. In contrast to albumin, $alpha_1$-acid glycoprotein concentrations in the serum are increased in the elderly patient and in the critically ill patient. Basic pH drugs are highly bound to $alpha_1$-acid glycoprotein, so drugs such as meperidine, propranolol, and lidocaine will be bound and less free fraction will be available to exert a pharmacological effect. Protein binding may also be affected by the affinity of the binding protein for the drug, but this does not appear to be significant.

C. Clearance

Clearance refers to the volume of blood or plasma cleared of drug within a given time. It is accomplished through hepatic metabolism, renal excretion, or a combination of both.

Drugs are metabolized or are biotransformed by way of the liver. The drug is changed into active or inactive metabolites that either exert a pharmacological effect or are eliminated by the kidneys. A decrease in liver mass in relation to body weight and a decline in hepatic blood flow are normally associated with aging (9). Disease states such as sepsis and congestive heart failure may also compromise blood flow to the liver. Thus, drugs that depend on blood flow to the liver may have reduced clearance. Liver function tests are typically unaltered with aging and do not reflect age-related alteration of the metabolism of drugs.

Certain pathways of liver metabolism are diminished in the aged, particularly the oxidative pathway, resulting in decreased clearance of drugs like diazepam.

Renal excretion of many drugs is diminished with aging (10). An average decline of 35% in glomerular filtration rate occurs between the ages of 20 and 90. Use of the measured serum creatinine concentration to assess renal function can be misleading in the elderly because a decrease in lean body mass is associated with aging and can result in decreased creatinine production. As a result, serum creatinine values may appear to be within the normal therapeutic range for younger adults but may in fact represent a decline in renal function. The creatinine clearance is a more accurate method to assess renal function. Measurement of endogenous creatinine clearances requires the collection of urine output over a defined period of time. Because of the time delay involved and problems with completeness of the urine collection, the creatinine clearance is usually calculated for initial drug regimens. The most commonly used equation to estimate creatinine clearance is the Cockcroft and Gault equation (11).

For men:

$$\mathrm{Clcr} = (140 - \mathrm{age})(\mathrm{wt\ in\ kg})/72 \times \mathrm{Scr\ (mg/dl)}$$

For women:

$$\mathrm{Clcr} = [(140 - \mathrm{age})(\mathrm{wt\ in\ kg})/72 \times \mathrm{Scr\ (mg/dl)}] \times 0.85$$

where Clcr = creatinine clearance; wt = lean body weight; kg = kilogram; and Scr = serum creatinine.

A caveat with this equation, however, is that the elderly patient may initially be seen with a serum creatinine less than 1 mg/dl. As stated earlier, this is attributed to a decrease in muscle mass and not an indicator of renal function. Patients 65 years of age and older with a serum creatinine less than 1 mg/dl should have their serum creatinine value rounded up to 1 mg/dl when using the Cockcroft and Gault equation. For example, when 0.5 mg/dl is used, a higher creatinine clearance will be calculated than when 1 mg/dl is used. A patient with a serum creatinine of 0.5 mg/dl will appear to have renal function superior to another patient who has a serum creatinine of 1 mg/dl; however, that may not be the case.

III. PHARMACODYNAMIC CHANGES

The interaction of a drug on its receptor organ may produce a desired beneficial therapeutic effect or a negative toxic effect. The elderly appear to be more sensitive to medications. This is due to age-related changes in receptor selectivity and changes in homeostatic control mechanisms (12–13). Drug response with aging may therefore be increased, decreased, or unchanged because of these multifactorial interactions. Among the changes that may occur include impaired sympathetic and parasympathetic response, thermoregulation, and postural stability; glucose intolerance; and reduced immune response and cognitive function (14). Impairment of the autonomic response may manifest as a decreased heart rate response to vasopressor agents and beta blockers. Evidence of an age-related decrease in response of the cholinergic receptors also exists. The effect of atropine on heart rate is less marked in the elderly (15). Specific disease states may also alter pharmacodynamic effects of the drug. Sedative and analgesic drugs have been observed to have more pronounced effects in those with renal, hepatic, and respiratory insufficiency. Changes in plasma electrolytes may depress or enhance drug action; for example, a decrease in serum potassium may potentiate digoxin effects (16). Low serum potassium and magnesium will potentiate amphotericin B nephrotoxic effects. The elderly also appear to require less warfarin to inhibit clotting factor synthesis, and thus anticoagulation should be initiated with lower doses of warfarin (17).

IV. DRUG DOSING IN THE CRITICALLY ILL GERIATRIC PATIENT

Multiple organ system dysfunction along with normal physiological changes in the critically ill elderly patient pose a challenge to drug dosing. Patients with renal and hepatic insufficiency require intense monitoring and dosage adjustment. Therapeutic drug monitoring is available for many medications with a narrow therapeutic index. Drugs that can be monitored include aminoglycoside antibotics, vancomycin, cyclosporine, digoxin, lidocaine, procainamide, theophylline, and phenytoin. For many other drugs, such as diuretics, anticoagulants, and cardiovascular agents, the dose is titrated to a set desired outcome or therapeutic effect.

A. Examples of Monitoring Drug Dosing

1. Aminoglycosides

Aminoglycoside antibiotics are commonly used to treat gram-negative bacilli bacterial infections in the critically ill patient (18). Because of their (gentamicin, tobramycin, amikacin, netilmicin) narrow therapeutic range and risk for causing nephrotoxicity and ototoxicity, serum concentrations of aminoglycosides must be monitored for efficacy and toxicity (19). Serum levels must be monitored more frequently in the critically ill geriatric patient because of the potential for altered pharmacokinetic parameters observed in this population. The critically ill geriatric patient is often hemodynamically unstable and requires aggressive fluid therapy. Renal function is often compromised. These parameters may influence aminoglycoside pharmacokinetics by altering the volume of distribution and elimination half-life. Many studies have shown that the volume of distribution is much larger in patients in the critical care unit than those on a general medical ward (20–22). Such pharmacokinetic change necessitates a larger than usual loading dose be given early in therapy (within the first 24 hours) to achieve a therapeutic drug concentration. Achieving a high concentration is particularly important in serious systemic infections, such as bacteremia, because of the high mortality rates when treatment is inadequate (23).

2. Vancomycin

Vancomycin is another commonly prescribed antibiotic in the critically ill geriatric patient. Vancomycin is indicated for the treatment of gram-positive infections resistant to penicillins or first-generation cephalosporins or in some instances in patients who are allergic to beta-lactam antibiotics. However, patients who are in a hypermetabolic state may require a higher dose. Vancomycin trough levels should be routinely monitored in critically ill patients to validate that therapeutic concentrations are achieved (24). The bacteria-killing activity of vancomycin depends on maintaining a concentration greater than the minimum inhibitory concentration of the organism; therefore, a trough level is useful to validate a therapeutic concentration (5–15 mg/L).

3. Digoxin

Digitalis glycosides, primarily digoxin, are commonly used to treat congestive heart failure and supraventricular tachyarrhythmias such as atrial fibrillation. Its primary mechanism of action is to increase the heart's force of contraction (i.e., positive inotropic action), thereby increasing cardiac output. Indirect pharmacological effects include a decrease in conduction and prolongation of refractoriness in the atrioventricular node, resulting in a decreased ventricular rate.

Intravenous digoxin will most likely be used in a patient with sudden-onset atrial fibrillation. Loading doses must be cautiously used in elderly patients because the volume of distribution is decreased in older patients as a result of an age-related decrease in muscle mass and alterations in tissue binding. Diminished renal function in the elderly along with decreased volume of distribution leads to an increased serum digoxin level, thereby resulting in cardiac toxicity such as ventricular tachycardia, premature ventricular contractions, and atrioventricular block. Serum levels should be monitored after a loading dose and maintenance dose to achieve the desired clinical effect. The usual therapeutic range is 0.5–2.0 ng/ml. Blood samples should be obtained at least 6 hours after a dose of digoxin to prevent erroneous interpretations of high levels. Monitoring serum creatinine is helpful because changes in creatinine clearance reflect changes in digoxin elimination rate.

Other laboratory parameters to monitor include serum potassium, magnesium, calcium, and thyroid function. Hypokalemia, hypomagnesemia, and hypercalcemia may contribute to digoxin toxicity with normal digoxin levels. Patients who are hypothyroid require less digoxin because less is excreted. Elderly patients concurrently taking diuretics and other drugs that increase digoxin concentrations, such as verapamil, quinidine, and amiodarone, should be monitored closely. Other adverse effects of digoxin include nausea, vomiting, diarrhea, confusion, weakness, insomnia, and color vision (green and yellow) changes.

Treatment of digitalis toxicity includes replacing potassium (with hypokalemia) and administering phenytoin and lidocaine. To correct a dysrhythmia when potassium is low, 40 to 80 mEq potassium chloride may be given intravenously at a rate of no more than 20 mEq/hr. Oral potassium may be necessary for prolonged suppression of dysrhythmias. Potassium should not be used when severe or complete heart block is due to digitalis. For dysrhythmias unresponsive to potassium, 0.5 mg/kg phenytoin may be given at a rate not exceeding 50 mg/min at 1- to 2-hour intervals. The maximum dose should not exceed 10 mg/kg/day. As an alternative, 1 mg/kg lidocaine over 5 minutes followed by 15–50 μg/kg/min infusion to maintain normal cardiac rhythm may be used. Digoxin-specific Fab antibodies (Digibind) reverse symptoms and signs of toxicity (25). It is indicated for life-threatening toxicity, including ventricular tachycardia or ventricular fibrillation or progressive bradydysrhythmias such as severe sinus bradycardia or second-degree or third-degree heart block not responsive to atropine. Ingestion of more than 10 mg digoxin by healthy adults or steady-state concentrations greater than 10 ng/ml may result in cardiac arrest. The dosage of Digibind is determined from a nomogram or calculated by means of the digoxin body load. It is given intravenously over 30 minutes, or if cardiac arrest is imminent, it may be given as a bolus.

4. Heparin and Warfarin

Deep vein thrombosis and pulmonary embolism are life-threatening complications that can occur after major trauma, abdominal, orthopedic or neurologic surgery, and in patients with congenital or acquired disorders of hypercoagulopathy. Other risk factors for deep vein thrombosis include those patients who are bedridden or debilitated, those with stasis caused by congestive heart failure, recent myocardial infarction, and malignancy (26–27). Heparin, low molecular weight heparins (LMWH), and warfarin are indicated for both the prophylaxis and treatment of deep vein thrombosis and pulmonary embolism. Heparin is an immediate anticoagulant and is usually given intravenously. The half-life of heparin is dose dependent and ranges from 30–150 minutes. Heparin binds to antithrombin III producing a conformational change that then inactivates thrombin, factor Xa, and factor IXa. The typical loading dose is 50–80 units/kg followed by a continuous infusion of 15–18 units/kg/hr. Various nomograms have also been developed by use of blood volume, weight, and adjusted body weight. Whichever regimen is used, it would be prudent to use lower doses for the elderly, especially if patients have had recent surgery. Clinical symptoms and signs of bleeding should be monitored, such as hematuria, bruises, tests for occult blood, decreased hematocrit, and thrombocytopenia. Partial thrombinplastin time should be monitored 6 hours after a loading dose and every 6 hours for the first 24 hours until desired results are achieved. Heparin should be discontinued if the platelet count drops to less than 100×10^9/L or a marked fall in platelet count occurs ($>200 \times 10^9$/L). If bleeding is suspected, the infusion may be temporarily stopped and packed red blood cells may be given.

Low molecular weight heparins are indicated for the treatment and prophylaxis of deep vein thrombosis with or without pulmonary embolism. Its advantages include ease of dosing and administration and less need for laboratory monitoring. The risk of heparin-induced thrombocytopenia (HIT) appears to be reduced with LMWH rather than unfractionated heparin; however, LMWH cannot be used in patients with HIT because of cross-reactivity (28).

In 1997 an FDA Public Health Advisory was issued alerting health care providers to the risk of hemorrhagic complications, including spinal hematomas, with LMWH use and concurrent spinal/epidural anesthesia or spinal puncture. The American Society of Regional Anesthesia has published recommendations to help minimize the risk of hemorrhagic complications with neuraxial anesthesia and anticoagulation (Table 2) (29). In reviewing reports of spinal hematoma cases, the consensus reached by the Conference panelists was that future cases of spinal hematomas can be averted through recognition of the increased risk with concurrent spinal/epidural anesthesia and LMWH.

Patients initated on heparin therapy are likely to be converted to warfarin therapy to complete their duration of treatment. The geriatric patient is at higher risk of warfarin-induced bleeding because of decreased mass and blood volume and increased receptor sensitivity. Geriatric patients initiated on warfarin should begin with lower doses than younger adult patients (17). The initial dose of warfarin should not exceed 5 mg. The prothombin time and international normalized ratio (INR) should be monitored daily at the onset of therapy and whenever a drug known to interact with warfarin is added or deleted from the patient's therapeutic regimen. Minor bleeding and high INR values (>3.0) may be treated by either withholding further doses of warfarin or, if necessary, by administering low doses of vitamin K (1 mg intravenously or 2.5–5 mg orally). For major bleeding or bleeding in central organs such as the brain, stomach, or eye, administration of

Table 2 Recommendations for Neuraxial Anesthesia and Low Molecular Weight Heparin

1. Monitoring of the anti-Xa level is not recommended. The anti-Xa level is not predictive of the risk of bleeding and is, therefore, not helpful in the management of patients undergoing neuraxial blocks.
2. Antiplatelet or oral anticoagulant medications administered in combination with low molicular weight heparin (LMWH) may increase the risk of spinal hematoma. Concomitant administration of medications affecting hemostasis, such as antiplatelet drugs, standard heparin, or dextran represents an additional risk of hemorrhagic complications perioperatively, including spinal hematoma. Education of the entire patient care team is necessary to avoid potentiation of the anticoagulant effects.
3. The presence of blood during needle and catheter placement does not necessitate postponement of surgery. However, initiation of LMWH therapy in this setting should be delayed for 24 hours postoperatively. Traumatic needle or catheter placement may signify an increased risk of spinal hematoma, and it is recommended that this consideration be discussed with the surgeon.
4. Patients receiving preoperative LMWH can be assumed to have altered coagulation. A single-dose spinal anesthetic may be the safest neuraxial technique in patients receiving LMWH preoperatively. In these patients needle placement should occur at least 10 to 12 hours after the dose of LMWH whereas patients receiving higher doses of LMWH (e.g., enoxaparin 1 mg/kg twice daily) will require longer delays (24 hours). Neuraxial technique should be avoided in patients administered a dose of LMWH 2 hours preoperatively (general surgery patients) because needle placement would occur during peak anticoagulant activity.
5. Patients with postoperative initiation of LMWH thromboprophylaxis may safely undergo single-dose and continuous catheter techniques. The first dose of LMWH is administered 2 hours after catheter removal.
6. The decision to implement LMWH thromboprophylaxis in the presence of an indwelling catheter must be made with care. Extreme vigilance of the patient's neurological status is warranted. An opioid or dilute local anesthetic solution is recommended in these patients to allow frequent monitoring of neurological function. If epidural analgesia is anticipated to continue for more than 24 hours, thromboprophylaxis may be selected (e.g., external pneumatic compression) on the basis of the individual patient's risk profile. These decisions should be made preoperatively to allow optimal management of both postoperative analgesia and thromboprophylaxis.
7. For any LMWH prophylaxis regimen, the timing of catheter removal is of paramount importance. Catheter removal should be delayed for at least 10 to 12 hours after a dose of LMWH. A true normalization of the patient's coagulation status could be achieved if the evening dose of LMWH was not given and the catheter was removed the following morning (24 hours after the last dose). Again, subsequent dosing should not occur for at least 2 hours after catheter removal.

Source: Ref. 29.

fresh frozen plasma and vitamin K (5–10 mg intravenous infusion over 10 minutes) is recommended.

B. Nonmonitored Drug Dosing

In cases in which therapeutic drug monitoring is not available, other methods for determining a dosage regimen are available. These methods include decreasing the usual dose of the drug and maintaining the same interval or maintaining the same dose while prolonging the dosing interval. Use of these methods depends on the clinician's goal for the drug, either obtaining a therapeutic peak or achieving an average steady-state concentration. Medications such as antihypertensive agents require a regimen that maintains an average steady-state concentration, therefore, a lower dose given without a change in interval is satisfactory.

Drugs metabolized to active metabolites should also be adjusted for renal insufficiency (Table 3). Metronidazole is primarily metabolized by the liver; however, its active metabolites may accumulate with renal insufficiency and cause neurological and gastrointestinal toxicity. Procainamide and theophylline produce active metabolites that may contribute to cardiac toxicity. Analgesics such as meperidine, morphine, and codeine have active metabolites and may cause prolonged central nervous system effects. Benzodiazepines such as diazepam also produce active metabolites and should be given cautiously. A shorter acting agent

Table 3 Drugs that Require Dose Adjustment for Renal Insufficiency

Antibiotics
Aminoglycosides
Beta-lactams
Sulfonamides
Vancomycin
Antifungals
Amphotericin B
Fluconazole
Cardiac glycosides
Digoxin
Histamine$_2$ (H_2) receptor antagonists
Famotidine
Ranitidine
Cimetidine

such as lorazepam is preferred and is more advantageous because it does not produce an active metabolite.

C. Adjustment of Drugs in Continuous Hemodialysis

Patients undergoing intermittent hemodialysis require unique drug-dosing regimens to stay as close to steady-state concentrations as possible. Problems with drug dosing and intermittent hemodialysis include unknown scheduling and duration of dialysis and the extent to which the drug is removed by dialysis. Drugs with significant removal must be replaced after hemodialysis, especially antibiotics. For example, metronidazole is effectively removed by hemodialysis, so a dose should be given after each session. Continuous hemodialysis and hemofiltration for the treatment of acute renal failure is also used and offers the advantage that it can be performed on hemodynamically compromised patients. The methods of use include continuous arteriovenous and venovenous hemofiltration or hemodialysis.

These differing procedures, along with membrane size and adsorbent properties, may all influence drug pharmacokinetics and hence clearance. Clearance of drugs depends on the flow rate of blood and dialysate, membrane characteristics, and filter size. For example, elimination of medications with large molecular weights such as vancomycin may vary with membrane pore size, or drugs such as aminoglycosides may be adsorbed onto the membrane itself (30). Thus, medication adjustment should be guided by obtaining serum concentration levels whenever possible. In general, the same loading dose given to patients with normal renal function may be given to those on intermittent hemodialysis and continuous hemofiltration or hemodialysis; however, a lower maintenance dose is required.

The volume of distribution for drugs may be either increased or decreased with end-stage renal disease. Alterations in the distribution volume may be due to increased or decreased protein binding. For example, phenytoin must be adjusted for patients with renal insufficiency and low serum albumin. Phenytoin is 90% bound to protein, and, therefore, patients with low serum albumin will have an increased free fraction available for therapeutic effect. Older patients tend to have decreased protein and renal insufficiency; therefore, renal function and serum albumin need to be considered when evaluating serum phenytoin levels. Therapeutic phenytoin concentrations are 10–20 mg/L for those patients with normal renal function (31). The free fraction is approximately 10% or 1–2 mg/L. The free fraction, however, rises to approximately 20% in patients who have end-stage renal disease, and thus, the total concentration is lower as a result of the increased volume of distribution. Consequently, a phenytoin level might appear to be subtherapeutic, despite the free concentration being in the therapeutic range. In elderly patients with hypoalbuminemia and end-stage renal disease receiving hemodialysis, the following equation is useful in predicting normalized phenytoin concentrations (31).

$$C\,(\text{normalized}) = \frac{C\,(\text{observed})}{\left[(0.48)\times(1-0.1)\times\dfrac{\text{patient serum albumin (g/dl)}}{4.4\ \text{g/dl}}\right]+0.1}$$

where C (normalized) = normalized phenytoin concentration and C (observed) = observed serum phenytoin concentration in hypoalbuminemic patients.

D. Adjustment of Medications in Liver Failure

Hepatic drug metabolism is altered in critically ill patients (32–33); however, the mechanisms of these alterations are not clearly understood and are difficult to address in clinical studies. Therefore, limited guidelines exist for determining the proper dose for patients with hepatic insufficiency or failure. At best, the clinician may make an educated guess on the basis of the drug's elimination profile, extent of protein binding, and degree of first-pass effect. Hepatic metabolism depends on hepatic blood flow, enzyme activity, and protein binding. Alterations to any one of these processes can result in variable hepatic drug metabolism. Hepatic drug metabolism can be classified into flow-dependent drugs and flow-independent drugs. Flow-dependent drugs have metabolism that is governed by the flow rate of blood to the liver. A reduction of blood flow to the liver will decrease clearance for these drugs. Blood flow to the liver may be affected by low cardiac output caused by sepsis, congestive heart failure, hemorrhagic shock, trauma, and mechanical ventilation. Morphine and midazolam have decreased clearance in patients who have septic shock. Lidocaine clearance has been shown to decrease as a result of decreased hepatic blood flow induced by mechanical ventilation. Drugs such as cimetidine, theophylline, and vasopressin have been shown to decrease liver blood flow. This may affect the clearance of other drugs such as lidocaine and propranolol (34–37). Conversely, drugs that increase hepatic blood flow by decreasing vascular resistance and increasing cardiac output, such as dobutamine, dopamine, and nitroglycerin, may increase the clearance of other drugs (38–40). Hepatic clearance is also affected by metabolic enzyme activity. Enzymatic reactions include phase I reactions and phase II reactions. Phase I reactions use oxidation, reduction, or hydrolysis to form a more polar substance that may be more active, less active, or inactive. Phase II reactions produce a bond between the drug or its metabolite and glucoronic acid, sulfuric acid, acetic acid, or other amino acids to form compounds that can be eliminated from the body. Induction or inhibition of these enzymes alters the hepatic clearance of drugs.

For patients with hepatic failure or insufficiency, drugs metabolized by the liver should be avoided if at all possible. If renal function is preserved, choosing an agent that is excreted predominantly by the kidneys is prudent. In the event a medication must be used and is cleared by the liver, choosing an agent that requires the least metabolism is essential.

REFERENCES

1. World Health Organization. International drug monitoring: the role of the hospital. Geneva, Switzerland: World Health Organization, 1966. Technical Report Series No. 425.
2. Lazarou J, Pomeranz BH, Corey PN. Incidence of adverse drug reactions in hospitalized patients: a meta-analysis of prospective studies. JAMA 279:1200–1205, 1998.
3. Lakshmanan MC, Hershey CO, Bresiau D. Hospital admissions caused by iatrogenic disease. Arch Intern Med 146:1931–1934, 1986.
4. Bates DW, Cullen DJ, Laird N, Peterson LA, Small SD, Servi D, Laffel G, Sweitzer BJ, Shea BF, Hallisey R, Vander VM, Nemesak R, Leape LL. Incidence of adverse drug events and potential adverse drug events: implications for prevention. JAMA 274:29–34, 1995.
5. Johnson JA, Bootman JL. Drug-related morbidity and mortality. Arch Intern Med 155:1949–1956, 1995.
6. Carbonin P, Pahor M, Bernabei R, Sgadari A. Is age an independent risk factor of adverse drug reactions in hospitalized medical patients? J Am Geriatr Soc 39:1093–1099, 1991.
7. Stevenson IH, Salem SAM, Sheperd AMM. Studies on drug absorption and metabolism in the elderly. In: Crooks J, Stevenson IH, eds. Drugs and the Elderly. Baltimore: University Park Press, 1979, pp 51–62.
8. Wallace S, Whiting B. Factor affecting drug binding in plasma of elderly patients. Br J Clin Pharmacol 3:327–330, 1976.
9. Bach B, Hansen JM, Kampmann JP, Rasmussen SN, Skovstad L. Disposition of antipyrine and phenytoin correlated with age and liver volume in man. Clin Pharmacokinet 6:389–396, 1981.
10. Epstein M. Effect of aging on the kidney. Fed Proc 38:168–172, 1979.
11. Cockcroft DW, Gault JH. Prediction of creatinine clearance from serum creatinine. Nephron 16:31, 1976.
12. Collins KJ, Dore C, Exton-Smith AN, Fox RH, MacDonald IC, Woodward PM. Accidental hypothermia and impaired temperature homeostasis in the elderly. BMJ 1(6057):353–356, 1977.
13. Feldman RD, Limbird LE, Nadeau J, Robertson D, Wood AJ. Alterations in leukocyte beta-receptor affinity with aging. A potential explanation for altered beta-adrenergic sensitivity in the elderly. N Engl J Med 310:815–819, 1984.

14. Feely J, Coakley D. Altered pharmacodynamics in the elderly. Clin Geriatr Med 6(2):269–282, 1990.
15. Kelliher GJ, Conahan ST. Changes in vagal activity and response to muscarinic receptor agonists with age. J Gerontol 45:842–849, 1980.
16. Prindle KH Jr, Skelton CL, Epstein SE, Marcus FI. Influence of extracellular potassium concentration on myocardial uptake and inotropic effect of tritiated digoxin. Circ Res 28:3337, 1971.
17. Gurwitz J, Avorn J, Ross-Degnan D, Choodnovskiy BS, Ansell J. Aging and the anticoagulant response to warfarin therapy. Ann Intern Med 116:901–904, 1992.
18. Masur H. Antimicrobials. In: Chernow B, ed. The Pharmacologic Approach to the Critically Ill Patient. 3rd ed. Baltimore: Williams & Wilkins, 1994, pp 685–699.
19. Zaske D. Aminoglycosides. In: Evans WE, Schentag JJ, Jusko JJ eds. Applied Pharmacokinetics. Spokane: Applied Therapeutics, Inc, 1986, pp 331–381.
20. Mann HJ, Fuhs DW, Awang R, Ndemo FA, Cerva FB. Altered aminoglycoside pharmacokinetics in critically ill patients with sepsis. Clin Pharm 6:154–159, 1987.
21. Mitchell MD, Wilson J, Dodek P, Russel J. Volume distribution in patients with gram negative sepsis in the ICU. Anesthesiology 67:A126, 1987.
22. Fuhs DW, Mann HJ, Kubajak CM, Cerra FB. Intrapatient variation of aminoglycoside pharmacokinetics in critically ill surgery patients. Clin Pharm 7:207–213, 1988.
23. Moore RD, Smith CR, Lietman PS. The association of aminoglycoside plasma levels with mortality in patients with gram-negative bacteremia. J Infect Dis 149(3):443–448, 1984.
24. Garaud JJ, Regnier B, Ingelbert F, Faurisson F, Bauchet J, Vachon F. Vancomycin pharmacokinetics in critically ill patients. J Antimicrob Chemother 14(suppl D):53–57, 1984.
25. Digibind® Digoxin Immune Fab (Ovine) Insert. The Wellcome Foundation Ltd., May 1994.
26. Weitz JI. Low-molecular-weight heparins. N Engl J Med 337(10):668–698, 1997.
27. Nanfro J. Anticoagulants in critical care medicine. In: Chernow B, ed. The Pharmacologic Approach to the Critically Ill Patient. 3rd ed. Baltimore: Williams & Wilkins. 1994, pp 666–683.
28. Warkentin TE, Levine MN, Hirsh J, Horsewood P, Roberts R, Gent M, Kelton J. Heparin-induced thrombocytopenia in patients with low-molecular weight heparin or unfractionated heparin. N Engl J Med 332:1330–1335, 1995.
29. Horlocker TT, Wedel DJ. Neuraxial block and low molecular weight heparin: balancing perioperative analgesia and thromboprophylaxis. Reg Anesth Pain Med 23(6 suppl 2):164–177, 1998.
30. Reetze-Bonorden P, Bohler J, Keller E. Drug dosage in patients during continuous renal replacement therapy. Clin Pharmacokinet 24(5):363–379, 1993.
31. Winter M. Phenytoin. In: Koda-Kimble M, Young L, eds. Basic Clinical Pharmacokinetics. 2nd ed Vancouver, Washington: Applied Therapeutics, Inc., 1988, pp 235–264.
32. Shoemaker WC, Szanto PB, Fitch LB, Brill NR. Hepatic physiologic and morphologic alterations in hemorrhagic shock. Surg Gynecol Obstet 118:828–836, 1964.

33. McKindley DS, Hanes S, Boucher B. Hepatic drug metabolism in critical illness. Pharmacotherapy 18(4):759–778, 1998.
34. Feely J, Wilkinson GR, Wood AJ. Reduction of liver blood flow and propranolol metabolism by cimetidine. N Engl J Med 304:692–695, 1981.
35. Feely H, Wilkinson GR, McAllister CB, Wood AJJ. Increased toxicity and reduced clearance of lidocaine by cimetidine. Ann Intern Med 96:592–594, 1982.
36. Kisor DF, Wooding-Scott RA. The effect of theophylline on estimated hepatic blood flow. Pharmacotherapy 10:406–409, 1990.
37. Silva YJ, Moffat RC, Walt AJ. Vasopressin effect on portal and systemic hemodynamics. JAMA 210:1065–1068, 1969.
38. Resii WG, Bauer LA, Horn JR, Zierler BK, Easterling TR, Strandness DE. Acute effects of sublingual nitroglycerin on hepatic blood flow in healthy volunteers. J Clin Pharmacol 34:912–918, 1994.
39. Maestracci P, Grimaud D, Livrelli N, Philip F, Dolisi C. Increase in hepatic flow and cardiac output during dopamine infusion in man. Crit Care Med 9:14–16, 1981.
40. Kawasaki T, Moriyasu F, Kimura T, Someda H, Hamato N, Okuma M. Effects of dobutamine on hepatosplanchnic hemodynamics in patients with chronic liver disease. Scand J Gastroenterol 29:1044–1054, 1994.

4

Acute and Critical Nursing Care

Terry Fulmer
New York University, New York, New York

Ellen Flaherty
Gitt Resource Center, Yorktown Heights, New York

Melissa M. Bottrell
New York University, New York, New York

Kathy Fletcher
University of Virginia Health Sciences Center, Charlottesville, Virginia

Mathy Mezey
New York University, New York, New York

I. CLINICAL RELEVANCE

A. Need for Acute Care Geriatric Nursing

The demographic trends that have swept the United States have had a profound effect on acute and critical care nursing of the elderly. In the 1970s, no journals were specifically focused on geriatric nursing, and within the existing journals, most geriatric nursing articles dealt with long-term care issues. Intensive care of the elderly was considered a nonissue. New treatments and equipment—ventilators, defibrillators, and bypass machines—were changing the nature of hospital nursing practice, but elderly patients were not routinely treated with these therapies. Lack of experience with how an older person might fare under such care may have contributed to the situation, but such scarcely available, extreme measures were also saved for younger more ''viable'' patients. Medical or societal taboos with regard to triaging out older patients were minimal, and policies for intensive care unit (ICU) admission, so named for the increased ratio of nurses to patients, openly reflected age biases. For example, as recently as 1970, age was used as an exclusion criterion for open-heart surgery (1). At present, such biases might exist, but they are certainly not stated overtly, and indeed might be the cause of litigation if they were. The reality today is that more than 65% of ICU beds are occupied by patients aged 65 years and older. More than one third of older adults in the United States are admitted and discharged from an acute care hospital each year, and between 6% and 45% of those people are likely to experience at least one untoward event while hospitalized (2). Despite the fact that so many critical care patients are elderly, nurses, including acute care and critical care nurses, have received little, if any, formal preparation in geriatrics. This chapter will discuss the importance of geriatric nursing knowledge in acute and critical care nursing. Information regarding nurses' current preparation to care for elderly patients in the critical care setting will be presented. Models of nursing care for geriatric patients in the acute and critical care setting that have been developed to meet the needs of elders in the hospital will be described. To support these models, institutional assessment strategies and care protocols will also be presented.

B. Background

The need to build a geriatric knowledge base has been recognized by the nursing field. At present, there are two major geriatric nursing journals, several interdisciplinary geriatric journals, and a growing body of knowledge as to what constitutes the best nursing practices in acute (hospital) and critical (ICU) care. Dramatic advances in technology and biotechnology revolutionized the treatments for infection, heart diseases, renal diseases, and degenerative age changes. Although hospital ethics committee's struggle with ethical questions about "when and under what conditions older people should receive treatment," America's ICUs have "aged," and the trend toward older individuals receiving extraordinary care continues. It is in response to this "natural experiment" and within this context that acute and critical care geriatric nursing practice began and continues to develop.

Early articles on acute care of the elderly primarily began appearing in the 1980s and primarily addressed assessment strategies to highlight important physiological and psychological differences between elders and younger adult patients (3,4). In one of the earliest geriatric nursing texts, Eliopoulis (5) reprinted the first set of *Standards of Gerontological Nursing Practice* developed by the American Nurses Association. Those seven standards focused primarily on special assessment parameters that were considered to be essential for the care of the elderly. Interestingly, although the terms "scientific principles" and "data" are used within the standards, the term "research" is never mentioned. With the establishment of the National Institute for Nursing Research (NINR) in 1986, then called the National Center for Nursing Research, grants from the National Institutes of Health (NIH) generated new opportunities to fund research questions related to acute nursing care of the elderly. Landmark investigations funded by NINR include Evans and Strumpf's studies in the area of restraints (6–8), Naylor's research on acute and posthospital follow-up for acutely ill elders (9), and Kleinpell's contribution on exploring outcomes after critical illness in the elderly (10–12). These studies have significantly advanced our knowledge of acute care issues as they relate to care for older adults.

C. Current Status of Acute and Critical Care

At present, persons aged 65 and older account for more than 47% of inpatient care days (13). The Health Care Finance Administration estimates that as much as 77% of Medicare expenditures in the United States are incurred for persons in the last 6 months of life and about one third of deaths occur in the hospital (14). The advances in technology that have accompanied the development of the critical care subspecialty have dramatically changed the approach and pace of care. The convergence of critical care nursing and geriatric nursing brought on by these demographic shifts and payment of care can only enhance patient care. Critical care nursing is an extremely popular specialty in the profession, with 70,000 members in the American Association of Critical Care Nurses (AACN). In stark contrast, the National Association of Gerontological Nurses has only 1741 members. The extraordinary difference in membership poses a number of questions. Is acute and critical care more highly valued than gerontological nursing care? Do those who deliver critical care of the elderly believe that they already have the needed knowledge base? Has the nursing leadership failed to make the bridge for those nurses who deliver critical care to the elderly? All may be true. Unfortunately, the data are absent, although badly needed.

The research grants program for the AACN has recently funded such important topics as ''communication needs during intubation,'' ''factors related to extubation,'' and ''psychosocial evaluation of trauma needs.'' It seems that the issues on any of these topics might vary drastically in the elderly compared with younger individuals. These are the questions for the next phase of critical care nursing research. Although many data tables in current publications break out samples by age, they do not provide the empirical data needed to guide nursing practice. The AACN is far ahead of the field in that it does feature a clinical column in every newsletter entitled, ''Geriatric Corner.'' But a column such as this alone will not provide the clinical knowledge or direction that critical care must embrace to fulfill the needs of older adults.

Generally, nurses, including acute and critical care nurses, are relatively unprepared to manage the needs of the geriatric client. Of the 63,191 master's-prepared nurse practitioners who responded to the 1997 National RN Sample Survey performed by the Division of Nursing of the Federal Bureau of Health Professions, only 4.7% stated that they had special preparation in geriatrics. Of respondents with post-master's preparation, only 4.2% had special preparation in geriatrics (Phillip Wilson, Bureau of Health Professions, Division of Nursing, personal communication). It is clear that many more nurses with geriatric specialty preparation are needed.

Despite the clear needs, new nurses coming out of baccalaureate programs have received little education in geriatric care issues. A national survey of baccalaureate nursing programs done by the John A. Hartford Foundation Institute for Geriatric Nursing examined geriatric content in the nursing curriculum (15). The study found that of the 480 schools surveyed (80% response rate) only 37% (n = 177) of schools have stand-alone courses in geriatrics and only 62% (n = 110) of those schools require the course be taken by their graduates. The remainder of schools (n = 303) state that geriatrics is integrated into the curriculum, but only 67% of schools state that geriatrics is integrated into their nursing fundamentals course. Most schools also reported that they had no faculty members, part-time or full-time, with an American Nurses Association certification in geriatrics: 58% report no full-time certified faculty members and 80% report no part-time faculty members (15). Given that 88.8% of nurses still get their first job in a hospital, it seems likely that in many schools, students are not being adequately prepared to confront and manage the needs of the geriatric client (16).

Given the scarcity of geriatric content in curricula, acute and critical care nurses welcome clinical practice guidelines and models of care that can support the care of the elderly in these settings. Although it is not our intent to change the orientation of each nurse from critical care to gerontology, the goal is to support practice with reasonable models that can help to enhance the care that is given. This enhancement model is already in place in medicine, in that specialty areas such as cardiology and pulmonology hold special courses on needs of the older patient, and textbooks increasingly add geriatric sections or chapters to their content. Similarly, the AACN has a special track in their annual meeting program that addresses geriatric issues. If the geriatrics field in nursing is serious about making a difference in the care of the elderly across settings, it will be necessary to go beyond the typical occasional lecture and support a variety of educational and clinical strategies, including organized models of nursing care that can be readily adapted (see next section).

II. MODELS OF NURSING CARE

Since 1992, the Nurses Improving Care to the Hospitalized Elderly (NICHE) Project has promulgated practice models for acute care geriatric nursing and developed adjunctive practice protocols targeted to common geriatric syndromes such as incontinence, pressure ulcers, restraint use, sleep problems, and pain management. Funded by the John A. Hartford Foundation, a substantial portion of NICHE stems from the Hospital Outcomes Project for the Elderly (HOPE), also funded by the John A. Hartford Foundation. The NICHE-recommended nursing care models have proven to be effective in improving care to hospitalized elderly, and these models can assist hospitals with redesigning their nursing care in ways that acknowledge hospitals' different capacities and resources. The models currently reflective of best practice in acute are described in the following.

A. The Geriatric Resource Nurse Model

The Geriatric Resource Nurse (GRN) model is a unit-based program that functions best in hospitals in which primary nursing is practiced. It has as its basis the premise that primary nurses know the most about the day-to-day patterns and problems of the elderly patients for whom they care. Thus, primary nurses, specifically educated to work as geriatric resource nurses, effectively integrate new practices into regular care patterns because they are highly visible and readily attain feedback from staff on their unit. The premise of the GRN model, as described elsewhere (17,18), revolves around staff nurses who self-select individuals who wish to be developed as resources for improving geriatric care on their respective units. Through a variety of continuing education activities, clinical rounds, and other unit-based practice initiatives supported by a geriatric nurse specialist, GRNs develop geriatric assessment and treatment knowledge and are then called on by other unit staff to apply their knowledge to specific patients. This model requires a geriatric advance practice nurse because when geriatric emergencies arise, the presence of a nurse who understands the fundamentals of geriatric care is essential.

B. The Acute Care of the Elderly Medical-Surgical Unit

The Acute Care of the Elderly Medical-Surgical Unit (ACE unit) model reallocates unused or underused hospital beds to create a specific unit targeted to improving clinical outcomes for elders (19,20). (See also Chapter 25.) The unit combines flexible nurse staffing and specific physical environmental adaptations to manage the problems of functional decline in the elderly. The benefit of an ACE unit is that best practice protocols can be developed and then disseminated throughout an entire hospital and health care system. Limitations include the need for a strong geriatric consultation team and physical space, which might be at a premium.

C. The Hospital-Wide Educational Model

In the hospital-wide educational model, an advance practice geriatric nurse provides consultation and education to improve nurses' accuracy and speed in detecting and managing a particular clinical syndrome, for example, delirium or restraint education. The advanced practice nurse might teach staff nurses to use and interpret simple bedside tests for assessing cognition and to recognize clinical features that distinguish delirium, dementia, and depression to accurately communicate patient symptoms to the team (21).

D. The Quality Cost Model of Transitional Care (Discharge Planning and Home Follow-up)

Developed by Naylor (9) the quality cost model of transitional care targets elderly at high risk for poor discharge outcomes. At the time of hospital admission, and through a period of weeks after discharge, an advanced practice geriatric nurse provides direct care and coordination of services to those at risk older patients. The advanced practice nurse adapts a general protocol to the specific needs of that elderly person and sees the patient soon after hospital admission. The nurse is available by telephone 24 hours a day, 7 days a week to the family and patient to help meet care needs and individualize care for that patient.

E. Multidisciplinary Case Management

The multidisciplinary case management model provides outcome-oriented patient care and ensures the appropriate use of resources for a wide variety of patients through the use of patient care pathways (22). The goal of this approach is to integrate and coordinate delivery of clinical services, to support collaborative practice and continuity of care, and to enhance patient and provider satisfaction. Patient care managers are educated about the complex conditions and comorbidities in the elderly so that they may target the care plan most effectively.

• • •

Each of the proceding models must be modified to accommodate institution-specific differences in resources and variations in philosophies. When selecting a model to implement, it is important to determine whether the model is consistent with the philosophy of the institution and the needs of the staff. New models of care include staff changes, staff mix, physical requirements, and institutional cost. All aspects of model implementation must be carefully examined, and managers should consider obtaining feedback from nursing staff about what type of model might best fulfill the needs and preferences as perceived by nursing staff. One way to begin the process of determining the staff's educational capacity to care for geriatric clients and institutional facilitators and barriers to best practice geriatrics is to survey the staff. The Geriatric Institutional Assessment Profile (GIAP) is one such available instrument (23).

III. THE GERIATRIC INSTITUTIONAL ASSESSMENT PROFILE

Before an institution initiates implementation of a nursing model, it is important to determine the institution's capacity to care for geriatric clients and how the institutional environment may impede or facilitate focusing care on the needs of the geriatric client. One approach to involve staff in the process of change and at the same time ascertain baseline capacity to care for geriatric patients is to survey the staff. The GIAP is a valid and reliable instrument administered to the staff that provides information about staff perceptions of, attitudes toward, and knowledge about common geriatric syndromes. The basis for the concept for the GIAP is the Institutional Assessment Profile developed by the Decisions Near the End of Life Model program, a product of the Educational Development Center and the Hastings Center (24). The GIAP consists of 62 items that help an institution reflect on its specific practice problems around the care of the elderly (23). Use of the GIAP enables institutions to obtain a baseline on practice issues in caring for the elderly before the initiation of new models, so that they might discern any changes in their environments once new practice models are fully engaged. The benefit of the GIAP is that it signals staff and other individuals affiliated with an institution that an interest in improving care to the elderly exists, and it sparks excellent discussion across disciplines regarding the best way to care for older patients. The GIAP uses four clinical areas—pressure ulcers, restraint management, incontinence, and sleep—as measures for best practice in geriatrics. Because these clinical issues run the gamut from areas about which the field of geriatrics has agreement on what best practice might be (i.e., restraints) to areas about which the field has yet to develop a consensus (i.e., management of sleep problems), these four clinical issues serve as proxy measures for overall capacity to provide best practice in geriatrics. Results from the GIAP allow an institution to identify in which clinical area(s) the institution excels and in which clinical area(s) the institution needs improvement, in terms of nursing knowledge, attitudes or environmental barriers, and facilitators. Such results then allow the institution to more appropriately target change in activities to actual needs. One limitation of the GIAP is that it reports only the perceptions of individuals who work in the environment rather than actual care practice. Once a geriatric institutional assessment is complete, the institution has data available to determine the appropriate focus for improvement—for instance, what educational programs would be most useful for staff and which clinical practice protocols should be implemented first in a setting.

A. Practice Protocols

All hospitals have nursing practice protocols as a Joint Commission on Accreditation for Healthcare Organizations (JACHO) standard. These protocols reflect the way that an institution's nursing department approaches particular care activities such as monitoring high blood pressure, assessing the confused patient, and intervening with the incontinent patient. If an institution is having difficulty in any of these settings, clinical groups can come together and re-evaluate the current practice protocols and improve them in a way that benefits the elderly patients. In ICUs, practice protocols that should especially be targeted for geriatric adaptation include pain management, skin care, and delirium. A variety of protocols are available for institutions to adapt and use in their settings, including those available from the Agency for Health Care Policy and Research. The NICHE Project has also developed a series of 13 protocols specifically targeted to provide care for syndromes commonly experienced by elderly patients. A number of these protocols, including those addressing management of pressure ulcers (25), depression (26), pain (27), and cognitive assessment (28), have been published in the journal *Geriatric Nursing*. A compilation of these protocols along with recommendations for adapting the protocols to various care environments is also available from Springer Publishing Company (29).

Implementation of any protocol should also be accompanied by educational in-servicing of staff, including nurses, physicians, and other professionals. Table 1 provides some sample lecture outlines that could be used by an advanced practice nurse or other clinical trainer to structure a lecture on common syndromes (Table 2) in the elderly client or a lecture on a specific geriatric syndrome. Lectures are especially enhanced when paired with geriatric nursing clinical rounds or teaching cases.

B. Use of Teaching Cases

Teaching cases can be especially useful in educating nurses on how to care for elders in intensive care environments. One of the authors (K.F.) of this chapter has compiled a set of cases that she uses routinely to help geriatric nurses think specifically about geriatric issues in that setting (K. Fletcher, personal communication).

Case 1

Mr. J. (80 years old) was admitted to the coronary care unit (CCU) for insertion of a temporary pacemaker after a series of falls at home. Mr. J. had been diagnosed with stage 2 Alzheimer's disease. His wife is his primary caregiver. After the insertion of the pacemaker, he frequently tried to climb out of bed in an attempt to find the bathroom, often leaving his pacemaker behind. Safety became

Table 1 Sample Lectures

Skin problems
Prevention is key
High morbidity and cost
Special flotation mattress
Careful nursing care
Team approach to intervention
Pain management
Problems with eating and feeding
Cold or unpalatable food
Restraints preventing eating
Poor dentition
Delirium
Nausea discomfort
Careful planning needed
Incontinence
50% institutionalized elders
15%–25% community elders
Prevention is key
Bowel and bladder guidelines
Treat the cause
Prevent symptoms
Confusion
Serious and potentially fatal
Delirium vs dementia
Baseline measure to compare
Team effort to prevent iatrogenesis
Management of disturbing behavior
Evidence of falls
Falls history
Nonrestraint as the best standard
Careful review of medication
Milieu theory
Special equipment/furniture
Sleep disorders
Common
Chronic pain dyspnea
Sedation may be unnecessary
Sleep hygiene program

Table 2 Common Geriatric Syndromes that Affect the Elderly in Acute and Intensive Care

SPICES
*S*kin problems
*P*roblems with eating and feeding
*I*ncontinence
*C*onfusion
*E*vidence of falls
*S*leep disorders

a serious concern because of his short-term memory deficits and impaired judgment. A geriatric resource nurse explored alternatives to restraint with the staff, and the patient was maintained in the CCU without a physical restraint and with minimal use of psychotropic medication.

During rounds with the advance practice nurse, it was noted that Mr. J. had nocturia and no documentation of a prostate examination existed. This was followed up and treated by the medical staff. Although Mr. J.'s primary problem was cardiac in origin, urinary incontinence is known to be a frequent precipitant of nursing home placement, and Mr. J.'s cognitive impairment already put him at risk for placement. Early identification and treatment of nocturia during hospitalization enabled him to return home with his wife.

Case 2

Mrs. K. (76 years old) was admitted to the medical intensive care unit (MICU) for acute gastrointestinal bleeding resulting from a combination of prescribed prednisone and excessive use of over-the-counter nonsteroidal anti-inflammatory drugs to control her pain from rheumatoid arthritis. Her physical condition was stabilized, but by the second day of hospitalization she was restless, agitated, and combative. The disruptive behavior was managed by the staff with physical and chemical restraints. The geriatric resource nurse explored all potential sources for the patient's delirious behavior and discovered that in the past medical history of the patient alprazolam was used long term for an anxiety disorder—something that was overlooked during the emergency admission of the patient. The MICU treatment team was informed of this finding and a psychiatric consultation was done. A tapering regimen of alprazolam was prescribed and the problem was resolved.

Case 3

Mrs. B. (92 years old) had a history of dementia and was brought into the emergency department (ED) from a local nursing home with a chief complaint that her "bra felt too tight." The initial response of the ED staff was that this was an inappropriate transfer. The geriatric resource nurse in the ED, appreciating the frequent atypical presentation of geriatric patients, responded quickly and performed a 12-lead ECG that revealed findings consistent with non-Q wave myocardial infarction. Mrs. B. received aggressive therapeutic management in the ED and was transferred to the CCU.

• • •

Case-based learning is a popular strategy for highlighting the multiple geriatric syndromes inherent in almost every geriatric patient presentation. Regular case presentations focused on geriatric syndromes as part of regular grand rounds held in any specialty will enhance the sensitivity that each nurse will have for geriatric issues. Once a case is discussed, a group leader can ask a variety of questions including (1) what are the geriatric syndromes imbedded in this case; (2) how does aging affect the way we assess this syndrome; (3) how does aging affect the way we treat this syndrome; and (4) how does discharge planning and advance directive discussion get modified by virtue of the age of the patient, if at all? Bringing out questions such as these sensitizes the clinician, uncovers any ageism that is present in the institutional culture, and helps develop an environment where age-related care becomes something to think about more specifically and rigorously.

IV. CONTINUITY OF CARE ACROSS SETTINGS

The changes described in the acute care setting have an impact on the continuum of care. Elders are discharged back home or to the long-term care setting faster than ever before, creating stress for those settings as they try to help the older person during the rehabilitative process. Excellent communication and continuity of care across settings has never been more important or necessary.

One way to begin the process of continuity of care, institutionalize awareness of geriatric care issues among nursing staff, and help develop advanced practice skills in staff nurses is through the use of a trigger card and anecdotal record keeping. The Geriatric Resource Nurse Program, as a part of the John A. Hartford Foundation's HOPE initiative (17), developed the SPICES mnemonic. SPICES (Tables 1 and 2) stands for *S*leep disorders, *P*roblems with eating or feeding, *I*ncontinence, *C*onfusion, *E*vidence of falls, and *S*kin breakdown (18). This is a simple approach in which the monthly collection of prevalence data on the preceding clinical problems helps focus the nursing unit on the common problems encountered in caring for older people and on what clinical guidelines need development or refinement for the elderly.

A. Sleep Disorders

Sleep disturbances, which are common in the elderly, are exacerbated by acute illnesses and hospitalizations. Symptoms that may cause or worsen the problem of insomnia, such as dyspnea, confusion, pain, depression, and anxiety, are often experienced by hospitalized elderly patients.

Nursing care of the patient with a sleep disorder should begin with a thorough history of sleep habits and previous successful and unsuccessful treatments for sleep used by the patient in the past. Initially, interventions should focus on the resolution of any etiological factors such as pain and other symptom management.

Nonpharmacological approaches to sleep disorders are preferable. Enabling routines and rituals that are associated with bedtime at home are encouraged whenever possible (30).

B. Problems with Eating and Feeding

Nearly 50% of persons aged 65 years and older are clinically malnourished at the time of admission to the hospital, and two-thirds are malnourished at the time of discharge (31). Institutional barriers that affect food intake may include food that is cold or unpalatable and not modified to a patient's cultural or ethnic preferences, newly imposed dietary restrictions, compromised dining experiences with frequent interruptions and minimal assistance available for patients with functional deficits, physical restraints that limit access or ability to eat, poor dental care, delirium, and discomfort associated with nausea and pain. In the acute care setting, additional factors such as ventilators, nasogastric tubes, profound illness, swallowing disorders, and depression can also contribute to anorexia (32).

Assessing dietary habits and obtaining a diet history will help to determine what interventions will be most effective. Nursing interventions to promote nutrition and increase food intake need to be individualized and may include serving smaller portions, understanding food preferences, and encouraging companionship during meals. Interventions that focus on pain reduction should be considered before meals for patients experiencing pain. Patients with cognitive impairments may need further assistance with caring and feeding. Careful planning is necessary to ensure that appropriate staff is available to provide eating assistance and that staff is well trained in how to feed patients with eating problems (32).

Nursing interventions in the acute care setting also include nutritional supplementation through the use of hyperalimentation feeding, tube feedings, and other supplements. Nutritional complications that are associated with acutely ill patients such as malabsorption syndromes, less physiological reserve, and weight loss may be clinically insignificant in a younger person but present a major barrier to the wellness of an older adult.

C. Incontinence

Incontinence, or the involuntary loss of urine sufficient to be a problem, occurs in more than 50% of institutionalized elders and in 15% to 25% of community-dwelling elders. Certain risk factors associated with incontinence such as immobility, increased confusion, medications, fecal impaction, low fluid intake, environmental barriers, and numerous disease processes are exacerbated during hospitalizations. Obtaining a history and identifying various risk factors is essential in determining the cause or type of incontinence the patient is experiencing. Causes should be determined and treated (33).

Urinary incontinence is categorized as urge, stress, overflow, or functional. Treatment for incontinence is varied and may include surgical interventions, pharmacological, and behavioral modalities.

Nursing interventions, which are part of the interdisciplinary team care plan, include scheduled toileting, the administration of medications such as anticholinergics, and monitoring side effects associated with the use of these medications. Products such as absorbent pads, diapers, and various skin barriers may also be part of the nursing care plan. Indwelling catheters are used in hospitalized elderly patients for various reasons, including the need to monitor output and to prevent incontinence in patients with severe skin ulcers. Nursing interventions with regard to monitoring and treating urinary tract infections associated with the use of indwelling catheters are essential (33,34).

D. Confusion

Changes in mental status are commonly seen in acutely ill elderly hospital patients. (See also Chapters 20 and 21.) Etiological factors that are associated with new onset confusion and or the worsening of an already existing dementia are varied. Initial nursing interventions need to focus on a thorough history from friends and family to determine baseline cognitive function of the patient. Assessment of cognitive status on admission and subsequently throughout the hospitalization is an essential component of nursing care. Use of the Mini-Mental State Examination (MMSE) provides a valid and reliable tool for screening cognitive impairments (35). It is easy to administer and requires only 5 to 10 minutes of nursing time.

Caring for confused elderly patients in the acute care setting requires a large amount of nursing resources. Physical and chemical restraints that are sometimes used to enable the care of these patients should be avoided. Nursing interventions should include all attempts to reduce environmental stress and should focus on individual communication and reassurance. Disturbing behaviors should not be allowed to interrupt appropriate care for older adults (36).

E. Evidence of Falls

A baseline assessment of all acutely ill hospitalized elderly patients with regard to falls risk is essential. Risk factors that are seen in many hospitalized elderly patients include cognitive impairments, depression, impaired mobility, gait and balance disturbances, history of previous falls, environmental factors, sensory impairments, elimination problems, postural hypotension, and the use of assistive devices.

Interventions that focus on falls prevention are an essential component to geriatric nursing in the acute care setting. Interventions such as easy access to call bells, low beds, proper lighting, appropriate footwear, elevated toilet seats with grab bars, and decreasing room clutter will help to prevent falls. Evaluating the cause of a history of falls is essential to prevent further incidents. A falls history should consist of determining the activity at the time of the fall, location of the fall, past medical history, medications and premonitory symptoms such as light-headedness and palpitations (29).

The use of restraints in acutely ill geriatric patients is no longer an acceptable standard. Alternatives to restraints need to be the focus of nursing care. This issue not only affects clinicians but also hospital administrators, who struggle with issues of liability, residents rights, and adequate staffing.

F. Skin Breakdown

The prevalence of pressure ulcers in acute care settings ranges from 2.7% to 32.1%, with an overall prevalence of 10% (37). In addition to the significant pain and altered levels of comfort associated with pressure ulcers, the cost burden to the health care system is also tremendous. Therefore, efforts targeted to prevention should be the focus of any initiative to solve this problem.

The prevention of pressure ulcers begins with assessing patients who are at risk for skin breakdown developing. Hospitalized patients who are bed or chair bound with an impaired ability to reposition themselves should be considered at risk. The use of valid and reliable risk assessment measures enables clinicians to develop individualized plans of care directly related to specific risk factors such as decreased mental status, incontinence, or nutritional deficits (38).

Interventions based on individualized assessment help to reduce specific risks. Nursing efforts should focus on reducing pressure and shear forces. Turning and positioning bed-bound patients at least every 2 hours should also use pillows or foam wedges to maintain alignment and keep bony prominences such as knees and ankles from direct contact with each other. Additional interventions related to prevention are individualizing bathing frequency and reducing injury resulting from friction and shear forces with the use of dry lubricants such as cornstarch. Nutritional interventions, including supplements, should be considered for those patients with compromised protein and calorie intake. The nursing care of incontinent patients consists of the assessment and treatment of incontinence, cleansing of the skin and the use of a topical moisture barrier, and the selection of underpads or briefs that are absorbent and provide a quick drying surface to the skin (25).

Nursing assessment of pressure ulcers uses staging of the lesion. Staging aids in the development of an appropriate treatment regimen and permits an ongoing evaluation of treatment success or failure. It is important to recognize that, according to the National Pressure Ulcer Advisory Panel (NPUAP), staging should occur only once because ulcers do not heal from stage IV to stage 1 (39). Limitations to the staging system include limited use with patients with darkly pigmented skin and the inability to stage an ulcer with an eschar present.

The treatment of pressure ulcers varies according to a patient's individual risk factors and the severity of the ulcer. However, the initial treatment objective of any pressure ulcer is to eliminate or to reduce pressure on the existing lesion and to new ulcers.

One of the NICHE projects was recently involved with a video supported by JCAHO that outlined JCAHO's perceptions of appropriate institutional response to skin problems and valuable resources for implementing skin treatment programs. Such a video may be a good source of information on appropriate medical and nursing care for prevention of skin breakdown. Overall, careful nursing care is the key to prevention of pressure ulcers (25).

REFERENCES

1. Skillman J. Surgical Intensive Care. Boston: Little, Brown, 1975, pp 1–7.
2. Jacelon CS. Preventing cascade iagrogenesis in hospitalized elders. J Gerontol Nurs 94:27–33, 1999.
3. Fulmer T, Ashley J, Reilly C. Geriatric nursing in acute settings. Annu Rev Gerontol Geriatr 6:27–80, 1986.
4. Ebersole P, Hess P. Toward Healthy Aging: Human Needs and Nursing Response. St. Louis: Mosby, 1981, pp 168–182.
5. Eliopoulos C. Gerontological nursing. New York: Harper & Row, 1979, pp 5–12.
6. Capezuti E, Evans L, Strumpf N, Maislin G. Physical restraint use and falls in nursing home residents (see comments). J Am Geriatr Soc 44(6):627–633, 1996.
7. Evans LK, Strumpf NE, Allen-Taylor SL, Capezuti E, Maislin G, Jacobsen B. A clinical trial to reduce restraints in nursing homes (see comments). J Am Geriatr Soc 45(6):675–681, 1997.
8. Siegler EL, Capezuti E, Maislin G, Baumgarten M, Evans L, Strumpf N. Effects of

a restraint reduction intervention and OBRA '87 regulations on psychoactive drug use in nursing homes (see comments). J Am Geriatr Soc 45(7):791–796, 1997.
9. Naylor M, Brooten D, Jones R, Lavizzo-Mourey R, Mezey M, Pauly M. Comprehensive discharge planning for the hospitalized elderly. A randomized clinical trial. Ann Intern Med 120(12):999–1006, 1994.
10. Daly K, Kleinpell RM, Lawinger S, Casey G. The effect of two nursing interventions on families of ICU patients. Clin Nur Res 3(4):414–422, 1994.
11. Kleinpell RM, Powers MJ. Needs of family members of intensive care unit patients. Appl Nur Res 5(1):2–8, 1992.
12. Minnick A, Roberts MJ, Young WB, Kleinpell RM, Micek W. An analysis of post-hospitalization telephone survey data. Nurs Res 44(6):371–375, 1995.
13. Palmer RM. Acute care. In: Hazzard WR, Blass JP, Ettinger Jr. WH, Halter JB, Ouslander JG, eds. Principles of Geriatric Medicine and Gerongology. 4th ed. New York: McGraw-Hill, 1999, pp 483–492.
14. Emanuel EJ, Emanuel LL. The economics of dying. The illusion of cost savings at the end of life (see comments). N Engl J Med 330(8):540–544, 1994.
15. Rosenfeld P, Bottrell MM, Fulmer TT, Mezey MD. Gerontological nursing content in baccalaureate nursing programs: findings from a national survey. J Prof Nurs. 15(2):84–94, 1999.
16. Louden D, Crawford L, Trotman S, eds. Profiles of the Newly Licensed Nurse. 3rd ed. New York: National League for Nursing Press, 1996, pp 49–75.
17. Fulmer T. Grow your own experts in hospital elder care. Geriatr Nurs 12(2):64–66, 1991.
18. Fulmer T. The geriatric nurse specialist role: a new model. Nurs Manage 22(3):91–93, 1991.
19. Landefeld CS, Palmer RM, Kresevic DM, Fortinsky RH, Kowal J. A randomized trial of care in a hospital medical unit especially designed to improve the functional outcomes of acutely ill older patients. N Engl J Med 332(20):1338–1344, 1995.
20. Palmer RM, Landefeld CS, Kresevic D, Kowal J. A medical unit for the acute care of the elderly. J Am Geriatr Soc 42(5):545–552, 1994.
21. The NICHE Project Faculty. Geriatric models of care: Which one's right for your institution? Am J Nurs 94(7):21–23, 1994.
22. Cohen EL, Cesta TG. Nursing Case Management: From Concept to Evaluation. St. Louis: Mosby, 1993, pp 117–125.
23. Abraham IL, Bottrell MM, Dash K, Fulmer T, O'Donnell L, Vince-Whitman C. Profiling care and benchmarking best practice in care of hospitalized elderly: the Geriatric Institutional Assessment Profile. Nurs Clin North Am 34(1):237–255, 1999.
24. Solomon MZ, O'Donnell L, Jennings B, Guilfoy V, Wolf SM, Nolan K, Jackson R, Koch-Weser D, Donnelly S. Decisions near the end of life: professional views on life-sustaining treatments. Am J Public Health 83(1):14–23, 1993.
25. Kresevic DM, Naylor M. Preventing pressure ulcers through use of protocols in a mentored nursing model. Geriatr Nurs 16(5):225–229, 1995.
26. Kurlowicz LH. Nursing standard of practice protocols: depression in elderly patients. Geriatr Nurs 18:192–200, 1997.

27. Fulmer T, Mion LC, Bottrell MM. Pain management protocol. NICHE Faculty. Geriatr Nurs 17(5):222–226, 1996.
28. Foreman M, Fletcher K, Mion L,and the NICHE Faculty. Assessing cognitive function. Geriatr Nurs 17:228–233, 1996.
29. Bottrell MM, Abraham I, Fulmer T, Mezey M, eds. Geriatric Nursing Protocols for Best Practice. 1st ed. New York: Springer, 1999.
30. Foreman MD, Wykle M. Sleep disturbances in elderly patients. In: Bottrell MM, Abraham I, Fulmer T, Mezey M, eds. Geriatric Nursing Protocols for Best Practice. New York: Springer, 1999; pp. 13–25.
31. Yoshikawa TT, Cobbs EL, Brummel-Smith K. Practical Ambulatory Geriatrics. 2nd ed. St. Louis: Mosby, 1998, pp 176–186.
32. Amella EJ. Assessment and management of eating and feeding difficulties for older people: A NICHE protocol. Geriatr Nurs 19(5):269–275, 1998.
33. Bradway C, Hernley S, and the NICHE Faculty. Urinary incontinence in older adults admitted to acute care. Geriatr Nurs 19(2):98–102, 1998.
34. U.S. Department of Health and Human Services. Urinary incontinence in adults: Acute and chronic management. Rockville, MD: AHCPR Publication No. 96-0686, 1996.
35. Folstein M, Folstein SE, McHugh PR. Mini-Mental State: a practical method for grading the cognitive state of patients for the clinician. J Psych Res 12:189–198, 1975.
36. Foreman MD, Fletcher K, Mion LC, Simon L, and the NICHE Faculty. Assessing cognitive function. Geriatr Nurs 17(5):228–233, 1996.
37. U.S. Department of Health and Human Services. Treatment of Pressure Ulcers. Rockville, MD: AHCPR Publication No. 95-0652, 1995.
38. Bergstrom N, Braden B, Boynton P. Using research based assessment scales in clinical practice. Nurs Clin North Am 30:539–551, 1995.
39. National Pressure Ulcer Advisory Panel. Proceedings of the national pressure ulcer advisory panel fifth national conference: Monitoring pressure ulcer healing, an alternative to reverse staging. Adv Wound Care 10(5):26–28, 1977.

5
Emergency Preoperative Evaluation

Edward H. Livingston
VA Greater Los Angeles Healthcare System, and UCLA School of Medicine, Los Angeles, California

Surgical emergencies in the elderly are among the most vexing problems clinicians have to manage. Frequently, disease processes that present as an acute illness in younger patients will evolve over a longer period of time in the elderly. The symptoms and signs of surgical disorders can be subtle. Consequently, surgical disorders are seen at a more advanced stage in elderly patients. These fragile individuals often have a severe disease burden, making their management difficult and outcomes poor.

In addition to the medical issues ethical considerations relevant to the elderly population must be considered. Not infrequently terminal events are first seen as surgical emergencies. Thus, before instituting aggressive surgical management clinicians must consider the patient's quality of life. Advance directives should be sought and family consulted.

Decision making for managing surgical emergencies in the elderly is complex. One must consider the overall physiological state of the patient, the disease burden, project the final outcome, and consider a variety of ethical issues when managing the elderly.

I. PLANNING

Elderly patients undergoing emergency surgery might have a prolonged and difficult hospital course after the intervention. The patient might be fully competent before an operation. Elderly patients are susceptible to loss of cognition after general anesthesia or from complications of the surgery. Therefore, if at all possible, discussion of the nature of the emergency, diagnosis, what intervention is planned, risks, informed consent, and advance directives, and an explanation of the most likely postoperative scenario should be held with the patient. Given these issues, the patient should identify procedures for medical decision making should he or she lose cognitive function. This discussion is best witnessed by another member of the medical team and documented in the medical record. One advisable practice is to write a note for the patient stating exactly on what has been agreed, then have the patient sign it while still awake and alert.

A. Diagnosis

Oftentimes elderly patients adapt to chronic pain, or pain is masked by other background conditions. For this reason diagnosing the cause of emergency problems is much more difficult in the elderly than in the young. The most common operative emergencies in the elderly are general surgical and orthopedic. Table 1 summarizes the most frequent indications for emergency general surgical procedures in the elderly (1).

B. Risk

The morbidity and mortality for surgery in the elderly are high. The mortality for elective operations in the elderly is approximately 10% but increases two-fold to three-fold for one-third of patients experiencing complications (1,2). The death rate is highest for patients undergoing laparotomy and is 50% to 60% (3,4). Mortality is associated with high American Society of Anesthesiologists (ASA) scores and significant bacterial contamination (1). Hypotension when the patient is initially seen, severe chronic disease factors, and lack of self-care ability strongly predict adverse surgical outcomes. When these factors are present, 57%

Table 1 General Surgical Causes for Emergent Operations in the Elderly

Diagnosis	%
Gallstone disease	22.1
Hernia	14.9
Colorectal cancer	13.7
Vascular disease	13.1
Peptic ulcer	6.5
Gastric cancer	5.9

of elderly patients undergoing laparotomy die compared with only 15% of those who do not have these features (4).

For the very old (i.e., greater than 90 years old) the most frequent operations are for hip fracture, lower extremity amputation, and abdominal problems. In this group 30-day and in-hospital surgical mortality total 36% for both elective and emergency surgeries. Poor outcomes are predicted when admission is from a nursing home and a major functional impairment is present preoperatively (5).

Serum albumin concentration, as an indicator of general health and nutrition, is the single most powerful predictor of outcome. In longitudinal studies of elderly patients serum albumin is highly correlated with all-cause mortality (6). In the largest prospective surgical risk assessment study performed, preoperative serum albumin levels of less than 3.7 g/dl were the single greatest predictor of postoperative complications and death (Figure 1 and Table 2) (7). When elderly patients are seen with an acute surgical emergency, careful attention must be paid to the patient's nutritional status. If patients are malnourished (defined as having an albumin level < 3.7 g/dL), the expected morbidity and mortality for surgical intervention are high. Under these circumstances, surgery should be delayed or minimized if at all possible until the nutritional status is improved.

Thus, the risks for surgery in the elderly are high and particularly so for

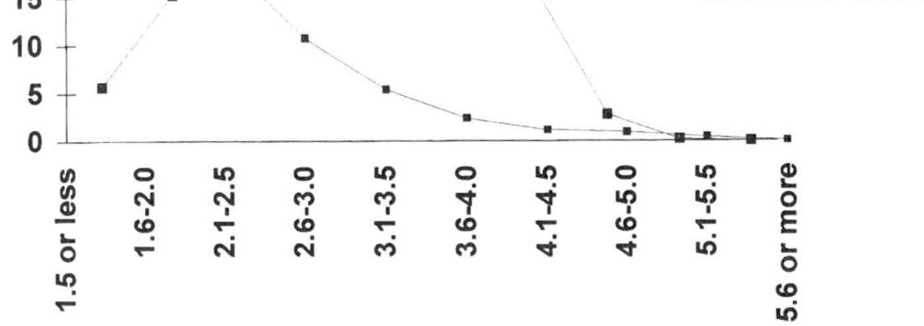

Figure 1 Univariate analysis: preoperative serum albumin. In the 103,342 surgeries prospectively evaluated in the VA Surgery Risk Assessment Study, serum albumin measurement (in grams per deciliter) correlated the closest to mortality. The larger square points represent the total number of deaths plotted against the serum albumin level on the abscissa. The smaller square points are the death rate that increases markedly for serum albumin levels less than 3.7 (S. Khuri, Personal communication).

Table 2 Frequency of Preoperative Variables in Nine Predictive Models[a]

Preoperative variable	No. of models	Average rank
Serum albumin	9	1.9
ASA class	8	3.6
Emergency status	8	5.4
DNR status	8	7.5
BUN >40	7	5.7
Disseminated cancer	7	6.0
Age	7	6.4
Weight loss >10%	7	8.1
Serum bilirubin >1.0	5	10.2
Dyspnea	5	11.0

ASA, American Society of Anesthesiologists; DNR, do not resuscitate; BUN, blood urea nitrogen.

[a] Analysis of risk factors for surgical mortality in 103,342 surgeries studied prospectively in the VA revealed that low serum albumin was the strongest correlate of mortality. Nine separate models were used, one for all operations and one for each surgical subspecialty. Low serum albumin predicted mortality in each of the nine models. (S. Khuri, Personal communication).

emergencies. Converting emergent situations to elective ones is a major benefit. This can be achieved by careful assessment of patients. If the surgery can be delayed and patients can undergo a thorough resuscitation, their expected mortality would be decreased. Careful screening of elderly patients to identify diseases frequently seen as emergencies might have substantial overall benefit. A case could be made for more aggressive elective removal of gallbladders or repair of the hernias to avoid these clinical problems being first seen as emergencies, with their attendant high surgical mortality.

C. Informed Consent

Elderly patients undergoing emergency operations are at risk for significant complications. A detailed description of the planned operation must be provided. The patient must be informed regarding expected side effects of an operation that will be permanent. For example, the presence of dumping syndrome and weight loss after gastric resection. Unanticipated complications such as infections, pulmonary embolus, and others should also be discussed with the patient. Complications are frequent in this population; they generally are severe, and the consequent loss of mental capacity is frequent. Because complications exact a high toll on the mental capacity of elderly patients it should be anticipated that patients will lose their ability to make decisions. A discussion of surrogate decision makers should be made and preferably a durable power of attorney form completed. Do-not-resuscitate (DNR) orders should be entertained and the exact nature and extent of resuscitative efforts be clearly delineated by the patient (see next section).

If a patient lacks the capacity to make health care decisions, a surrogate decision maker must be identified. The following can identify these decision makers:

Durable power of attorney for health care (See next section for definition).

Legal guardian or special guardian. These individuals are appointed by a court of law and retain the power to decide on the patient's behalf. A legal guardian retains the authority to make all forms of decisions for another individual. A special guardian only retains the authority to make medically related decisions on a patient's behalf.

Next of kin. This is an adult relative of the patient who can serve as a surrogate decision maker. Generally, it is accepted that the following priority be used in determining who should serve as the surrogate: spouse, adult child, parent, adult sibling, grandparent, and adult grandchild.

Close friend. Close friends are individuals who have shown care and concern for the patient's welfare and are familiar with the patient's activities, health, religious beliefs, and values. They may also be relatives not listed in the preceding section as next of kin. It is preferable that the individual designated as a close friend who retains medical decision-making authority provide a written statement agreeing to take responsibility and specifying the relationship to the patient.

No surrogate available. Should the patient not be competent to make decisions and no surrogate is identified, the treatment team must make decisions. Individual hospitals will have policies and procedures for authorizing emergency treatments. If time permits, the hospital Bio-Ethics committee may be consulted. Under these circumstances, documentation in the medical record is crucial explaining what the nature of the emergency was, who participated in the decision making, and what efforts were made to identify or find surrogate decision makers.

D. Advance Directives for Health Care

Advance directives are documents declaring a patient's health care choices or naming someone to make those choices should they become incapacitated. (See also Chapter 2.) Federal law requires that any patient receiving Medicare or Medicaid benefits be given information regarding advance directives. Explanations regarding the patient's legal rights in reference to medical decision making must be provided. There are two major types of advance directives: (1) a living will, which is a declaration regarding the use of life-sustaining procedures; and (2) a durable power of attorney for health care, which is a document designating another person responsible for making medically related decisions.

1. Living Will

A living will is a document directing the medical care team to withhold or withdraw various life-sustaining procedures in the event of a terminal illness and a patient becomes unable to make his or her own medical decisions. In many instances, living wills are not valid for withholding or withdrawing nutrition or hydration. The living will only takes effect when the terminal condition or patient's incompetence is present.

2. Durable Power of Attorney for Health Care

A durable power of attorney names another individual to make health care decisions for patients should they become incompetent. The document might provide certain guidelines for that decision making. In the absence of such guidelines, the surrogate retains the authority to make medically relevant decisions. Similar to a living will this document only becomes valid when the patient is unable to make his or her own health care decisions.

3. Do-Not-Resuscitate Orders

As part of the advance directive process DNR orders may have been written. If a DNR order has not been written, it is important to discuss this with the patient. Elderly patients undergoing emergency operations are highly susceptible to complications. Those complications are often poorly tolerated by the elderly. During the recovery process, it is likely that the patient's ability to make competent medical decisions will be compromised. Before this occurs, it is critically important to know what the patient's desires are regarding resuscitative efforts. The concept of DNR should be incorporated with the discussion of informed consent (see earlier section).

Surgery may be required in a patient who has a pre-existing DNR order. Under these circumstances, the DNR order may be rescinded or modified in the immediate perioperative period (8).

II. RESUSCITATION AND PREPARATION FOR SURGERY

A. Immediate Interventions

Many patients requiring emergency operations are hypovolemic when they first arrive at the hospital. The most common disorders resulting into emergency operations for elderly patients are abdominal problems, such as cholecystitis, or fractures. Either of these conditions can result in hypovolemia and shock. Failure to properly and adequately resuscitate patients will result in poor outcomes. The physiological stress of surgery is significant. If a patient enters the operating room while still in shock, the combination of physiological stress resulting from surgery with the underlying shock results in significant end organ injury. Resuscitation can be considered in terms of ABCDEF (i.e., *a*irway, *b*reathing, *c*irculation, *de*compression, *e*limination, and *fl*uids) (9).

1. **A**irway

Shock is defined as circulatory failure resulting in inadequate delivery of oxygen to the tissues. The quickest way to deprive tissue of oxygen is depleting the blood supply of oxygen by inadequate air exchange in the lungs. For this reason ensuring adequate airway function is the first priority in resuscitation. The clinician must first assess the airway patency and ensure that the patient is breathing adequately. In the lethargic patient who is at risk for the airway being obstructed by a lax tongue, an oral airway should be placed. Any patient at risk for shock should have oxygen administered. This is to ensure that the blood is maximally saturated with oxygen to minimize the risk of inadequate tissue oxygenation. Care must be taken with elderly patients suspected of having chronic obstructive pulmonary disease; oxygen potentially decreases the respiratory drive, resulting in hypoventilation.

Endotracheal intubation must be considered in any patient with respiratory compromise or severe shock. One of the greatest errors in critical care management with the most dramatic consequences is the failure to intubate a patient when it is needed. This is especially true for the elderly patient. Older patients have some degree of organ degeneration by virtue of their age. Lesser degrees of tissue hypoxia result in injury in the elderly than would be the case for younger patients. Thus, the damaging effect of failure to promptly intubate elderly patients who need it is substantial. A low threshold must be present for intubation in the elderly patient with any degree of respiratory distress or shock. The consequences of unnecessary intubation with subsequent extubation are minimal compared with those related to failure to intubate on a timely basis.

2. **B**reathing

Once the airway is secured, attention must be directed toward breathing. The patient's respirations are observed, and if tachypnea is present, intubation should be considered. Breath sounds should be auscultated. If breath sounds are diminished and a pneumothorax or pleural effusion is suspected, a needle can be placed into the pleural cavity through the second intercostal space and the pleural cavity emptied. In the critically ill elderly patient in whom any question exists regarding hemodynamic or respiratory compromise resulting from a pneumothorax, a chest tube should be placed. This is easily performed by making an incision on the anterior chest wall at the fourth intercostal space. This corresponds to the thinnest portion of the chest wall just beneath the breast. The pleural cavity can be entered and a chest tube inserted. If the patient is wheezing, bronchodilators should be given to ensure maximal airflow through the respiratory system.

3. Circulation

Establishing adequate intravenous (IV) access is important. Patients requiring emergency operations generally require large volumes of fluid. Obtaining an IV access in the elderly can be difficult because of fragile veins. Ideally, two large-bore catheters are placed in each antecubital fossa. If this cannot be achieved, it is usually best to place a central venous catheter in the jugular or subclavian vein. In the elderly, this can be hazardous because of anatomical distortion of the relationship between the major vessels and chest wall that occurs with aging. In younger patients, the saphenous vein cutdown provides excellent access. However, in the elderly these vessels may have been harvested for coronary or peripheral vascular reconstructions. In the very elderly, these vessels tend to be small and friable, making the cut-down technically difficult. In the acute setting, it is probably better to insert a femoral vein catheter. Although this line is highly susceptible to infection, it is relatively easy to place with little risk of complications. When the patient has stabilized, other forms of IV access can be pursued and the femoral line discontinued.

In the process of obtaining IV access, blood can be collected for the hematocrit determination and other laboratory tests. Blood should be sent to the laboratory for blood type and cross match.

4. Decompression

Nasogastric tube insertion is critical for almost any elderly patient undergoing emergency surgery. Certainly if the cause of the emergency is an intra-abdominal process, a nasogastric tube must be placed. Moreover, elderly patients tend to have reduced gastric emptying. The added stress of a serious medical problem requiring emergency surgery will result in the development of an ileus. In fact, one of the most common causes of ileus is orthopedic surgery of the hip (10). Aspiration pneumonia is highly lethal in postoperative elderly patients. For these reasons any elderly patient undergoing urgent surgery or being resuscitated should have a nasogastric tube placed as early as possible.

5. Elimination

Foley catheter placement is essential. In the absence of renal failure, monitoring the urine output provides the most accurate measurement of the resuscitation.

Before any patient goes to the operating room, fluid resuscitation must be as complete as possible. If the urine output responds to fluid resuscitation, the patient's shock is being effectively reversed. In the absence of urine output, shock or ongoing renal failure is present and more aggressive monitoring might be indicated before surgery.

6. Fluids

Fluids must be given in large volumes for patients who either are bleeding or in shock. One common mistake is to give too little fluid to elderly patients. Because of their susceptibility to congestive heart failure, some are reluctant to give significant amounts of fluids to the elderly. However, the damaging effects of untreated shock exceed those of congestive heart failure. Elderly patients who have congestive heart failure develop generally respond to diuretics. Under the worst circumstances they may require intubation and dialysis. However, the patient with untreated shock will have end organ damage. This can result in acute respiratory distress syndrome, renal failure, hepatic failure, other end organ damage, and death. (See also Chapter 11.)

Blood is the best resuscitative fluid. Patients with hemorrhagic shock or those initially seen with anemia with shock from other causes should have blood administered. For extremely critical patients type O negative blood may be given before blood typing. Once the patient's blood is typed, specific blood can be adminstered until cross-matched blood is available.

Normal saline is the next best resuscitative fluid. Colloids are theoretically attractive because they increase plasma oncotic pressure and, therefore, retain intravascular fluid. However, numerous trials comparing colloid to saline resuscitation have found these two modalities to be equivalent (11). Thus, liberal amounts of normal saline should be given to patients in shock. With a Foley catheter in place the response to fluid administration is easily determined. Saline should be given as rapidly and safely as possible until urine output is restored. In the absence of renal failure, recovery of the urine output in response to fluid administration is the most sensitive indicator of adequate resuscitation.

Until all the steps outlined in the preceding are completed, other diagnostic tests or therapeutic interventions are of no added benefit. Frequently, when patients are being resuscitated, the first steps taken are acquisition of blood gases, ordering x-ray films, and so on. Until a patient is resuscitated by the interventions previously outlined, these additional maneuvers simply waste time (9). The results from added diagnostic tests will make little difference unless the patient is well underway to being resuscitated. Time is of the essence for patients who are in shock. Each minute of delay can translate into significant end organ damage and a prolonged intensive care unit stay.

7. Antibiotics

Infection is a major cause of morbidity and mortality after emergency surgery. Early administration of antibiotics will help reduce the risk of an infection developing. In the presence of active infection, parenteral antibiotics reduce the magnitude of sepsis. Broad-spectrum antibiotics should be administered early with conversion to more organism-specific agents should a specific pathogen be identified later in the hospital course.

When all the resuscitative maneuvers have been completed and the resuscitation is well under way, other tests can be pursued.

B. Laboratory Testing

Although few laboratory tests are required for younger patients undergoing emergency surgery, extensive evaluation is warranted in the elderly. Not infrequently, the elderly patient has several chronic degenerative diseases and may be taking multiple medications. For these reasons virtually all organ systems need evaluation before emergency surgery.

1. Electrolytes (See also Chapter 16)

Elderly patients frequently are taking medications that may have an impact on the serum electrolytes. Use of diuretics is common with concomitant potassium loss. Hypokalemia must be corrected before anesthetic induction. Hyperkalemia should be treated with insulin and glucose or by other measures as clinically appropriate. If hyponatremic patients require volume resuscitation, hypertonic saline can be used. Hypernatremic patients will require additional free water.

Serum chloride is measured along with the other electrolytes, although serum chloride abnormalities are not directly treated. In combination with the other electrolytes, the anion gap may be determined, which is important in differentiating among the various types of acidosis. In patients who have been vomiting, hypochloremic, hypokalemic acidosis may be present and is corrected by administering large volumes of normal saline and IV potassium.

The serum bicarbonate (CO_2) value accompanying serum electrolyte measurements closely approximates the bicarbonate levels obtained with an arterial blood gas. Thus, the CO_2 provides a good determination for acidosis. The degree of acidosis is important because it is one indicator of how sick the patient is and how vigorous resuscitation must be implemented. Acidosis is treated primarily by volume replacement. Controversy exists regarding the infusion of bicarbonate to treat acidosis. Good evidence exists that for lactic acidosis, the most common form of acidosis in patients in shock, administration of bicarbonate may be harmful (12).

Measurement of blood urea nitrogen (BUN) and serum creatinine provides information regarding renal function status. Basal determinations of these values are important in the event the patient has postoperative renal failure develop. By establishing baseline renal status, the clinician is better able to gauge postoperative treatment and monitor recovery.

Serum glucose should be determined. Hyperglycemia can be significant in septic diabetic patients and requires aggressive treatment with insulin.

2. Complete Blood Count

A complete blood count (CBC) is extremely useful. The hematocrit or hemoglobin concentration must be determined in all patients before undergoing surgery. It is essential to know the baseline value of the hematocrit in the event of intraoperative bleeding. In addition, patients with low hematocrit should be resuscitated with blood before surgery. When patients present with anemia and an operation with substantial blood loss is anticipated, the treatment team should plan for blood transfusions during surgery. For patients with suspected bleeding, monitoring serially determined hematocrits gauges the amount of bleeding, potential need for blood transfusions, or the need for emergency surgery.

The white blood cell (WBC) count may be a useful indicator of infection. However, in malnourished or very sick patients the WBC count can be misleading. It is not uncommon for elderly patients with profound sepsis to have normal WBC counts.

3. Liver Function Tests

Liver function tests provide a baseline on the status of the liver should the patient become ill postoperatively. Patients with severe, prolonged shock have hepatic failure develop. Thus, establishing the basal parameters for liver function before emergency surgery enables the clinician to follow abnormalities of the liver and assess prognosis should the patient remain in shock after surgery. As indicated in the section on risk, serum albumin concentration is particularly useful for assessment of surgical risk. Patients with low serum albumin, which is indicative of malnutrition, have predictably high morbidity and mortality. If the patient is malnourished, surgery should be delayed if at all possible until the patient's nutritional status is improved.

4. Coagulation

Prothrombin time (PT) and partial thromboplastin time (PTT) should be obtained. Elderly patients are not infrequently placed on anticoagulation regimens for a variety of disorders. Patients with chronic liver disease or malnutrition may also have coagulation factor deficiencies. Before surgery it is important to know whether an easily correctable coagulopathy is present. If the PT or PTT is abnormal, fresh frozen plasma (FFP) should be administered. Vitamin K administration is not advisable because it might be necessary to anticoagulate the patient postoperatively. Exogenous vitamin K complicates the process of anticoagulation for several days after its administration. FFP can be given to correct a coagulopathy and should further anticoagulation be required heparin is titrated to the degree of targeted anticoagulation. Typically, FFP is given 2 units at a time and its effect is measured by repeat PTT determinations. However, I have found this method of FFP administration to be ineffective. Rather, FFP is given as a continuous infusion until the coagulopathy is resolved clinically. For the hypovolemic patient FFP is a good resuscitation fluid, although it cannot be given quickly.

Platelet counts can be obtained with a CBC. A coagulopathy resulting from thrombocytopenia can be treated with platelet infusion. However, many elderly patients take aspirin or other nonsteroidal anti-inflammatory drugs (NSAIDs) that decrease platelet function. Patients can have a clinically significant coagulopathy with normal platelet count. The diagnostic test of choice is a bleeding time; however, this is impractical in the emergency setting. For patients with clinically evident bleeding and a history of aspirin or NSAID use, platelet infusions should be given.

5. Arterial Blood Gas

Arterial blood gas should be measured as early as possible. Important decisions can be made from the results of blood gases. If the pH is less than 7.2, the P_{CO_2} >50, or the P_{O_2} <50, endotracheal intubation should be performed. Metabolic acidosis is treated by vigorous fluid resuscitation. Oxygenation is best monitored by noninvasive pulse oximetry. Respiratory acidosis is treated by intubation.

6. Drug Levels

Many elderly patients are taking potentially toxic medications such as digoxin, procainamide, and phenytoin. Often, elderly patients will initially be seen with less than therapeutic levels of these important medications. Serum levels should be obtained to help guide the resumption of these medications in the perioperative period.

7. Urinalysis

Urine specimens should be sent for urinalysis to determine whether pyuria is present, suggesting a urinary tract infection. Microscopic analysis should also be performed to look for casts indicative of renal parenchymal disease.

8. Chest Radiography

A chest radiograph is helpful to evaluate for underlying congestive heart failure and pulmonary disease. As with the other tests, establishing a baseline is important should the patient have a difficult postoperative course.

9. Electrocardiogram

Electrocardiography is important to ensure the patient does not have a serious dysrhythmia, recent myocardial infarction, or myocardial ischemia. If the patient is having myocardial infarction concomitant to the surgical emergency, prioritization for treating the most life-threatening condition must be made. For example, a patient with simultaneous myocardial infarction and massively bleeding gastroduodenal ulcer requires surgery despite the high risk. Alternatively, in a patient with a fracture it might be best to delay the surgery if possible until the cardiac status has been optimized. Dysrhythmias need to be assessed given that they are frequent in acutely ill elderly patients. Atrial fibrillation must be rate controlled and hopefully converted to a sinus rhythm. Ventricular ectopy must be minimized or eliminated. Supraventricular tachydysrhythmias other than atrial fibrillation must be differentiated from sinus tachycardia and treated if present.

C. Invasive Monitoring

1. Arterial Line

Placement of an arterial line can assist greatly in the management of the acutely ill patient. The major advantage is instantaneous measurement of systemic blood pressure. In the very critically ill patient, the blood pressure generally must be monitored in this manner so as to avoid too low or too high a blood pressure during diagnostic and therapeutic intervention. Because elderly patients frequently have diffuse atherosclerotic disease, the pressure needed to perfuse various organ beds is often higher than in younger patients. For this reason hypotension can be devastating in elderly patients and must be avoided. Arterial line monitoring is useful to avoid this problem.

The prevalence of lung disease is high in the elderly. Blood gas determination may be needed on a frequent basis for critically ill elderly patients. Arterial line placement facilitates repeated acquisitions of arterial blood.

2. Central Venous Pressure

Because elderly patients frequently have veins that are difficult to cannulate, central line placement is often needed for access purposes. Once in place, the central venous pressure (CVP) line is useful for assessing the resuscitative effort by measuring the CVP. In general, measurement of the pulmonary artery pressure is superior to the venous pressure; however, CVP measurement is adequate for most circumstances.

3. Pulmonary Artery Catheters

Placement of a pulmonary artery (Swan-Ganz) catheter remains controversial. For elderly patients with stiff hearts and a propensity for cardiopulmonary failure, these catheters may be useful. Measurement of pulmonary artery pressure is another method of assessing the effectiveness of resuscitative efforts when large amounts of fluids are given over a short period of time. Monitoring pulmonary artery pressure is essential for patients in renal failure when the urine output will not adequately reflect resuscitation. Swan-Ganz catheter monitoring in the perioperative period is also useful because dramatic fluid shifts are anticipated after emergency surgery. Despite their apparent usefulness, data exist suggesting that placement of Swan-Ganz catheters is more harmful than good (13,14).

REFERENCES

1. Di Palo S, Giangreco L, Vignali A, Carlucci M, Staudacher C. Surgery in the very old patient: evaluation of factors linked to postoperative morbidity and mortality. Aging Milano 1995; 7:110–116.
2. Linn BS, Linn MW, Wallen N. Evaluation of results of surgical procedures in the elderly. Ann Surg 1982; 195:90–96.
3. Cook TM, Britton DC, Craft TM, Jones CB, Horrocks M. An audit of hospital mortality after urgent and emergency surgery in the elderly. Ann R Coll Surg Engl 1997; 79:361–367.
4. Kennedy RH, al-Mufti RA, Brewster SF, Sherry EN, Magee TR, Irvin TT. The acute surgical admission: is mortality predictable in the elderly? Ann R Coll Surg Engl 1994; 76:342–345.
5. Ackermann RJ, Vogel RL, Johnson LA, Ashley DW, Solis MM. Surgery in nonagenarians: morbidity, mortality, and functional outcome. J Fam Pract 1995; 40:129–135.
6. Corti MC, Guralnik JM, Salive ME, Sorkin JD. Serum albumin level and physical disability as predictors of mortality in older persons (see comments). JAMA 1994; 272:1036–1042.
7. Khuri SF, Daley J, Henderson W, Hur K, Gibbs JO, Barbour G, Demakis J, Irvin G, Stremple JF, Grover F, McDonald G, Passaro Jr. E, Fabri PJ, Spencer J, Hammermeister K, Aust JB. Risk adjustment of the postoperative mortality rate for the comparative assessment of the quality of surgical care: results of the National Veterans Affairs Surgical Risk Study. J Am Coll Surg 1997; 185:315–327.
8. Cohen CB, Cohen PJ. Do-not-resuscitate orders in the operating room (see comments). N Engl J Med 1991; 325:1879–1882.
9. Livingston EH, Passaro EJ. Resuscitation. Revival should be the first priority. Postgrad Med 1991; 89:117–120, 122.
10. Livingston EH, Passaro EJ. Postoperative ileus. Dig Dis Sci 1990; 35:121–132.
11. Roberts JS, Bratton SL. Colloid volume expanders. Problems, pitfalls and possibilities. Drugs 1998; 55:621–630.
12. Graf H, Leach W, Arieff AI. Evidence for a detrimental effect of bicarbonate therapy in hypoxic lactic acidosis. Science 1985; 227:754–756.
13. Connors AJ, Speroff T, Dawson NV, Thomas C, Harrel Jr. FE, Wagner D, Desbiens

N, Goldman L, Wu AW, Califf RM, Fulkerson Jr. WJ, Vidaillet H, Broste S, Bellamy P, Lynn J, Knaus WA. The effectiveness of right heart catheterization in the initial care of critically ill patients. SUPPORT Investigators (see comments). JAMA 1996; 276:889–897.
14. Dalen JE, Bone RC. Is it time to pull the pulmonary artery catheter? (editorial; comment) (see comments). JAMA 1996; 276:916–918.

6
Emergency Anesthesia

Calvin Johnson, Sharon Anita Ashley, and Stephen N. Steen
Charles R. Drew University of Medicine and Science, and Martin Luther King, Jr.–Charles R. Drew Medical Center, Los Angeles, California

Aging itself only minimally increases operative risk. The primary risk factors for geriatric patients undergoing surgery are listed in Table 1. The operative risk increases for the geriatric patient with increasing severity of concomitant diseases according to the American Society of Anesthesiologist (ASA) classification (Table 2), complexity of surgery, length of surgery and whether the surgery is an emergency. The operative risk in the geriatric patient increases from 1% for elective cases to 45% for emergency surgeries (1). Therefore, precise assessment and appropriate management of the geriatric surgical patient represent a great challenge when administering anesthesia for emergency surgery.

I. PHYSIOLOGICAL CHANGES WITH AGING

The aging process may affect all organ systems. With aging, the maximal functional capacity of many organ systems decreases along with the organ system functional reserve capacity. This has significant impact on the anesthesia management of the geriatric patient. Geriatric individuals who appear to be physiologically ''young'' or ''old'' have lesser or greater rates of decline, respectively, than average, but they may also have had significantly different maximal capacities as young adults (2). There is an increase of 20% to 40% in body fat, a decrease of 10% to 15% of body water, and a decrease in lean muscle, all of which result

Table 1 Primary Surgical Risk Factors for Geriatric Patients

Number of associated disease states
Severity of associated disease states
The type of surgery
The length of surgery
Patient's ASA classification
Whether surgery is elective or emergent

ASA, American Society of Anesthesiologists.

in changes in volume of distribution of drugs. Also, a 10% to 15% decrease in effective protein binding is an important factor; for example, meperidine (Demerol) for a 70-year-old is 70% unbound to serum proteins, whereas 30% of the drug is unbound for a 20-year-old. Thus, for most elderly, many drugs should be given in smaller doses with dosages increased slowly; in the case of neuromuscular blockers, the doses are generally similar as with a younger individual, but the rate of the transfer (from protein bound to unbound state) is slower (about 35% less). (See also Chapter 3.) As age increases, not only do organ functions decrease but disease also increases, with an increase in medications; thus, we may expect more adverse reactions. Only one in five elderly patients has no preoperative problem. The assessment of organ system functional reserve, along with the identification of specific disease processes within each organ system, remains the primary objective of the process of preoperative assessment of geriatric patients (3). (See also Chapter 5.)

Table 2 American Society of Anesthesiologists Classification

Status	Disease state
ASA Class 1	No organic, physiological, biochemical, or psychiatric disturbance
ASA Class 2	Mild to moderate systemic disturbance that may or may not be related to the reason for surgery
ASA Class 3	Severe systemic disturbance that may or may not be related to the reason for surgery
ASA Class 4	Severe systemic disturbance that is life threatening with or without surgery
ASA Class 5	Moribund patient who is expected to die within 24 hours and has surgery as a last resort
Emergency	Any patient in whom an emergency operation is required

A. Cardiovascular Changes with Aging

With aging, the cardiovascular system undergoes both functional and anatomical changes (Table 3). Data from the Framingham longitudinal study (4) suggest that progressive loss of peripheral vascular elasticity and increases in collagen cross-linking combine to stiffen the arterial tree, which increases systolic pressure and widens arterial pulse pressure with aging. Increasing mechanical stiffness of the arterial system reduces compliance and causes progressive enhancement of the size of the pulsatile components of arterial afterloading to which the left ventricle is subjected. Secondary adaptive changes include ventricular hypertrophy produced by progressive increases in impedance to ventricular ejection (5). However, increases in ventricular wall thickness reduce myocardial wall tension, making these changes self-limiting in the absence of arterial hypertension (6). Aging alters ventricular hemodynamics by greatly increasing dependence on atrial contraction for the maintenance of normal stroke volume. Moreover, short-term increases in cardiac output (CO) are accomplished in the geriatric patient initially by modest increases in heart rate and then by progressively larger stroke volumes. However, inotropic and chronotropic responses to stress decrease with aging. Passive ventricular filling, which normally occurs during the early phase of diastole, is decreased in geriatric patients (stiffer and less compliant ventricle). This decrease in diastolic function makes geriatric patients more dependent on synchronous atrial contraction for complete ventricular filling. These changes greatly magnify the negative hemodynamic consequences that follow the loss of normal sinus cardiac rhythm, with diastolic dysfunction playing a greater role in the cause of ventricular failure in elderly patients than previously recognized. In addition, small decreases in venous return resulting from positive pressure ventilation, anesthetic drugs, hemorrhage, and vasodilators may significantly compromise stroke volume, especially when cardiac dysrhythmias are present. As a result, perioperative arterial hypotension associated with anesthetic agents is predictably more common in elderly than in young patients.

Systolic arterial hypertension, which is caused by increases in systemic

Table 3 Cardiovascular Changes with Aging

Cardiac physiology	At rest effect	Exercise effect
Heart rate	No change or slight decrease	Less increase
Systolic blood pressure	Increased	Greater increase
Diastolic blood pressure	No change	Slight increase
Cardiac output	No change	Slight increase
Ejection fraction	No change	No change or slight increase
Stroke volume	No change or slight increase	Greater increase

vascular resistance, reflects fibrotic replacement of elastic tissues within the cardiovascular system (produces the ''overshoot'' characteristics of radial artery waveform tracings in elderly patients and the discrepancies between blood pressure measured invasively versus by cuff). This decreased compliance of the vascular system results in the elderly patient being volume sensitive and volume intolerant.

B. Pulmonary Changes with Aging

The respiratory system undergoes anatomical and functional alteration with aging (Table 4). (See also Chapter 14.) Aging increases residual volume (RV) and compromises vital capacity (VC) in both men and women. These changes in VC and the decline in physical stature associated with aging are responsible for the ''typical'' age-related loss of total lung capacity (the sum of RV and VC). These changes, coupled with weakened respiratory muscles, cause closure of small airways, resulting in a decrease in all lung volumes except functional residual capacity.

Important causes of hypoxemia, apart from failure of delivering sufficient oxygen to the patient or equipment failure, are intubation of the esophagus or of a bronchus; bronchospasm (after drugs); aspiration; pulmonary edema; pulmonary embolism; pneumothorax after surgical procedures of the head, neck, or thorax; tracheal suctioning; and airway obstruction, which may be due to the patient's tongue, bronchospasm, damaged teeth, dentures, a throat pack, foreign body, or endotracheal tube kinking. Many anesthesiologists do not advocate the use of

Table 4 Pulmonary Changes with Aging

Pulmonary function test	Effect of aging
VC	Decreased 20 mL/yr
FEV_1	Decreased
FEV_1/FVC	Unchanged or slight decrease
CC	Increased
FRC	Increased
RV	Increased
TLC	Unchanged or slight decrease
DL	Decreased
Pao_2	Decreased

VC, Vital capacity; FEV_1, forced expiratory volume in the first second; FVC, forced vital capacity; FRC, functional residual capacity; CC, closing capacity; RV, residual volume; TLC, total lung capacity; DL, diffusing capacity; Pao_2, arterial oxygen partial pressure.

the laryngeal mask airway for emergency anesthesia because a reduced risk of aspiration after its use has not been demonstrated; in fact, aspiration is known to occur after endotracheal tube placement with an inflated cuff. Hypoxemia (low arterial oxygen partial pressure [Pa_{O_2}] may be due to either reduced alveolar oxygen partial pressure [PA_{O_2}] or, if PA_{O_2} is normal or increased [patient breathing supplemental O_2] an increase in the alveolar-arterial P_{O_2} difference. This difference between Pa_{O_2} and PA_{O_2} is termed venous admixture. This venous admixture may be due to a diffusion defect, an abnormal distribution of ventilation-perfusion ($\dot{V}/\dot{Q}$) ratios, or an absence of ventilation of perfused parts of the lung (i.e., $\dot{V}/\dot{Q} = O$); this last condition (called a ''shunt'') is resistant to correction by increasing the fraction of inspired oxygen (FI_{O_2}).

The relationship of arterial oxygen partial pressure to age may be represented as $Pa_{O_2} \simeq 100 - 0.5$ age (in years) for a supine subject at sea level with a normal carbon dioxide partial pressure ($P_{CO_2} \simeq 40$ mm Hg).

During intubation for general anesthesia, geriatric patients are susceptible to hypoxemia, thus preoxygenation is required before induction of general anesthesia. Geriatric patients have diminished response to hypercarbia and hypoxia, making them prone to respiratory depression resulting from the residual effects of anesthetic drugs and narcotics in the postoperative period. In addition, both general anesthesia and the supine position increase the incidence of atelectasis and pneumonia in the postoperative period.

Other cardiorespiratory changes such as hypoventilation, hyperventilation, hypovolemia, hypervolemia, hypotension, hypertension, tachycardia, bradycardia, and dysrythmias are discussed in detail elsewhere.

C. Renal Changes with Aging

Renal function declines with age as a result of anatomical and functional alterations. (See also Chapter 15.) Renal blood flow, glomerular filtration rate, and creatinine clearance decline. These decreases result in the geriatric patient being more susceptible to acute renal failure if ischemia or nephrotoxic insult occurs during the perioperative, intraoperative, or postoperative period. Most geriatric patients who are seen for emergency surgeries are dehydrated; thus, careful fluid resuscitation is required to preserve renal perfusion and avoid fluid overload, which could result in congestive heart failure. In addition, geriatric patients have an impaired renin-angiotensin-aldosterone system, which also predisposes them to fluid overload after and during emergency anesthesia and surgery.

D. Hepatic Changes with Aging

Liver tissue mass decreases about 40% by the 80 years, and hepatic blood flow is proportionally decreased. Loss of hepatic tissue mass is thought to be the primary explanation for slowed metabolism and prolonged clinical effects of anesthetic drugs (especially opioids) after emergency anesthesia in geriatric patients.

E. Neurological Changes with Aging

Aging leads to progressive functional changes in the nervous system. (See also Chapter 20.) Brain size decreases with aging, with most of the loss reflecting attrition of neurons, particularly in the gray matter. Neurons that synthesize neurotransmitters (dopamine, norepinephrine, tyrosine, serotonin) seem to be most affected. Cerebral blood flow decreases in proportion to decreased brain tissue mass. Autoregulation of cerebrovascular resistance in response to changes in arterial blood pressure is well maintained, and the cerebral vasoconstrictor response to hyperventilation remains intact. Aging results in loss of neuronal substance (decrease in size and number of axons) with a decrease in synaptic transmission. Aging can be thought of as a progressive beta-blockade. In the absence of cerebrovascular disease, the conventional guidelines for controlled hypotension during neurosurgical procedures may be appropriate for elderly patients.

II. ANALGESIC AND ANESTHETIC CHANGES WITH AGING

The anatomical and physiological changes associated with aging affect the dosing, potency, and duration of anesthetic drugs (Table 5).

Table 5 Changes in Anesthetic Drugs in Geriatric Patients

Drug group	Adjustment needed
Inhalational agents	Decrease inspired concentration
Barbiturates, etomidate, and propofol	Small to moderate decrease in initial dose; smaller maintenance infusion rate
Opioids	Marked decrease in initial dose; anticipate increased duration of systemic and epidural effects; greater incidence of rigidity; increased respiratory depression
Local anesthetics used for spinal/epidural anesthesia	Small to moderate decrease in segmental dose requirement; anticipate prolonged effects
Benzodiazepines	Modest decrease in initial dose; anticipate marked increase in duration (except midazolam)
Succinylcholine	Slightly reduced dose in elderly men
Nondepolarizing muscle relaxants	Same or slight increase in initial dose; anticipate increased duration (except atracurium or mivacurium)

A. Regional Anesthesia

Higher levels of sensory blockade occur in the geriatric patient undergoing spinal anesthesia. In addition, segmental dose requirements are reduced for local anesthetics during epidural analgesia in geriatric surgical patients.

B. General Anesthesia

The effect of aging on the nervous system reduces the dose requirements for general anesthesia. With increasing age, the relative minimum alveolar concentration (the dose of anesthetic required to prevent 50% of patients from moving after painful stimuli), of inhaled anesthetic gases declines progressively by as much as 30% from young adult values, with virtually the same decrement seen for the newest agents, desflurane and sevoflurane, as for traditional drugs such as halothane and isoflurane. The reason for this age-related increase in sensitivity to anesthetic agents is unknown, but the consistency of this phenomenon for anesthetic agents with markedly different chemical characteristics suggests that it is the result of fundamental neurophysiological rather than purely pharmacological processes. Aging would appear to produce a progressive, age-related decline in nervous system functional reserve. Thus, the concentration of inhaled anesthetic gases must be reduced in emergency anesthesia in geriatric patients.

C. Narcotics and Sedatives

The data for the effect of aging on the pharmacodynamics or dose requirements for opioids, barbiturates, and benzodiazepines are less consistent than those for inhalational anesthetics. (See also Chapter 3.) Considerable controversy exists as to whether the clinically apparent age-related increase in the potency of these drugs is truly a pharmacodynamic phenomenon or whether it simply reflects age-related changes in pharmacokinetics because in elderly subjects plasma drug concentrations immediately after drug injection are usually higher than in young adults. Clinical experience and traditional measurements demonstrate significant age-related reductions in the dose requirements for thiopental and virtually all other agents that depress consciousness. In addition, the aging process increases brain sensitivity to narcotics. This results in the need to reduce the doses of these agents when used for emergency anesthesia in geriatric patients.

D. Neuromuscular Blocking Drugs

The plasma and extracellular fluid concentrations of competitive neuromuscular blocking drugs that produce interruption of neuromuscular transmission are determined primarily by the dynamics of interaction between acetylcholine released from motor neurons and the quality and quantity of cholinergic receptors at the muscle end plate. The dosages of nondepolarizing neuromuscular blocking drugs do not simply decline in parallel with the age-related atrophy of skeletal muscle mass. Rather, their median effective doses (ED_{50}) and steady-state plasma concentrations remain virtually unchanged or may actually increase slightly in the elderly patient. The clinical duration of their effects is markedly prolonged if their elimination from plasma depends on organ function. Rates of plasma clearance for almost all neuromuscular blocking drugs, including the newest agents such as rocuronium, actually decline dramatically with increasing age and are inversely proportional to the duration of neuromuscular blockade produced by these agents.

III. PERIOPERATIVE MANAGEMENT AND OUTCOME

Morbidity and mortality rates are higher in elderly patients undergoing emergency anesthesia largely because this surgical patient subpopulation has a greater average incidence and severity of underlying comorbid conditions and diseases than that found in younger adults. The high prevalence of polypharmacy associated with chronic disease and its treatment also produces an age-related increase in adverse drug reactions that complicate perioperative management. In general, however, no patients are probably ''too old'' for anesthesia, even for surgical procedures to be done on an ambulatory basis. The probability of a serious pulmonary or hemodynamic complication after surgery in the elderly, as in the young adult, is largely determined by the site of operation and by the patient's physical status. In the absence of severe cardiac dysfunction or incapacitating lung disease, an elderly patient may be an excellent candidate for any kind of surgery.

The choice of anesthetic agent or technique itself does not appear to be a major determinant of overall outcome when assessment of total morbidity and mortality for any type of surgery encompasses both immediate and long-term complications. The most common cause of failure to emerge promptly from anesthesia, in fact, is simply the use of too much anesthesia or too many anesthetic agents.

The physical management of elderly patients in the operating room and afterwards requires specific precautions. Aged skin and bones are fragile and joints are stiff and their range of motion is limited, especially if they are compromised by age-related arthritic processes. The elderly surgical patient requires gentle and expert routine care if traumatic injuries from improper positioning, bandaging, or enforced bed rest are to be avoided. Active heating devices in contact with poorly perfused skin or connective tissue pressure points can quickly produce ischemic lesions requiring surgical treatment, and prolonged lithotomy positioning is a particular hazard in this patient population. In all elderly patients, postoperative bleeding diatheses or hypercoagulable states and bacterial infection are more frequent than in younger adults, perhaps because sustained sympathoadrenal stress responses evoked during a protracted and difficult recovery are undiminished in magnitude in aged patients. For this reason, an anesthetic plan that includes postoperative epidural sympathectomy and analgesia appears to be of special value in the elderly surgical patient. In addition, the anesthetic plan should seek to promote healing, reduce cardiovascular and pulmonary demands, and eliminate the long periods of stress caused by the inadequate analgesia sometimes imposed on geriatric patients because of exaggerated fears of narcotic side effects. If complications are to be minimized in the elderly, their perioperative care simply requires the highest standards of preparation, sensitivity to clinical issues, vigilance, and meticulous execution of all details of anesthetic and postoperative management.

IV. PREOPERATIVE EVALUATION OF GERIATRIC PATIENTS

Preoperative evaluation of the geriatric patient will be discussed in depth in a another chapter. (See Chapter 5.) In brief, appropriate preoperative evaluation of geriatric patients should focus on the organ-based assessment of function and physical status, and, therefore, assessment requires directed testing rather than simple screening for unsuspected disease. The protocol for preoperative laboratory assessment for emergency anesthesia is thus driven largely by the clinical history, mechanism of injury, and severity of underlying medical disease processes.

V. SPECIFIC EMERGENCY SITUATIONS

Frequently, geriatric patients reach the operating room in suboptimal condition for emergency anesthesia. A thorough preanesthetic evaluation may be difficult to obtain, but each patient should be seen before entering the operative suite.

The elderly patient may be afflicted with arthritis (rheumatoid or degenerative), bone disease, paraplegia, endocrine dysfunction, and a host of other maladies (for example, of the cardiovascular and respiratory systems). Accordingly, correct patient positioning before the induction of anesthesia and intraoperatively is of prime importance. If the operative site is above heart level, precautions should be taken to recognize and treat air embolism.

Monitoring techniques for acute emergencies, in particular in cases of persistent or massive blood loss, should use simple, noninvasive blood pressure monitoring, pulse oximetry, capnography (especially after insertion of an endotracheal tube), urine output, and careful clinical observation. Large-bore venous catheters (two or more) are placed in preference to time-consuming invasive procedures. A double-lumen, large-bore (2 × 12 gauge) catheter should be inserted into the jugular or subclavian vein if access to peripheral veins is unavailable or inadequate. Obviously, in the case of neck trauma, catheters should not be inserted distal to sites of possible vessel injury (such as subclavian or innominate veins). Improved bioimpedance monitoring, a relatively new technology, appears to obviate the need for insertion of a Swan-Ganz catheter, but limitations include some operations on the neck, open-heart surgery, and, at this time, in patients whose weight is less than 20 kg or more than 170 kg.

Induction of anesthesia is of the rapid-sequence type: preoxygenation, cricoid pressure, IV agent (thiopental or propofol, for example), and succinylcholine (if not contraindicated; if so, rocuronium or atracurium may be used because their effect wears off when their administration is discontinued). If desired, the patient may be placed in the left lateral head-down position, which displaces the tongue and frequently improves laryngeal exposure. This technique is for the right-handed physician using the laryngoscope in the left hand; otherwise for a left-handed physician with the appropriate scope, a right lateral head-down position may be used. A neuromuscular blockade transmission monitor should be used to determine full recovery, and an antagonist combination (such as neostigmine plus atropine) should be avoided if possible because dehiscence of anastomoses of the bowel may occur.

Maintenance of anesthesia may be with any of the presently used inhalational anesthetic agents. After abdominal surgery, upper chest physiotherapy with positive-pressure breathing should be instituted as soon as feasible to manage basal collapse of the lungs, which occurs early in the postoperative period. If infection occurs postoperatively, a wound dehiscence may occur. Such cases should be treated as emergencies with the anesthetic technique described previously.

A. Abdominal Anesthesia

In elderly patients initially seen with an acute condition of the abdomen, age-related neurological disease may co-exist, as well as respiratory, cardiovascular, hepatic, renal, and endocrine problems. Myocardial infarction (<6 months old) presents a greater anesthetic risk, as does the risk of infective endocarditis from pre-existing valvular heart disease for which appropriate antibiotics should be prescribed preoperatively. Electrolyte imbalance needs correction with proper fluids and circulating volume before anesthesia. For example, a patient with an acute condition of the abdomen may be suffering loss of extracellular fluid and circulating volume; thus, crystalloid and colloid solutions should be administered. The usual crystalloid replacement is approximately 110 mL/h for a 70-kg person;

if tissue trauma is more than minimal, additional fluid will be needed. A preoperative chest film is essential; respiratory function tests are rarely feasible under these emergency conditions.

B. Burn Anesthesia

Burns are most commonly thermal in nature, and each year in the United States more than 1 million individuals sustain such an injury, with 100,000 being admitted to the hospital, of which 50% become disabled or deformed and 7000 die.

Burn size is estimated by use of "the rule of 9" (i.e., 9% for each arm, 18% for each leg, 36% for the front and back of the trunk, and 9% for the head and neck). Intra-arterial blood pressure monitoring is indicated if an extremity is not available for noninvasive blood pressure measurements. Electrocardiogram (ECG) tracings are feasible because adhesive leads do not have to stick for a recording to be obtained. Silver sulfadazine is a cream and an excellent conductor, and leads merely need to be placed on it. Moreover, the forehead or other nonstandard sites can be used; needle electrodes can also be used on burned areas if patient electrical grounding is adequate.

Edema occurs within minutes at the site of injury, and patients with a ≥ 50% burn surface area (BSA) may lose one-third of their total plasma volume in a few hours and go into shock. An increase in metabolic rate occurs, which may last for months, depending on the extent of the burn, resulting in increased caloric requirements. The frequent need for repeated anesthetic administrations and blood transfusions impairs immune functions, which increases susceptibility to infection. Many formulas have been promulgated for fluid resuscitation, which are beyond the scope of this chapter, but all patients should be titrated to maintain a normal urinary output of 0.5 to 1.0 mL/kg/h.

All patients with major burns (>18% BSA) require the placement of an endotracheal tube. Fixation of the tube in burns of the face and neck is difficult, and the endotracheal tube may be fixed in place with twill tape or a soft bandage (if possible). If the burn is >8 hours old, succinylcholine should not be administered because hyperkalemia may result and lead to cardiac arrest; accordingly, a rapid-acting, nondepolarizing muscle relaxant should be used. For maintenance, all muscle relaxants should be given slowly in increments, with a peripheral nerve stimulator as a guide to the depth of blockade.

Pressure ulcers are usually ischial ulcers and are frequently urgent in nature. Before surgical intervention, culture of the ulcer, treatment of any medical problems, and sepsis should be considered.

C. Anesthesia for Head Injury

Head injury in the elderly patient may occur from trauma (violence, a fall) or a space-occupying lesion (neoplasm, hemorrhage). The anesthetic management goals are to optimize intracranial dynamics, to maintain cardiovascular stability, and to ensure an impeccable airway; fluid therapy is mandatory for adequate cerebral perfusion and tissue oxygenation because hypovolemic shock increases morbidity and mortality. Time should not be wasted in search of a ''correct'' IV fluid; any solution (within reason) should be administered.

Intraoperative fluid administration is based on the vital signs, blood loss, urinary output, and the maintenance requirements of the patient. Glucose and water, a commonly administered IV solution during the intraoperative period, may have adverse effects that outweigh the benefits; for example, if brain ischemia is present, it has been recommended that the blood glucose level be maintained at <200 mg/dL because hyperglycemia increases glycolysis and the production of lactate. Intravenous mannitol (0.25–0.50 g/kg), an osmotic diuretic, is used to reduce brain edema, and intravenous phenytoin (20 mg/kg) is frequently used prophylactically to prevent seizures. Hypothermia (at 32–33°C) has been used to protect the brain from ischemia. Corticosteroids are of no value.

D. Ophthalmic Anesthesia

Ophthalmic emergencies may be minor or major. Minor eye emergencies are conjunctival lacerations or corneal foreign bodies for which local anesthetics usually suffice. Major emergencies include a perforated eye or one that will be opened during surgery, eyelid repair, or a lacrymal drainage procedure; these generally require general anesthesia. The anesthesiologist should avoid any increase in central venous pressure (CVP) (from bucking on the endotracheal tube or straining) because changes in CVP produce like changes in the intraocular pressure (IOP) (because there are no valves between the orbit, the veins, and heart). Hyperventilation to an end-tidal carbon dioxide (CO_2) of 25 to 30 mm Hg is used because a reduction in arterial carbon dioxide partial pressure ($PacO_2$) reduces IOP. Ketamine is contraindicated because it raises IOP.

Corneal transplantation may be performed after severe ocular trauma. Patients >30 years of age are usually operated on with local infiltration with an anesthetic agent containing epinephrine plus anesthesia standby for sedation.

E. Orthopedic Anesthesia

The geriatric patient commonly is seen by an orthopedic surgeon because of fracture(s) of extremities (from a fall, trauma), peripheral vascular disease, tumors, and infections, or for reconstructive surgery (as in the case of rheumatoid arthritis). Eighty percent to 90% of hip fractures occur in the geriatric population. (See also Chapter 8.)

Major lower extremity amputations are generally performed with the patient under general anesthesia or a regional block (epidural or subarachnoid). In an older patient who is to undergo a lower limb amputation, psychological stress plays an important role in that the patient assumes that he or she will become dependent postoperatively.

Of the postoperative complications (joint contraction, flap neurosis, wound infection, phantom limb/pain) encountered, thromboembolism is a serious threat to the elderly patient who is partially immobilized, and cardiovascular monitoring is necessary to prevent complications caused by the higher energy demands of ambulating with a prosthesis. Patients older than 70 undergo prosthetic replacement surgery for displaced femoral neck fractures because such fractures will not heal without surgery.

F. Otorhinolaryngeal and Faciomaxillary Anesthesia

Otorhinolaryngeal and faciomaxillary emergencies in the elderly patient are of real concern for the anesthesiologist in that co-existing injuries and medical problems are frequent, in addition to a difficult airway. Prior planning is essential so that if alternative methods of airway management have to be adopted, all necessary equipment is functional and readily available. In addition to oxygen (a *sine qua non*) and suction, endotracheal tubes, laryngeal mask airway, forceps (Magill or another type), a tracheal tube changer, a jet ventilator, fiberoptic bronchoscope, a cricothyrotomy kit (including 14-gauge IV cannulas), and a tracheostomy tray should be immediately available.

Subsequent to securing an airway and ventilation, the circulation must be considered because considerable blood may be lost or possible cardiac tamponade or contusion, tension pneumothorax, or shock may occur. Thus, before the induction of anesthesia, restoration of the intravascular volume is necessary to avoid subsequent circulatory collapse.

In the case of many dental emergencies, patients may not need to be hospitalized. However, facilities for overnight admission should be available in case the dental condition affects co-existing disease (e.g., an acute infection that has an impact on the management of diabetes mellitus). Such patients may have taken analgesics or alcohol (if not already having imbibed alcohol and been involved in a traumatic incident) to allay pain, and thus the possibility of potentiation of anesthetic agents may occur.

G. Urologic Anesthesia

Urologic surgery may be indicated for neoplasm, tumor, renal calculi, and prostatic hypertrophy and may be performed with the patient under general anesthesia or regional anesthesia.

H. Vascular Anesthesia

Major vascular surgery generally refers to procedures requiring aortic cross-clamping in which resection of an abdominal aortic aneurysm, replacement of vascular segments during bypass, or endarterectomy of occluded kidney or bowel vessels is done. Anesthetic management of this type of surgery requires close cooperation between the anesthesiologist and the surgeon because hemorrhage may be profuse and sudden. Awareness of pre-existing vascular disease is important because perfusion of brain, kidneys, and heart will probably be impaired; cross-clamping will increase hydraulic stress to the left ventricle. The elderly patient frequently has underlying pre-existing vascular diseases (i.e., myocardial ischemia, congestive heart disease, renal insufficiency, and hypertension). (See also Chapter 10.)

A 30% risk of death or myocardial infarction (peaks postoperatively at days 3 to 5) is present in patients operated on within 6 months of a myocardial infarction; this risk is four times greater for emergency operations compared with elective procedures.

VI. POSTANESTHESIA CARE UNIT

The elderly patient who has undergone anesthesia for an emergency surgical procedure may have increased morbidity and mortality in the postanesthetic period. The following categories indicate the problems that are more frequently encountered by the elderly in the postoperative period.

A. Respiratory Complications

Many elderly patients have alterations in pulmonary function or gas exchange after anesthesia for emergency surgery. Many of these problems occur intraoperatively; however, co-existing medical conditions may increase the risk of these complications. The following respiratory complications are commonly encountered in the immediate postoperative period: hypoventilation, hypoxemia, hyperventilation/hypocapnia, hypercapnia, airway obstruction, pulmonary edema, pulmonary embolus, aspiration, and atelectasis.

1. Hypoventilation

Hypoventilation may be a result of pain, fear, inadequate reversal of muscle relaxants, opioid depression, and the volatile anesthetics. Anesthetic agents can cause a decrease in cardiac output, which can increase alveolar dead space if ventilation is constant. When ventilation remains constant, the $\dot{V}/\dot{Q}$ ratio increases, which leads to a decrease in flow through nondependent lung areas.

2. Hypoxemia

Hypoxemia is a common and serious complication in the postoperative period. Because of the effects of normal aging and pulmonary diseases, the elderly patient tends to become hypoxic more easily. Ventilation-perfusion mismatch is exaggerated in the elderly and is commonly caused by decreased oxygen delivery, hypoventilation, pre-existing right-to-left intrapulmonary shunts, areas of low ventilation-to-perfusion, shivering, hypothermia, and myocardial depression.

Extra care should be taken to provide supplemental oxygen to patients during regional anesthesia with sedation, during transport from the operating room to the recovery room, and in the recovery room. The liberal use of arterial catheters for the measurement of blood gases is encouraged. Postoperative mechanical ventilation may improve the outcome for patients with severe lung disease or other major risk factors, especially after emergency abdominal surgery. Treatment should be further aimed at evaluation of the patient, and the cause of the hypoxemia should be investigated with appropriate studies: arterial blood gas, chest x-ray films, and when indicated $\dot{V}/\dot{Q}$ scan.

3. Hyperventilation/Hypocapnia

High tidal volumes (10–15 mL/kg) are frequently used to ventilate patients during an anesthetic. The average tidal volume is 5 to 7 mL/kg. End-tidal and arterial carbon dioxide levels are usually lower than 35 mm Hg. Large tidal volumes produce a decrease in venous return and reduce cardiac output (CO). Myocardial depression occurs as a result of hypocapnia, and in combination with the depressant effects of the anesthetic agents this may lead to a decrease in dead space. A decrease in CO may further aggravate existing intrapulmonary shunts (atelectasis, pulmonary edema, aspiration) and lead to hypoxia.

4. Airway Obstruction

Airway obstruction may occur in the postoperative period. The most common cause of obstruction is the tongue in patients who are not fully awake and poorly positioned. Other causes include laryngospasm and unremoved throat packs. Patients should receive supplemental oxygen. Obstruction can be relieved with backward head tilt and anterior displacement of the mandible (jaw thrust). Laryngospasm can be approached by use of the head-tilt/jaw-thrust maneuver and by administering supplemental oxygen with positive pressure. If this maneuver is not successful, small doses of succinylcholine (10–20 mg IV) may be administered by skilled personnel to relieve the obstruction.

5. Thromboembolus

Pulmonary embolus may account for 3% to 4% of deaths after total joint replacement (7). The incidence of deep vein thrombosis (DVT) has been reported as high as 70% after total hip or knee replacement (8). If invasive monitoring is initiated during the induction and maintenance of anesthesia, careful attention to the hemodynamic variables should be continued in the postoperative period. Any standard mode of DVT prophylaxis is acceptable.

B. Circulatory Changes

Changes in the circulatory system in the elderly after emergency surgery include alterations in blood pressure, congestive heart failure, and myocardial ischemia or infarction.

1. Alterations in Blood Pressure

Hypotension and hypertension are the major circulatory changes in the elderly after surgery. Hypotension may be a result of inadequate flow to the heart, decreased pump function, and decreased vascular resistance.

Inadequate flow to the heart may be diagnosed by use of a CVP or Swan-Ganz catheter. The most common cause of inadequate flow to the heart is decreased venous return, which may be caused by blood loss, translocation of fluid (''third spacing''), or poor preoperative fluid intake (9).

Decreased pump function may be a result of the myocardial depressant effect of drugs (volatile anesthetic agents, beta-blockers, calcium channel blockers, propofol, barbiturates, and lidocaine). These effects are dose dependent. The decrease in cardiac function may also be a result of worsening of pump function or failure of the heart to increase CO in the presence of decreased vascular resistance. Dysrhythmias are common in the elderly and may persist or become exacerbated in the postoperative period. Sinus tachycardia, sinus bradycardia, premature ventricular beats, ventricular tachycardia, and atrial fibrillation are the more common dysrhythmias seen in the elderly. All of them may be responsible for a decrease in pump function. Treatment, if necessary, is aimed at maintaining normal perfusion pressures. Other causes of dysrhythmias included hypoxia, hypercarbia, metabolic alkalosis and acidosis, electrolyte imbalance, and preexisting heart disease.

Hypotension may be caused by a decrease in vascular resistance if no appropriate increase in CO occurs. Factors responsible for a decrease in vascular resistance include sympathetic blockade after spinal or epidural, neurogenic (spinal cord trauma or transection), drugs (excessive use of nitroprusside or nitroglycerin), preoperative use of antihypertensive drugs, sepsis, anaphylaxis, and vasomotor paralysis after removal of an aortic cross-clamp or a tourniquet.

2. Myocardial Ischemia

In the elderly population, patients older than 70 have a 10-fold increase in the risk of myocardial infarction and cardiac death compared with younger persons.

Perioperative ischemia is related to perioperative myocardial infarction (10). Postoperative infarction may be difficult to diagnose. Postoperatively, several factors may confuse the clinical presentation. Substernal pain may be absent as a result of analgesics, residual regional blockade, and painful stimuli from the surgical incision. Tachycardia may be caused by a variety of factors including pain, hypotension, anxiety, and medications. Shivering and hypertension can increase myocardial oxygen consumption. Hypoxemia or hypoventilation may lead to ischemia, despite adequate coronary perfusion. Cardiac dysrhythmias, which may have been present in the preoperative period, should be evaluated if hypotension and other ECG changes persist. The ECG and changes in creatine kinase isoenzyme MB (CK-MB) fraction are the most useful for diagnosing perioperative ischemia. CK-MB may be released by tissues other than the heart. Levels of >5% may be present after cesarean section, gastrointestinal resection, and transurethral resection of the prostate. The serum CK-MB/CK ratio may be a sensitive and specific test after 10 to 24 h of the postoperative period (11). Therapy of postoperative myocardial ischemia must be individualized. Appropriate monitoring must be initiated.

C. Neurological

Common neurological conditions that may be seen early in the postoperative recovery of the elderly include delirium, agitation, worsening of dementia, and cerebral dysfunction. Less common are perioperative stroke and failure to regain consciousness.

1. Delirium

Delirium may be characterized as abnormalities in attention span, memory, cognition, perception, and thinking. (See also Chapter 20.) Postoperative delirium may be an ominous sign of a treatable underlying disease. The most common causes of delirium include cerebral hypoxia, anesthetic agents, organic brain disease, psychiatric disorders, endocrine and acid-base imbalance, postoperative pain, or covert drug abuse. The anesthetic agents that may be implicated include ketamine (hallucinations and agitation) and anticholinergic agents (atropine and scopolamine cross the blood-brain barrier). Antidepressant and antipsychotic drugs with significant anticholinergic activity that may contribute to postoperative mental confusion are amitriptyline (Elavil), doxapram (Sinequan), imipramine (Tofranil), nortriptyline (Aventyl), and chlorpromazine (Thorazine).

2. Perioperative Stroke

The incidence of a new focal neurological deficit during the perioperative period may have a frequency that is 10-fold higher in the elderly. This is presumably a result of co-existing cerebral or carotid vascular disease. Hypotension has been implicated as a cause of perioperative stroke and thrombotic and embolic events. A small study of patients with transient ischemic attacks showed that a transient period of hypotension, which was sufficient to produce global ischemia (about a 60% decrease in systolic pressure), did not unmask focal deficits nor did it produce a stroke. A retrospective study found that 42% of perioperative strokes were cardiogenic in origin (i.e., related to a myocardial infarction or atrial fibrillation) (12).

D. Nausea and Vomiting

Regardless of age, nausea and vomiting is the most common morbidity in the recovery period. Factors associated with nausea and vomiting include female gender, obesity, history of motion sickness, anxiety, type of induction, type of maintenance agent, operative procedure, opioid analgesics, duration of surgery, food or alcohol intake, postoperative pain, motion on transport, and a previous history of postoperative emesis.

Treatment may be prophylactic or after the problem has occurred. Multiple regimens exist to manage this complication (13). Several classes of drugs are used to treat nausea and vomiting, including anticholinergics, antihistamines, serotonin antagonists, benzamides, butyrophenones, and phenothiazines.

VII. POSTOPERATIVE PAIN MANAGEMENT

The pharmacological and pharmacodynamic changes associated with aging must be considered when choosing an appropriate postoperative pain management intervention in the elderly.

Modalities for pain control include intrathecal and epidural narcotics in a bolus or continuous infusion route, patient-controlled analgesia (PCA), intercostal nerve blocks, skin infiltration with local anesthetics, and intramuscular injections.

A. Patient-Controlled Analgesia

In the elderly, the loading dose and lockout time for PCA may need to be decreased. All initial drug dosages should be titrated with careful observation of the patient with subsequent doses. The patient should be monitored with a pulse oximeter and should also be placed near the nursing station.

B. Epidural and Spinal Analgesia

Epidural opioid analgesia produces segmental analgesia without the concomitant motor, sensory, or autonomic changes associated with the use of local anesthetics

(14). However, dilute concentrations of local anesthetics may be added to the opioid and given as a continuous infusion. The dilute local anesthetic decreases the amount of hypotension, motor block, and sensory block associated with a more concentrated solution. The combination also allows for a decrease in the amount of opioid use and decreases the adverse risks of pruritus, respiratory depression, urinary retention, nausea and vomiting. The side effects of epidural and spinal narcotics can be reversed with naloxone.

C. Wound Infiltration and Nerve Blocks

The use of wound infiltration and nerve blocks to decrease postoperative pain are advantageous and help to decrease the amount of parenteral analgesics that may be required. Limitation is related to restriction to single application. Catheter techniques associated with nerve blocks allow for reinjection of the local anesthetic.

D. Intramuscular Injections

The intramuscular route (IM) is the most common route of pain control after surgery; however, it is not the most effective. Factors that influence the absorption of drugs include site of injection, muscle perfusion, sex, age, temperature, pH of drug, drug formulation, hypotension, and the use of vasoconstrictors. The elderly have a decrease in muscle mass and a decrease in perfusion in the periphery. Absorption is variable after IM meperidine, which is the most commonly used drug for this route of pain management. In the first 24 h after IM injections of meperidine are instituted, at a dosage range of 100 mg given IM every 3 to 4 hours, the drug concentrations are in the therapeutic range for only 35% of the time (15).

VIII. POSTOPERATIVE COMPLICATIONS

The management of the postoperative geriatric patient requires meticulous attention so that complication may be avoided that might contribute to the death of the patient. The mortality is 1.9% in the 7 days postoperatively for all surgical patients; however, for 80-year-olds, it is 8.2%.

Complications may be preoperative, intraoperative, or postoperative. Postoperative complications that may be life threatening, and an appreciation of the symptoms and signs thereof with appropriate treatment, are essential for safe emergency anesthesia and have been briefly discussed under specific emergency situations.

The incidence of postanesthetic mental problems appears to be the same for general anesthesia or regional anesthesia. General anesthesia is the norm when multiple injuries and bleeding require emergency surgery.

Failure to regain consciousness may be due to hypoxemia, severe hypercapnia, inadequate cerebral perfusion (e.g., from severe hypertension or head injury), drug overdose, and so forth.

Postoperative nausea and vomiting, itching, urinary retention, infection, or neurological complication (from pressure or stretching of a nerve, regional blocks) should be treated appropriately as soon as possible and documented in the anesthesia record as for all complications.

REFERENCES

1. Townsend E, Thompson C. Organ physiology of aging. Surg Clin North Am 1994; 74:23–39.
2. Hayflick L. Biologic and theoretical perspectives of human aging. In: Katlic MR, ed. Geriatric Surgery: Comprehensive Care of the Elderly Patient. Baltimore: Urban and Schwarzenberg, 1990, pp 3–21.
3. Williams ME. Clinical implications of aging physiology. Am J Med 1984; 76:1049–1054.
4. Kannel WB, Gordon T. Evaluation of cardiovascular risk in the elderly: The Framingham Study. Bull NY Acad Med 1978; 54:573–591.
5. Wei JY. Aging and the cardiovascular system. N Engl J Med 1992; 327:1735–1739.
6. Geokas MC, Lakatta EG, Makinodan T, Timiras PS. The aging process. Ann Intern Med 1990; 113:455–466.
7. Conventry MB, Nolan DR, Beckenbaugh RD. ''Delayed'' prophylactic anticoagulation: a study of results and complications in 2,012 total hip arthroplasties. J Bone Joint Surg 1973; 55A:1487.
8. Salzman EW, Hirsch J. Prevention of venous thromboembolism. In: Coleman RW, Hirsch J, Marder V, Salzman EW, eds. Haemostasis and Thrombosis. Philadelphia: JB Lippincott, 1987, pp 1252–1257.
9. Gravenstein N. Manual of Complications During Anesthesia. Philadelphia: Lippincott, 1991, pp 189–190.
10. Slogoff S, Keats AS. Does perioperative myocardial ischemia lead to perioperative myocardial infarction? Anesthesiology 1985; 62:107–114.
11. Bendz R, Strom S. Diagnostic significance of serum CK-MB elevations during surgical damage to skeletal muscles. Scand J Thorac Cardiovasc 1981; 15:199–204.
12. Hart R, Hindman B. Mechanisms of perioperative cerebral infarction. Stroke 1982; 13(6):766–773.
13. Haynes GR, Bailey MK. Postoperative nausea and vomiting: review and clinical approaches. South Med J 1996; 89:940–949.
14. Cousin MJ, Mather LE. Intrathecal and epidural administration of opioids. Anesthesiology 1984; 61(3):276–310.
15. Austin KL, Stapleton JV, Maher LE. Multiple intramuscular injections: a major source of variability in analgesic response to meperidine. Pain 1980; 8:47–51.

7
Traumatic Injuries

Arthur W. Fleming and Jo E. Linder
Charles R. Drew University of Medicine and Science, and Martin Luther King, Jr.–Charles R. Drew Medical Center, Los Angeles, California

I. CLINICAL RELEVANCE

A. Definition

Physicians, epidemiologists, researchers, and other health care professionals use the words *trauma* and *injury* interchangeably. The term *injury* seems to be more easily understood by the community at large. The word *trauma* derives from the Greek meaning ''bodily injury'' (1).

In medicine, the term trauma was long applied to any serious body wounds or injuries, such as severe bone fractures or losses of blood or tissue as a result of accidents. A more clinical definition of trauma is a wound or injury, characterized by a structural alteration or physiological imbalance resulting from acute exposure to mechanical, thermal, electrical, or chemical energy, or from the absence of such essentials as heat or oxygen (2).

B. Epidemiology

Injury is the principal public health problem in the United States today (3). Injury causes almost half the deaths in children aged 1 to 4 years, more than half the deaths in children aged 5 to 14, and nearly four-fifths of the deaths of persons aged 15 to 24 years (4).

Because trauma is the most frequent cause of death in persons less than 44 years of age, several authors have acknowledged that a perception exists that trauma is a young person's ''problem'' (5,6). However, for injury victims aged 65 to 74, the rate of unintentional deaths (motor vehicle crash, falls, poisoning, burn, drowning) per 100,000 population is greater than that for all younger age groups, including the 15- to 24-year-old group. In injury victims aged 75 years and older, the unintentional death rate is three times that of victims aged 65 to 74 or 15 to 24 (7). More deaths occur from falls among individuals age 85 and older than motor vehicle deaths among men 18 to 19 years old (3700 vs 2900) (8).

Trauma is a heterogeneous disease occurring across all age groups with varying degrees of severity. Chronological age raises the index of suspicion for higher risk of complications and death; physiological age plays a significant role as well (9). In 1995, injuries were responsible for 147,891 deaths, 2.6 million hospitalizations, and more than 36 million emergency department visits (10). Thus, injury (unintentional injury, suicide, and homicide) is the leading cause of lost years of potential life before age 75. Injury and its consequences accounted for 12% of all medical spending. The cost of injury, estimated at $260 billion in the United States in 1995, was about the same amount as the combined cost of cancer and heart diseases. (The cost estimates included hospital and related services, physicians' services, prescription drugs, professional medical services, and medical care services.) (11) Despite the magnitude and cost of injury, society benefits from early and aggressive treatment to reduce the number of deaths and complications caused by traumatic injuries(12,13).

Elderly patients live longer and are more active than in the past (14). As our population becomes more health and exercise conscious, these active elderly sustain more injuries that are traumatic (15). In 1991, the elderly made up approximately 12.7% of the population and 29% of the deaths caused by trauma (5).

The posttrauma potential for mortality is higher in the elderly compared with young adults (15%–30% vs 4%–8%). Four factors influence mortality after major injury: (1) injury severity, (2) host factors, (3) time to definitive care, and (4) the quality of care (16). Emergency operations in the elderly greatly increase the operative risk of complications—from approximately 1% for elective cases to 45% for emergency procedures (17–20). Aggressive care in the older injured person is warranted for the following reasons: (1) errors in triage may underestimate the magnitude of injury for a given impact in older persons; (2) good outcomes are often influenced by early care; (3) the extent of underlying disease in the elderly cannot be quantified early; and (4) no reliable predictors exist of who will have a poor or favorable response to injury (8,21).

In a study group of 199,737 trauma admissions to California acute care hospitals in 1986, age and gender influenced mortality and hospital admission rates. Severity of injury was the most specific determinant of overall mortality. As early as age 40, mortality rates started to rise in severely injured men. Patients 65 years of age and older were more likely to die with minor injury regardless of sex. Mortality rates increased in both middle age (40–64 years) and elderly (65 years and older) groups of patients with injuries of moderate severity (16).

C. Essential Factors of Aging

Three major factors influence the care needs of the injured geriatric patient: known pre-existing disease, diminished physiological capacity, and occult disease. In the younger trauma victim, in whom pre-existing diseases are infrequent, the injury may be the sole cause of a clinical problem. In contrast, the geriatric patient may have one or more pre-existing diseases that may have varying levels of influence on physiological reserves, host resistance, and diagnosis and management of injuries. Second, a reduction in physiological function that would not qualify as a disease requiring treatment but is age-related may nevertheless reduce the available physiological reserve capacities. Third, many diseases or disorders may become manifest during stress. Certainly, the stress of trauma can bring to the forefront a specific disease entity that had previously been silent or undetected.

The presence of pre-existing conditions adversely influence outcome in patients admitted for traumatic injuries. The prevalence of pre-existing conditions increases significantly with age. More than 13% of trauma patients 55 to 64 years old and approximately 25% of trauma patients older than 75 have at least one pre-existing condition. Depending on the nature of the pre-existing medical condition (PEC), the relative odds of dying increase by as much as 30% with one PEC; the odds are twice as high (60%) in patients with two or more PECs. The types of conditions with the greatest effect on mortality are cirrhosis, congenital coagulopathy, chronic pulmonary or cardiac disease, and diabetes mellitus (22).

A thorough understanding of age-related physiological changes is critical for the diagnosis and management of diseases and injuries in older patients (23). Age-related physiological changes may alter responses to trauma (which may confound or delay the diagnosis of injury), mask certain vital signs, or influence an older person's response to treatment and the complications that may occur. Descriptions of various physiological changes of aging (by organ system) are found throughout other chapters of this textbook.

II. SELECT CAUSES OF INJURIES IN THE ELDERLY

A. Falls

1. Clinical Relevance

Falls are the most common mechanism of injury in the elderly, resulting in immobility, morbidity, and mortality. They account for 41% of the injuries in patients 65 and older (24). Extended care facilities report between 0.6 and 3.6 falls per nursing home bed, and up to one-third of elderly persons living at home fall (25). The underlying reasons for the fall may play a greater role in the outcome than the actual injuries. Several studies have demonstrated the presence of significant

Table 1 Factors Predisposing Elderly to Falls

Degenerative joint disease
Impaired sensation and proprioception
Near-syncope
Neuromuscular disorders
Predisposition to syncope
Unsteady gait and balance
Visual disturbances
Weakness of musculature

pre-existing medical problems or decreased physiological reserve in older persons who fall (16, 25, 26). The decreased physiological reserve, along with the development of significant complications, is often responsible for increased mortality in this population. Eight major factors predispose elderly patients to falls (Table 1). The possible causes for loss of consciousness in the elderly patient can be grouped according to cardiac and noncardiac causes (Table 2) (27). In one study, the three most prevalent causes of falls in the elderly were generalized weakness, environmental hazards, and orthostatic hypotension (25).

2. Clinical Manifestations

Elderly patients who fall exhibit findings that may be due to the mechanical fall or may have caused the fall in the first place. Acute changes in orientation may indicate trauma to the central nervous system, including, most commonly, acute or chronic subdural hematoma. Aging of the brain results in cerebral atrophy and increased venous fragility. Subdural hematoma should be considered in an elderly patient presenting with changes in mental status, headache, disturbances in ambulation, or nonfocal neurological findings. Spontaneous intracranial bleeding, stroke, or other cerebrovascular event may have caused the fall. Other findings in the patient 65 and older with acute changes in mental status may include cardiac dysrhythmia, acute myocardial injury, or metabolic disorders.

Musculoskeletal injuries are another class of common clinical manifestations in the older patient who may have experienced a fall. Any chest wall injuries can be fatal in the elderly patient, ranging from chest wall contusion to rib fractures to flail chest. Trauma to the underlying chest organs may cause pulmonary contusion, cardiac contusion, and injury to the major vessels of the chest. Hip fractures and other extremity fractures are common and primarily caused by osteoporosis. A fall may be the initial presentation of pathological fractures caused by primary or metastatic tumors. Spinal fractures may cause significant injury to

Table 2 Reasons for Loss of Consciousness in the Elderly

Cardiac causes
Dysrhythmias
Bradyarrhythmias
Tachyarrhythmias
Pacemaker failure
Anatomical or mechanical causes
Aortic stenosis
Other valvular dysfunction
Hypertrophic cardiomyopathy
Pulmonary embolism
Myocardial ischemia or infarction
Atrial myxoma
Pericardial tamponade
Aortic dissection
Vasomotor tone dysfunction
Vasovagal syncope
Carotid sinus hypersensitivity
Cough/micturation/defecation syncope
Orthostatic hypotension caused by
Medication
Volume loss
Autonomic dysfunction
Noncardiac causes
Cerebrovascular disease
Transient ischemic attack
Stroke
Seizure
Occult head trauma
Metabolic diseases
Intoxication
Alcohol
Sedative or hypnotic related
Other medications
Hypoglycemia
Pre-existing anemia
Chronic anemia
Sudden occult blood loss
Gastrointestinal hemorrhage
Abdominal aortic aneurysm
Psychogenic
Uncertain cause

the spinal cord and peripheral nerves. Clinical findings may include subtle findings of constipation or incontinence and obvious paralysis.

3. Immediate Diagnostic Approach

In all patients with traumatic injuries, assessment of the airway (A) is the first priority. Elderly patients may have upper airway obstruction caused by relaxed musculature of the oropharynx and may have displaced dentures impairing airflow. Once a patent airway is assured, checking for breathing (B) and circulation (C) includes looking for chest trauma. Is the chest expanding symmetrically? Are there any signs of flail chest? Evaluation for circulation of the extremities may reveal deformities compromising blood flow.

Elderly patients who fall commonly have neurological or musculoskeletal injuries. As in all trauma patients, immediate assessment and intervention is guided by Advanced Trauma Life Support (ATLS) protocol and dictated by the acute injuries and underlying physiological compromise. Once the ABCs (airway, breathing, circulation) are secure, secondary evaluation and management are guided by known pre-existing conditions and suspicion for injury on the basis of the mechanism of injury.

4. Intervention

Aggressive immediate intervention in the elderly is warranted regardless of age, unless the patient is known to have an advance directive limiting aggressive intervention or have pre-existing disorders or severe injuries that are shown to be associated with low probability of survival. Stabilization may require fluid resuscitation, which must be used with caution in the elderly patient, especially with underlying cardiovascular disease. Judicious use of crystalloid fluid is recommended, preferably Ringer's lactate in the older patient, to avoid hyperchloremia in the older patient with impaired renal capacity. If significant blood loss is a complication, after 1 to 2 L of crystalloid infusion, blood (packed red blood cells) should be infused. Geriatric patients may need platelets and fresh-frozen plasma earlier than younger patients in the resuscitation, especially if underlying liver dysfunction or hematological compromise is present.

5. Follow-up Management

A thorough history will help determine the cause of the fall and direct interventions that may prevent subsequent falls. Information regarding the height of the fall, associated loss of consciousness, and agility before and after the fall are important historical factors. The remainder of the evaluation can be targeted from the history combined with a complete physical examination. Blood tests and urinalysis are indicated in patients with signs of anemia, dehydration, or infection.

Cardiac assessment, including a Holter monitor, is useful only in symptomatic patients. Radiographic and other imaging studies should be completed when appropriate.

Identification and treatment of illnesses, adjustment of medications, and reduction of risks associated with falls result in long-term health benefits for these patients. Rehabilitation to increase muscle strength, joint mobility, and balance after a fall should be coupled with equipment to assist with ambulation and stability. Additional environmental interventions to consider are improved lighting; handrails in the bedroom, bathroom, hallways, and stairs; and removal of potential hazards.

Rehabilitation therapy increases mobility and may actually increase the potential for subsequent falls in the elderly fall survivor. However, postintervention follow-up has shown fewer numbers of falls of less severity in the treated patients (26).

B. Motor Vehicle Crashes

1. Clinical Relevance

Motor vehicle crashes account for 28% of all injuries, the second most common mechanism of injury, in the age group 65 years and older (24). Of note, motor vehicle crashes are the most common type of ''fatal'' event in the elderly through age 80 (28). Risk of motor vehicle trauma is higher in the aged driver because of underlying medical disorders, changes in depth perception, decreased visual and auditory acuity, and increased reaction times. Alcohol, reckless driving, and speed play a minor role in this age group compared with younger drivers.

Automobile versus elderly pedestrian injuries are the third most common mechanism of injury in the geriatric patient, representing 10% of all injuries for persons aged 65 years and older. Factors contributing to auto-pedestrian injuries seen in the elderly include the following: (1) impaired visual acuity and decreased peripheral vision, (2) postural kyphosis, (3) progressive deafness, (4) altered gait and strength owing to arthritis, (5) muscle atrophy, and (6) chronic neurological disease that can lead to marked decreases in ambulatory speed (29).

2. Clinical Manifestations

Altered mental status is the most common clinical manifestation in the elderly patient involved in a motor vehicle collision as a driver, passenger, or pedestrian. The physician must determine whether the mental status findings are due to intracranial injury, injuries to other sites causing system complications (e.g., hypotension, hypoxia) or acute excerbation of underlying diseases (e.g., heart failure), or whether the altered mental status was the primary cause of the trauma.

The injured elderly patient exhibits a combination of decreased physiological reserve and a high incidence of pre-existing medical conditions that cause a comparably worse outcome, more complications, longer hospital stays, and greater costs (30–32). An awareness of the importance of pre-existing medical conditions and a coordinated, directed approach to the management of the injuries and the concomitant diseases leads to the most effective care and patient outcome (32). Trauma care in the United States has evolved into local, county, and state trauma systems. By design, these systems offer a continuum of care that extends from the prehospital arena to acute care and through rehabilitation. Trauma triage criteria do not include age and can seriously underestimate the severity of injury in the geriatric patient (Table 3) (26).

Unstable vital signs are ominous, and signs of shock (e.g., hypotension, tachycardia, and tachypnea) may be irreversible in the injured patient 65 years

Table 3 Trauma Score (1–16)

Parameters	Points
Respiratory rate (per minute)	
10–24	4
25–35	3
>35	2
<10	1
0	0
Systolic blood pressure (mm Hg)	
>90	4
70–90	3
50–69	2
<50	1
0	0
Glasgow Coma Scale score	
14–15	5
11–13	4
8–10	3
5–7	2
3–4	1
Respiratory effort	
Normal	1
Shallow/retractive	0
Capillary refill	
Normal	2
Delayed	1
None	0

and older. Older patients with what appear to be normal vital signs after a motor vehicle crash may have other complications develop because of their compromised physiological reserve or may subsequently die because of the acute trauma.

Respiratory insufficiency often develops early after trauma in the elderly patient. Differentiation between acute pulmonary or cardiovascular injury and underlying chronic respiratory disease is important. Respiratory failure can develop later in the course of treatment and recovery from traumatic injury as a result of pulmonary infection or pulmonary embolus caused by immobility.

3. Immediate Diagnostic Approach

The diagnosis and treatment of the geriatric multiple trauma victim should follow standard trauma guidelines including a primary survey to assess critical injuries requiring immediate intervention and stabilization and a secondary survey for more complete patient assessment. Understanding the mechanism of injury, the condition of the vehicle, and the status of others involved in the collision helps guide treatment recommendations. It is prudent to assume that all geriatric trauma patients have some level of pre-existing illness or inadequate reserves (Table 4) (28).

In the prehospital arena, an appreciation of the fragility and limited physiological reserve of the geriatric patient is essential for the emergency medical service provider, the receiving trauma center surgeons, and emergency department personnel. A combination of known factors and a high index of suspicion regarding the unknown factors form the basis of management of acute traumatic emergencies and critical care of the elderly. In the elderly patient with an initial trauma score of 7 or less, the expected mortality is 100%. However, a high initial trauma score of 14 to 16 does not necessarily correlate with final morbidity or mortality (33, 34). Older patients are more likely to die than younger patients involved in motor vehicle crashes, and the most common cause of death in both groups is severe head trauma (14, 35).

With mechanism of injury and physical examination as a major guide, these diagnositic studies should be performed on the basis of the following criteria.

(a). Abdominal Ultrasonography or Peritoneal Tap/Lavage. In the presence of hypotension in the prehospital setting, not completely explained by a quantitative amount of blood loss in the chest, external blood loss, or other proven causes, the patient must undergo either a peritoneal tap (to determine whether gross blood is in the peritoneal cavity) or abdominal ultrasonography (preferred method). This is done to ensure that the patient will not suddenly decompensate from blood loss while undergoing other diagnostic studies outside the immediate resuscitation area. Patients with gross intra-abdominal bleeding go directly to the operating room for exploratory laparotomy.

Table 4 Treatment Guidelines for Geriatric Trauma

Age 55 to 64 years

1. Assume some mild decrease in physiological reserve.
2. Suspect the presence of some common diseases of middle age (diabetes, arteriosclerotic cardiovascular disease, hypertension, previous surgery, previous transfusion).
3. Suspect the use of prescription or over-the-counter medications.
4. Assume the patient is competent to provide an accurate medical history.
5. Look for subtle signs of organ dysfunction, especially cardiovascular and respiratory systems; obtain pulse oximetry, arterial blood gas measurements, and electrocardiograms if indicated.
6. In the presence of a history of loss of consciousness or abnormalities of cognitive function or personality, assume a serious brain injury is present until proven otherwise; CT scan is appropriate.
7. Proceed with standard diagnostic and management schemes unless contraindicated by information collected during history.

Age 65 to 74 years

1. Accept the presence of age-related and acquired disease–induced physiological alterations of organ systems.
2. Accept the presence of acquired diseases and medications to correct or control them; assume a higher incidence of previous surgery and transfusion.
3. Decide whether the patient is competent to give a reliable medical history; review the history as soon as possible with the patient's relatives or personal physician.
4. Aggressively monitor the patient and control the physiological characteristics to optimize cardiac performance and oxygen metabolism.
5. Assume that any alteration in mental status or cognitive or sensory function indicates the presence of a brain injury; imaging of the brain is mandatory.
6. Proceed with standard diagnostic and management schemes, including early, aggressive operative management.
7. Be aware of poor outcome, especially with severe injury to the central nervous system or marked physiological deterioration resulting from injury; check for advance directives.

Age 75 years or older

1. Proceed as in items 1 through 5 for patients 65 through 74 years of age.
2. Assume a poor outcome with moderately severe injury, especially in the central nervous system or for any injury causing physiological dysfunction.
3. After aggressive initial resuscitation and diagnostic maneuvers, examine item 2 and discuss appropriateness of care with the patient (if competent) and family members.

Source: Ref. 28.

(b). Computed Tomography. Computed tomography (CT) imaging of the head, chest, or abdomen when indicated is appropriate once the patient is hemodynamically stable. Intracranial injury is often the cause of death in the elderly patient. Abdominal CT is useful to determine retroperitoneal hematomas and solid organ injuries without free blood in the peritoneal cavity.

(c). Vascular Imaging Including Angiography. A relatively minor injury might be life threatening in an individual with limited physiological reserve. When necessary, appropriate studies may detect significant vascular injuries.

(d). Other Studies. Knowledge of the mechanism of injury involved will help guide the diagnostic evaluation. Studies should be obtained on the basis of clinical manifestations and suspicion of injury.

4. Intervention

The ABCs (airway, breathing, circulation) of trauma management, established by the American College of Surgeons Committee on Trauma-Advanced Trauma Life Support (ATLS) Course, offer an essential guideline for the initial management of the trauma victim. Once the patient's airway is protected, a search for blood loss, even in the face of normal vital signs, must be initiated. In the geriatric patient, commonly used parameters to assess hemodynamic status can be misleading; therefore, continuous monitoring of vital signs, cardiac activity, and oxygen saturation is essential. Following an established protocol for evaluation and treatment of the patient with complex trauma increases the suspicion for occult bleeding in the older patient who appears ''clinically stable.''

5. Follow-up Management

Early monitoring and optimization of cardiac output, oxygen delivery, and consumption are particularly important in elderly trauma patients if they require general anesthesia or intensive care (36). An aggressive approach to evaluation, monitoring, and treatment is warranted in all geriatric trauma patients. Admissions to critical care units with invasive monitoring to guide therapy for trauma victims 75 years or older with injuries that are moderate to more serious increase the potential for survival. In fact, the chance of survival at an independent functional level is significant if the patients are discharged from the acute hospital setting (12).

C. Elder Abuse

1. Clinical Relevance

Physical abuse of dependent older adults requires special consideration and is discussed extensively in another chapter. (See Chapter 24.) However, a few salient points are worth re-emphasizing. With a growing elderly population, geriatric abuse is on the rise. To identify and effectively treat these victims of domestic violence, physicians must have an awareness of the problem and include the suspicion of abuse in their patient evaluations. The potential for domestic violence is increased in the following settings: family use of alcohol or illicit drugs, significant life stresses in the primary caregiver, unemployed caregiver financially dependent on elder, underlying progressive conditions requiring high level of care (dementia, parkinsonism, stroke), family history of mental illness or domestic abuse, or inadequate or unsafe housing (37).

2. Clinical Manifestations

Elder abuse can manifest in several ways, most commonly as physical abuse. Soft tissue injuries and broken bones may result from beatings, deliberate burns, physical restraints, or other cruelties. Personality or behavioral changes may indicate abuse, especially in the absence of objective neurological findings and negative diagnostic studies. Medication side effects or new onset of dementia may be related to abusive treatment by the caregiver.

3. Immediate Diagnostic Approach

Diagnostic evaluation of all trauma patients should include questions about the circumstances surrounding the injuries. It is important to ask alert patients whether they can recall instances of rough handling or being struck. For dependent individuals, ask the caregivers what their care schedule is like. Does the patient live at home or in a facility for the elderly? Do the stories match, and if not, why not?

4. Intervention

Protection must be provided to the abused older person. Admission to an acute care facility for monitoring and intervention may be necessary to prevent further abuse. Treatment should be appropriate to the injuries sustained.

5. Follow-up Management

Social services should be involved early in the evaluation and assist with placement needs if needed. Suspicion and intervention to prevent further injury are key to long-term survival of all survivors of violence.

D. Other Causes of Traumatic Injuries in the Elderly

Stabs and gunshot wounds represented 8.1% of injuries in the elderly (12). Burns represent approximately 8% of all elderly trauma deaths (38). Other chapters in this book cover fractures of the hip, acute vascular emergencies, neurological emergencies, and cardiac emergencies and offer additional insights into the management of trauma in the elderly. Evaluation and treatment should follow ATLS guidelines as noted previously.

III. FOLLOW-UP MANAGEMENT OF THE INJURED ELDERLY

Although traumatic injuries result in a higher incidence of mortality in geriatric patients, the outcome for survivors looks promising. A review of outcome studies demonstrated that most discharged patients 65 years and older were living independently 1 to 2 years later (20, 39). In one study of patients 75 years and older, one-third of the patients studied survived more than 5 years and most of those in independent living situations (12). Recognizing and treating the injuries aggressively increase survival and discharge rates. Rehabilitation improves mobility and independence. Providing assistive devices and implementing preventive measures after discharge may prevent recurrent injuries. As the aging population continues to grow, trauma systems must continue to meet the special needs of the injured elder.

REFERENCES

1. Committee on Trauma, American College of Surgeons. Resources for optimal care of the injured patient: 1999. Chicago: American College of Surgeons, 1998.
2. Committee on Trauma, American College of Surgeons. Resources for optimal care of the injured patient: 1993. Chicago: American College of Surgeons, 1993.
3. Fleming AW, Sterling-Scott RP, Carabello G, Imari-Williams I, Allmond B, Foster RS, Kennedy F, Shoemaker WC. Injury and violence in Los Angeles: Impact on access to health care and surgical education. Arch Surg 1992; 127(6):671–676.
4. Committee to Review the Status and Progress of the Injury Control Program at the Centers for Disease Control. Injury control. Washington, DC: National Academy Press, 1988.
5. Santora TA, Schinco MA, Trooskin SZ. Management of trauma in the elderly patient. Surg Clin North Am 1994; 74(1):163–186.
6. Goldschmidt MJ, Castiglion CL, Assael LA, Litt MD. Craniomaxillofacial trauma in the elderly. J Oral Maxill Surg 1995; 53(10):1145–1149.
7. National Safety Council: Accident Facts, 1994. Chicago: National Safety Council, 1994.
8. Baker SP, O'Neill B, Haddon W Jr., Long WB. The injury severity score: a method for describing patients with multiple injuries and evaluating emergency care. J Trauma. 1974; 14(3):187–196.

9. Martin RE, Teberian G. Multiple trauma and the elderly patient. Emerg Med Clin North Am 8:411, 1990.
10. Fingerhut LA, Warner M. Injury chartbook. Health, United States, 1996–97. Hyattsville, MD: National Center for Health Statistics, 1997.
11. Bonnie RJ, Liverman CT, Fulco CE, eds. Reducing the burden of injury: advancing prevention and treatment. Committee on Injury Prevention and Control, Division of Health Promotion and Disease Prevention, Institute of Medicine. Washington DC: National Academy Press, 1999:1–16.
12. Battistella FD, Din AM, Perez L. Trauma patients 75 years and older: Long-term follow-up results justify aggressive management. J Trauma 1998; 44(4):618–623.
13. Johnson C, Margulies DR, Kearney TJ, Hiatt JR, Shabot MM. Trauma in the elderly: an analysis of outcome based on age. Am Surg 1994; 60:899–902.
14. Levy DB, Hanlon DP, Townsend RN. Geriatric trauma. Clin Geriatr Med 1993; 9(3):601–620.
15. Scalea TM, Kohl H. Geriatric trauma. In: Feliciano DV, Moore EE, Mattox KL, eds. Trauma. 3rd ed. Stamford, Ct: Appleton & Lange, 1996, pp 899–915.
16. Morris JA, Mackenzie EJ, Damiano AM, Bass SM. Mortality in trauma patients: The interaction between host factors and severity. J Trauma 1990; 30(12):1476–1478.
17. Adkins R, Scott H. Surgical procedures in patients aged 90 years and older. South Med J 1984; 77:1357–1364.
18. Greenburg A, Saik R, Farris J, Peskin GW. Operative mortality in general surgery. Am J Surg 1982; 144:22–28.
19. Evans L. Risk of fatality from physical trauma versus sex and age. J Trauma 1988; 28(3):368–378.
20. Chelluri L, Pinsky MR, Grenvik AN. Outcome of intensive care in the oldest-old critically ill patients. Crit Care Med 1992; 20(6):757–761.
21. Kauder DR. The elderly trauma patient. Post-graduate course, Chicago: American College of Surgeons, 1988, 17–19.
22. Morris JA, Mackenzie EJ, Edelstein SL. The effect of preexisting conditions on mortality in trauma patients. JAMA 1990; 263(14):1942–1946.
23. Rowe JW. Aging and geriatric medicine. In: Wyngaarden JK, Smith LH, Bennett JC, eds. Cecil textbook of medicine. Philadelphia: W.B. Saunders, 1992, pp 21–26.
24. Champion HR, Copes SW, Buyer D, Flanagan ME, Bain L, Sacco WJ. Major trauma in geriatric patient. Am J Public Health 1989; 79(9):1278–1282.
25. Rubenstein LA, Robbins AS, Josephson KR, Schulman BL, Osterweil D. The value of assessing falls in an elderly population. A randomized clinical trial. Ann Intern Med 1990; 113:308–316.
26. Finelli FC, Jonsson J, Champion HR, Morelli S, Fouty WJ. A case control study for major trauma in geriatric patients. J Trauma 1989; 29(5):541–548.
27. Mandavia D, Newton K. Geriatric trauma. Emerg Med Clin North Am 1998; 16(1): 257–274.
28. Schwab CW, Kauder DR. Trauma in the geriatric patient. Arch Surg 1992; 127: 701–706.
29. McCoy GF, Johnstone RA, Duhie RB. Injury to the elderly in road traffic accidents. J Trauma 1989; 29(4):494–497.

30. DeMaria EJ. Evaluation and treatment of the elderly trauma victim. Clin Geriatr Med 1993; 9(2):461–471.
31. Knies RC Jr. Assessment in geriatric trauma: what you need to know. Int J Trauma Nurs 1996; 2(3):85–91.
32. McMahon DJ, Schwab CW, Kauder D. Comorbidity and the elderly trauma patient. World J Surg 1996; 20(8):1113–1119.
33. Knudson MM, Lieberman J, Morris JA Jr, Cushing BM, Stubbs HA. Mortality factors in geriatric blunt trauma patients. Arch Surg 1994; 129(4):448–453.
34. Pellicane JV, Byrne K, DeMaria EJ. Preventable complications and death from multiple organ failure among geriatric trauma victims. J Trauma 1992; 33(3):440–444.
35. Van der Sluis CK, Duis JH, Geertzen JHB. Multiple injuries: An overview of the outcome. J Trauma 1995; 38(5):681–686.
36. Wilson RF. Trauma in patients with pre-existing cardiac disease. Crit Care Clin 1994; 10:461–501.
37. Jones J, Dougherty J, Schelble D, Cunningham W. Emergency department protocol for the diagnosis and evaluation of geriatric abuse. Ann Emerg Med 1988; 17:1006–1015.
38. Osler T, Hales K, Baack B, Baer K, His K, Pathak D, Demarest G. Trauma in the elderly. Am J Surg 1988; 156(6):537–543.
39. Zietlow SP, Capizzi PJ, Bannon MP, Farnell MB. Multisystem geriatric trauma. J Trauma 1994; 37(6):985–988.

8

Critical Care of the Hip Fracture Patient

William T. Long
Charles R. Drew University of Medicine and Science, and Martin Luther King, Jr.–Charles R. Drew Medical Center, Los Angeles, California

Earl Warren Brien
Orthopaedic Hospital, Los Angeles, California

I. CLINICAL RELEVANCE

A. Epidemiology

Hip fractures are the most common fractures that affect survival and the quality of life of the geriatric patient. More than 300,000 hip fractures occur per year in the United States, and this number is expected to double by the year 2050 (1). Two-thirds of the patients will not return to their previous functional level, and approximately 40% will not survive more than 2 years after the fracture (2,3). Under the most favorable circumstances, a displaced hip fracture will lead the geriatric patient to a course that includes an immediate operation, ambulation on the first postoperative day, and a 3- to 12-month program of rehabilitation. Too often the hip fracture patient becomes engulfed by staggering problems, including perioperative complications, prolonged hospitalization, and expensive long-term supportive care. It has been estimated that the direct medical costs of hip fractures amount to more than $8 billion per year in the United States (4,5). A patient who survives the fracture but loses independent function will often have an immeasurable loss of self-esteem, especially when the patient perceives that they are a burden to loved ones and family.

Internists and geriatricians are frequently called on to evaluate whether patients are medically stable for surgery and then to follow-up to prevent and treat medical complications in the perioperative period. Both pre-existing illness and disorders uncovered during the preoperative evaluation may require the attention of a medical specialist or the anesthesiologist. Internal fixation or hip replacement is the preferred treatment. No current literature supports routine nonoperative treatment of hip fractures. The orthopedic surgeon must consider a variety of procedures and select the one operation that offers the best chance for rapid recovery along with the lowest incidence of complications. Zuckerman and colleagues demonstrated the efficacy of a multidisciplinary approach that decreases complications and improves function and independence (6,7).

B. Pathogenesis

1. Osteoporosis

Primary osteoporosis is an age-related disease characterized by normal bone composition with a decrease in the quantity of osseous tissue per unit volume. Age, gender, and race determine bone mass. Peak bone mass is attained during the third decade of life followed by a slow phase of bone loss. This bone loss continues equally in men and women at a rate of 0.3% to 0.5% per year. An accelerated phase of bone loss, which occurs at the rate of 2% to 3% per year, begins after menopause and is related to decreased estrogen levels. This phase continues for 6 to 10 years, after which bone loss returns to a basal slow-phase level of 0.3% to 0.5% per year. Peak bone mass is 30% higher in men, and the accelerated phase of bone loss is an uncommon occurrence in men. This helps to explain the increased prevalence of osteoporosis in women compared with men. The incidence of osteoporosis in white women is two to three times higher than that reported for black and Hispanic women (8). Osteoporosis by no means occurs in all women who have undergone menopause or in all persons who have reached advanced age. However, approximately 30% of women and 20% of men who live to be 90 years old will sustain a hip fracture associated with osteoporosis.

Normal adult proximal femur is composed of marrow, trabecular bone, cortical bone and periosteum. A healthy trabecular lattice is a bridging network of densely packed cancellous bone. In patients with osteoporosis, this trabecular lattice is thinned and sparse (Figure 1B). The cortical bone of the diaphysis of patients with osteoporosis is thin, and the medullary canal is wide (Figure 2B). This occurs in osteoporosis by the process of endosteal bone erosion, coupled with periosteal bone deposition. The diaphysis compensates for loss of bone by expanding the remaining osseous material. Progressive enlargement of diaphyseal bone dimensions decreases bending stresses, leads to greater moments of inertia, and helps to mitigate worsening fracture risks (9,10) (Figure 2). Trabecular bone has no such mechanism to compensate for mineral loss. Bones that are primarily trabecular include the vertebral bodies, distal radius, and proximal femur. Fifty percent of trabecular bone density in the lumbar spine may be lost between the

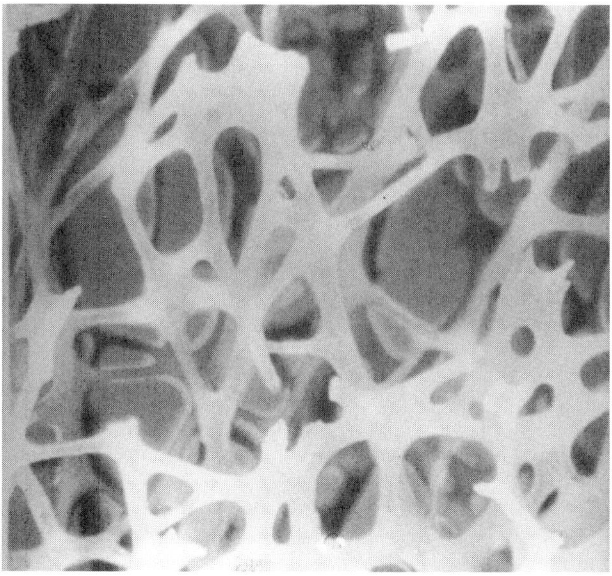

(A)

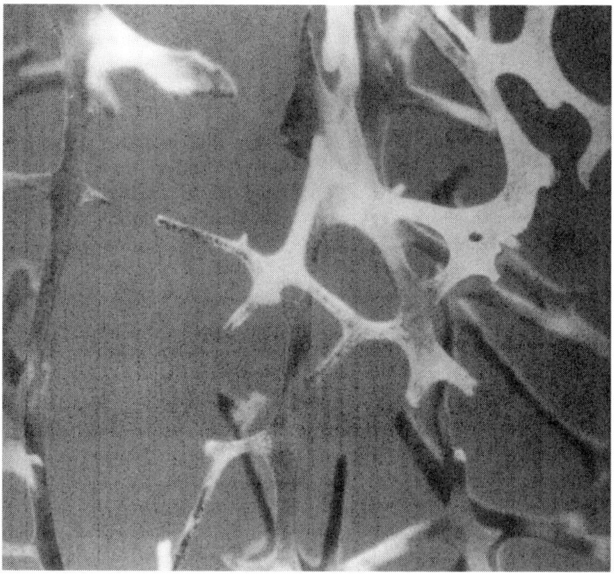

(B)

Figure 1 (A) Section through normal adult trabecular bone demonstrates an interconnected network of bridging bone. (B) Trabecular bone in osteoporosis is thin and sparce.

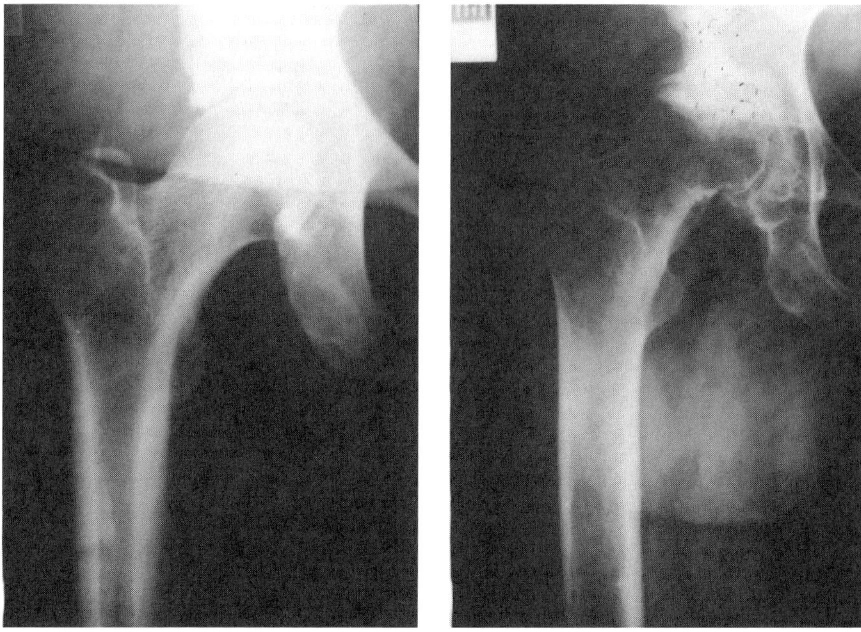

(A) (B)

Figure 2 (A) Radiograph of the proximal femur of a 38-year-old man demonstrates the thick cortical bone of the diaphysis. (B) The diaphysis of an 83-year-old woman is thin and the medullary canal is wide.

ages of 20 and 80. This is consistent with the observation that vertebral compression fractures are the most common, followed by hip fractures, and fractures of the wrist (11,12). Some degree of osteoporosis is seen in approximately 85% of patients with femoral neck fractures, and numerous authors have shown that intertrochanteric fractures commonly occur through osteoporotic bone (13–15). A reduction in bone mass may result in fracture after being subjected to lower stresses than those required to fracture normal bone (16–19). Such fractures are termed *fracture of insufficiency*. Similarly, the relative hip fracture risk and the risk of other osteoporotic fractures are increased in patients who have reduced bone density (20,21). Although osteoporosis is the single most important factor, the physician who encounters these patients should be familiar with other important causes of hip fractures in the elderly.

2. Osteomalacia

The roentgenograph of a patient with a hip fracture and osteomalacia may be indistinguishable from that of a patient with a hip fracture and osteoporosis. The term *osteopenia* describes the radiographic finding of decreased bone density without indicating the underlying cause. Osteomalacia is a metabolic bone disorder in which mineralization of newly formed organic matrix (osteoid) is inadequate. Osteomalacia may occur in the elderly because of vitamin D deficiency or renal phosphate wasting. Risk factors include nutritional deficiency, gastric or small bowel resection, chronic steatorrhea, lack of sunshine (ultraviolet light), and the use of anticonvulsants. Approximately one-third of the patients with osteomalacia come to medical attention because of a fracture or because of an abnormal biochemical profile. Fractures in patients with osteomalacia usually occur in the neck of the femur (22). Wilton et al. performed iliac crest biopsies in more than 1000 elderly patients with femoral neck fractures. Osteomalacia was found in only 2% of the specimens, and osteoporosis was the predominant bone disease associated with hip fractures in that population sample (23). The physician must examine clinical risk factors and the biochemical profile. These findings accompanied by characteristic radiographic evidence such as Looser's lines or biconcave vertebral bodies will help to make the diagnosis of osteomalacia. In some patients a transiliac bone biopsy after tetracycline labeling is necessary to confirm the diagnosis.

3. Bone Tumors

The incidence of metastatic bone disease increases with advancing age and so does the index of suspicion that a hip fracture is related to a metastatic or primary bone cancer. The proximal femur is a common site for metastatic lesions that result in pathological fractures or impending fractures. Common malignancies that spread hematogenously to the bone include lung, breast, prostate, renal, and thyroid cancers. Primary bone tumors including multiple myeloma, Paget's sarcoma, sarcomas associated with bone infarct, and carcinomas of the bone must also be suspected. An incisional biopsy may be required to identify a tumor before definitive surgical treatment. The specimen must be of ample size, taken from the appropriate region of the lesion, and preserved properly to give the pathologist the best opportunity to make the correct diagnosis. It is important to avoid contamination and the spread of tumor cells. The orthopedic bone tumor specialist and pathologist can provide useful recommendations if they are consulted before a biopsy specimen is taken.

When a tumor is suspected, a thorough history and physical examination will guide the evaluation. A more extensive preoperative evaluation may be required to identify a primary malignancy or determine the origin and extent of metastatic disease. In addition to routine preoperative hip and chest radiographs, a skeletal survey may be necessary. Multiple myeloma, renal and thyroid malignancies frequently demonstrate metastatic lesions on radiographs but may not reveal significant uptake with bone scan (Figure 3). Computed tomography (CT) scan of the head, chest, abdomen, and pelvis may be necessary to identify a

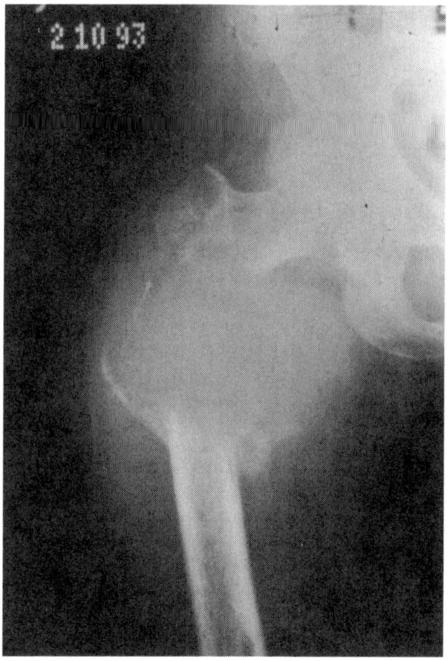

(A)

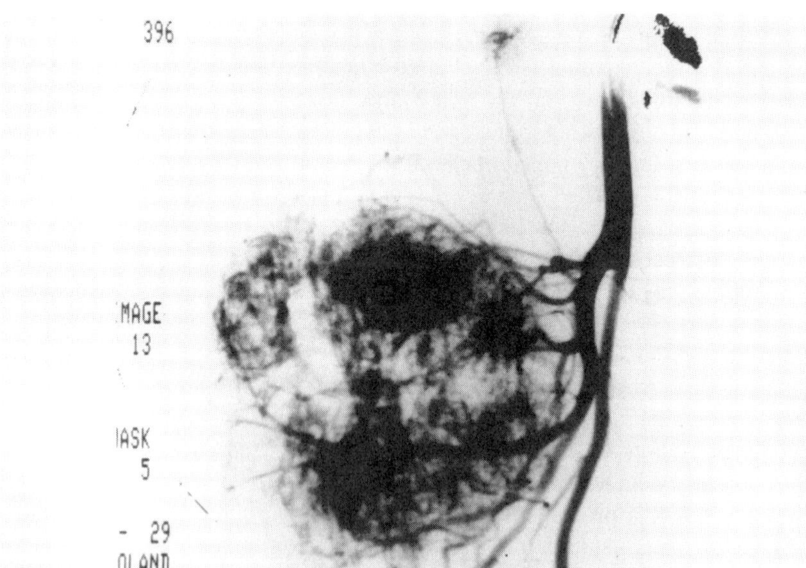

(B)

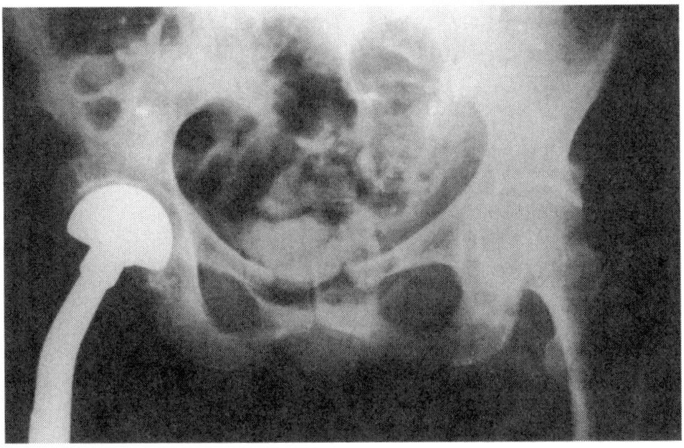

(C)

Figure 3 (A) The large lytic lesion and destruction of the subtrocanteric region of the proximal femur are the result of metastatic renal cell carcinoma. (B) Hypervascularity seen on an arteriogram of the common femoral artery and its branches is characteristic of renal cell carcinoma. (C) En-bloc resection and hemiarthroplasty was the treatment of choice in this case.

primary lesion or evaluate distant spread of disease. Laboratory studies include a complete blood cell count and erythrocyte sedimentation rate (commonly abnormal in multiple myeloma or chronic diseases including malignancy), blood chemistry (evaluating serum calcium, liver enzymes, alkaline phosphatase, and acid phosphatase), urinalysis (for proteinuria and occult blood), thyroid function studies, and prostate specific antigen in men. Serum and urine protein electrophoresis, carcinoembryonic antigen, and urinary pyridinoline may be useful if multiple myeloma, carcinoma, or Paget's disease is suspected, respectively.

II. IMMEDIATE DIAGNOSTIC APPROACH

Patients who sustain hip fractures can be divided into two major groups: elderly women and young adult men. Ninety-five percent of hip fractures occur in patients older than 50 (24). Women experience 70% to 80% of the hip fractures in the older age group. Men make up as much as 80% of patients in the young adult group. The presenting symptoms of a patient with a femoral neck fracture vary widely. The elderly patient with an impacted, incomplete, or nondisplaced femoral neck fracture may have mild complaints. Symptoms may be limited to groin pain during full weight bearing or hip pain while rising from a chair. In contrast, the elderly patient with a displaced hip fracture will usually describe an acute onset of severe hip pain and the inability to walk after a fall. The young trauma patient with a hip fracture complains of severe hip or groin pain with any movement of the hip, unless these symptoms are masked by altered mental status or the pain of associated injuries. In all high-risk patients special attention to the patient's symptoms will alert the physician to the unrecognized or nondisplaced hip fracture.

It is not always possible to determine the mechanism of injury from the history given by the patient. Extremely brittle bone can fracture during normal daily activities and cause the patient to fall. Stronger bone will not fracture during ambulation, but the force of impact with the ground from a fall can cause a fracture of the hip. The close association between low-energy falls and hip fractures in the elderly has led some authors to conclude that approximately 90% of hip fractures in the elderly occur as the result of a fall (25). Medical conditions that predispose to falls include cardiac dysrhythmia, seizures, and cerebrovascular insufficiency; disorders of vision, gait, and balance; and deficits of muscular strength and coordination. Home safety hazards also cause falls. A patient who sustains a hip fracture after an unexplained fall should be carefully evaluated for predisposing conditions. In contrast, environmental hazards in young hip fracture patients consist mainly of fast-moving automobiles and low-energy projectiles fired from handguns (26).

A patient with a nondisplaced or impacted fracture may walk into the physicians office with only a subtle limp. The limb will not be short and pain may be elicited only at the extremes of internal and external rotation. This explains how a hip fracture may be overlooked or misdiagnosed as a ''groin pull'' by the initial examining physician. The physical findings become obvious once the fracture becomes displaced. Physical examination of a patient with an acute, displaced, unstable fracture of the hip will reveal a patient who cannot walk or bear weight on the affected lower extremity. When compared with the contralateral side, the limb will be short and externally rotated in most patients. Pain will be elicited by alternately internally and externally rotating or ''log rolling'' the thigh while keeping the knee extended. Painful pistoning may be observed at the hip joint when the extremity is axially loaded.

Special effort should be taken to examine the patient for associated problems, including deep venous thrombosis, pressure ulcers, and osteoporotic fractures of the spine and wrist. The physical examination should include a comprehensive search for pre-existing illness, especially cardiovascular, pulmonary, and central nervous system disorders. Associated disorders can have a serious impact on the timing of surgery and limit the available treatment options.

A plain anteroposterior (AP) radiograph of the pelvis and an AP and lateral radiographs of the affected hip will clearly demonstrate the displaced femoral neck or intertrochanteric femur fracture. The plain AP radiograph of the pelvis is important because it provides an image of the contralateral hip. Routine preoperative planning requires measurement of the unaffected hip because an important goal of hip surgery is to restore lower extremities that are equal in length.

Femoral neck and intertrocanteric femur fractures occur with about equal frequency. However, intertrochanteric fractures occur in patients who are approximately 10 years older than patients with femoral neck fractures. The most widely used classification scheme for femoral neck fractures is that proposed by Garden (27). Garden I and II fractures are grouped together as ''nondisplaced,'' whereas Garden III and IV fractures are said to be ''displaced.'' Femoral neck fractures are also described by the anatomical location of the fracture as subcapital, transcervical, and basilar neck. Subcapital fractures carry the highest incidence of avascular necrosis and basilar neck fractures the lowest. The prognosis for survival of the femoral head can influence the decision to perform hip fixation or femoral head replacement. Agreement on a classification system for intertrocanteric fractures is not universal. The classification by Evans provides an anatomical description of the most common fracture patterns (28,29). Many internal fixation systems are designed to address the common fracture patterns described by Evans.

When a hip fracture is suspected and standard radiographs do not confirm the presence of a fracture, several imaging options are available. A T1-weighted magnetic resonance imaging (MRI) scan is an excellent imagining technique to diagnose occult hip fractures. Quinn and McCarthy found the T1-weighted MRI scan to be 100% predictive of hip fractures in 20 patients studied prospectively (30). The CT scan yields excellent bone detail and can reveal fractures not seen on plain radiographs. The CT scan also provides valuable information about the amount and location of comminution. The CT scan should be ordered with 2- to 3-mm slices through the region in question because larger slices increase the chance of missing the fracture completely. Further diagnostic testing for occult fractures includes the technetium (Tc 99m) bone scan, which has a high sensitivity (93.3%) and specificity (95.0%) for identification of nondisplaced fractures (31).

Laboratory tests are an important part of the preoperative evaluation. Published studies have shown that broad, nonselective testing is not an effective approach for finding clinically important abnormalities (32). For the initial evaluation of an older patient complete blood cell count, blood urea nitrogen, serum creatinine, electrolyte and glucose determinations, electrocardiography, and chest radiography are generally adequate. A urinalysis is important because urinary tract infections are common in this group of patients, and effective treatment can be initiated before surgery. Tests of prothrombin time or partial thromboplastin time are obtained routinely to evaluate coagulopathy. These tests are not likely to yield clinically useful information in an asymptomatic patient with no history of bleeding problems. However, it is the practice of most physicians to obtain these studies before any major operation because unanticipated perioperative bleeding period can have devastating consequences. Routine liver function testing is most likely not warranted because elevated serum transaminase values occur in only 0.5% to 3% of preoperative patients, and minimal elevations do not have a significant impact on surgery (33). Patients who have major elevations in preoperative liver function tests will in all likelihood give some indication of liver disease by history or will present signs of liver damage during physical examination.

III. THERAPEUTIC INTERVENTION

A. Immediate Medical Stabilization

Most elderly patients with an acute hip fracture will initially be seen with coexisting underlying medical conditions and perhaps chronic disabilities. The immediate concern is to stabilize the cardiovascular and pulmonary status of the patient. Hypotension may be a result of blood loss related to the hip fracture or exacerbation of an underlying condition (e.g., myocardial infarction from coronary artery disease). Respiratory distress seen in association with the hip fracture may be related to cardiac disease, pulmonary embolus, fat embolus, aspiration, or an underlying pulmonary disorder. Appropriate management of these conditions will require assistance from an internist, cardiologist, pulmonologist, or geriatrician. Finally, an assessment should be made of the acid-base, electrolyte, and renal status of the patient before consideration for surgical intervention. Elderly persons often have renal dysfunction and hypertension, which can complicate the perioperative management of the hip fracture patient. Medical problems that can be rapidly corrected must be distinguished from chronic stable conditions to determine whether immediate surgical intervention for the hip fracture should be implemented.

B. Nonsurgical Management

1. Unacceptable Surgical Risks

Nonsurgical management is expected to delay, compromise, or eliminate the patient's ability to ambulate. Decreased mobility and physical activity jeopardizes the patient's ability to participate in leisure activities and social functions. Within days of being placed on complete bed rest, the elderly patient can develop deep venous thrombosis, thromboembolism, pneumonia, pressure ulcers, and nosocomial infections. Prolonged decreased activity can lead to accelerated loss of bone and muscle mass, joint contractures, and deterioration of the cardiovascular and respiratory systems. Each day that the patient remains hospitalized the cost of care rises along with the potential for iatrogenic problems. Despite these compromises, a small group patients will be best suited for nonsurgical management.

The most common reason to select nonoperative treatment is that the risks of surgery are considered unacceptably high by the treating physician, the patient, or the patient's family. Cardiovascular instability, pulmonary failure, and septicemia are among health problems that can derail plans to perform a major operation. In these cases, it is advisable to consult with medical specialists and the anesthesiologist early in the patient's course. Appropriate interventions can often stabilize or improve some condition, making the patient an acceptable surgical candidate. A referral to social service or a family conference can enhance communication and help the patient and family come to a decision regarding surgery. Every consideration should be given to correcting the underlying problem before relegating the elderly hip fracture patient to a nonoperative status.

A patient may be considered a poor surgical candidate in the absence of an unstable, critical medical condition. The failure rate of an operation can become unacceptably high in the presence of unusual anatomical variations or pre-existing musculoskeletal disease. Morbidly obese patients have been shown to be at high risk when they are managed with general surgical and gynecological operations (34–37). General consensus is that excessive weight increases the risk of complications associated with hip fracture surgery (38). Additional challenges such as pressure ulcers near the proposed incision site, severe osteoporosis, or infections of the affected limb can combine to make nonoperative management the safest course of treatment.

2. Low Patient Benefit

Nonoperative treatment is certainly indicated in any patient who cannot benefit from the proposed operation. The goal of most hip fracture operations is to relieve pain and restore mobility. Individuals with hip fractures who do not experience pain include patients with spinal cord injury or peripheral nerve disease. In cases in which pain relief is not among the goals of surgery, the clinician must carefully contemplate the goals of the operation. The patient with an insensate lower extremity rarely uses the extremity to ambulate. These patients can be mobilized from the bed to the chair safely and comfortably without an operation. When mobility cannot be improved by an operation and pain is not a significant factor, nonoperative management of the hip fracture is the treatment of choice.

Frequently the patient who sustains a hip fracture was previously nonambulatory or the fractured lower extremity had poor motor function but intact sensation to pain. Hip fractures occur in patients with pre-existing hemiparesis, muscle disease, or severe lower limb deformity. Motion of the fracture fragments results in continued bleeding, excessive soft tissue swelling, and severe pain. These patients can often be successfully managed with pain medication and assisted bed-to-chair transfers. In many cases severe fracture pain will subside within 2 to 4 weeks. Internal fixation or hip replacement can also benefit nonambulatory patients by decreasing fracture pain during routine nursing care and patient transfers. The risks of surgery must be weighed against the potential side effects of acute and possible long-term management with pain medication.

Life expectancy has been used to determine the appropriateness of surgical intervention. It is not uncommon for a terminally ill patient to have a relatively short life expectancy and stable medical problems. When such a patient sustains a hip fracture, the decision to operate takes into consideration the patient's life expectancy. Some authors have recommended a life expectancy of at least 90 days and others have suggested as little as 30 days (39). Although agreement is not universal, nonsurgical treatment is indicated when the pain and disability caused by the operation is expected to persist throughout the patient's remaining lifespan. The physician cannot always accurately predict whether the quality of a relatively short life will be enhanced by an operation. However, it is the responsibility of the treating physician to advise the patient and recommend the best treatment on the basis of the available information. Every effort must be made to avoid treatment that will leave the terminally ill patient to spend the remaining lifetime hospitalized and recovering from hip surgery or its complications.

3. Nonoperative Treatment Protocol

Successful nonsurgical treatment is labor intensive, and the management must be individualized to fulfill the needs of each patient. The number of unnecessary days that the elderly patient remains on bed rest must be kept to a minimum. Control of pain is predictably at the top of the patient's list of priorities. The physician will generally place mobilizing the patient at the top of the priority list, with the intention of minimizing morbidity and mortality. In the case of the impacted or nondisplaced fracture, an additional goal is to maintain satisfactory fracture alignment until the fracture unites. This will allow the patient to return to independent ambulation in a short time, such as within 6 weeks. The objectives of nonoperative treatment mirror those of surgical treatment. Unfortunately, in the absence of rigid internal fixation, control of the fracture fragments becomes unpredictable. Displacement, nonunion, and chronic pain are too often the result of nonoperative treatment.

When the decision is made to proceed with nonsurgical treatment and the routine course of pain medications is not effective, consultation with a pain management specialist should be considered. Narcotic analgesics are initially given intravenously or intramuscularly. Spinal or epidural anesthetics are effective for short-term pain control. The physician must seek a balance between effective pain relief and the side effects of pain medication. Pain relief will not help the patient to accomplish bed-to-chair transfers if central nervous system depression incapacitates the patient. Early success with nonoperative treatment becomes a long-term treatment failure if the fracture heals but the patient has a lifelong addiction to narcotics.

Once pain is successfully controlled, the focus can shift to achieving independent mobility. A patient who accomplishes independent bed-to-chair transfers achieves both an upright chest position and increased independence. Depending on the fracture pattern, the patient's preinjury condition, and the clinical course, it is possible for some patients to advance from a walker, to crutches, to a cane, and eventually to unassisted ambulation with nonoperative treatment.

Patients who are confined to bed should be placed on a regimen to protect them against deep venous thrombosis. Compressive stockings and dynamic compression devices have a demonstrated degree of effectiveness along with a low incidence of complications (40). The wide assortments of anticoagulant regimens each have been reported to demonstrate effectiveness and each has an associated incidence of complications (41–43). Selection of the ideal anticoagulant regimen for a patient should take into consideration the standard of care in the community, the experience of the physician monitoring and managing the anticoagulant, and the patient's risk factors. Consultation with a internal medicine specialist or a geriatrician can be extremely helpful regarding anticoagulant selection and monitoring of the elderly patient. Physical and occupational therapy personnel should be consulted for transfer training, gait training, and use of assistive devices. Social services and the discharge planners help to determine whether the patient has the indications and resources to receive help at home or if admission to a rehabilitation facility is appropriate. Nonsurgical treatment requires a coordinated team approach.

C. Surgical Management

1. Operative Approach

Once the preoperative evaluation has determined that the patient is an acceptable surgical risk, attention turns to selection of the ideal surgical procedure. Modern surgical technology provides the orthopedic surgeon with a myriad of reliable methods to repair or replace the fractured hip. Internal fixation techniques retain and stabilize the fractured hip fragments. Internal fixation systems are designed with instruments and implants to achieve maximum fixation in each of the well-recognized fracture patterns. Hemiarthroplasty discards and replaces the fractured head and neck, whereas total hip replacement reconstructs the head and the acetabulum.

The minimally invasive screw fixation methods require an incision measuring less than 2 cm long and can be completed with blood loss of less than 50 mL. Fluoroscopically assisted, percutaneous screw fixation is usually reserved for patients with incomplete or complete nondisplaced fractures (Garden I and II). The technique applies the least amount of internal fixation to poor-quality bone in a location that experiences tremendous biomechanical forces. This method is indicated when stability is provided primarily by bone fragments that are compressed, impacted, and locked together. For basilar neck fractures and intertrochoteric fractures sliding compression screws, fixed angle plates, and cephalomedullary nails are larger implants that offer greater bone purchase. Each of these requires a larger incision, more extensive dissection, and a surgical technique that is more demanding than percutaneous screw fixation. With every form of internal fixation, the bone and implant construct does not provide maximum strength until more than 6 weeks after implantation and fracture union occurs. The high union rate and a low incidence of avascular necrosis makes internal fixation the preferred treatment for most intertrochanteric fractures. Internal fixation devices for intertrochanteric fractures are designed to allow early weight bearing and prevent loss of fixation and malunion (44–49). Arthroplasty is reserved for use as a salvage procedure in the treatment of intertrochanteric femur fractures (50,51).

With femoral neck displacement (Garden III and IV), hemiarthroplasty provides the most predictable outcome because it eliminates the risk of nonunion, malunion, and failure of fixation within the femoral head and neck (52,53). Hemiarthroplasty allows immediate full weight bearing, and the risk of dislocation is lower than the risk after total hip replacement. To understand the limitations of hemiarthroplasty, it is essential to realize that the metal head of the femoral component articulates directly with living hyaline cartilage of the acetabulum. Once the acetabular cartilage erodes, it does not regenerate, and contact between the hemiarthroplasty and acetabular bone causes pain. Hemiarthroplasty is an excellent option in the sedentary or low-demand patient with a displaced femoral neck fracture (Figure 4). It will provide predictable pain relief and allows immediate full weight bearing; the procedure is less extensive than total hip replacement, and the risk of dislocation is low.

Primary total hip arthroplasty offers active patients and patients with preexisting hip arthritis a single operation that provides lasting pain relief while eliminating the need for revision surgery caused by acetabular cartilage erosion. Total hip arthroplasty allows otherwise healthy patients to resume an active lifestyle. Total hip arthroplasty is considered by many surgeons to be a more technically demanding operation because the acetabulum must be exposed and resurfaced. Greenough and Jones reported a 19% revision rate at 1.7 years in a series of 37 elderly patients with displaced subcapital fractures treated with total hip arthroplasty (54). Other authors have demonstrated excellent results treating acute femoral neck fractures with total hip arthroplasty (55). Surgeons with special training and experience with joint replacement surgery often prefer total hip arthroplasty and consider the incidence of acetabular erosion with hemiarthroplasty unacceptable. The general orthopedist may favor the predictably sat-

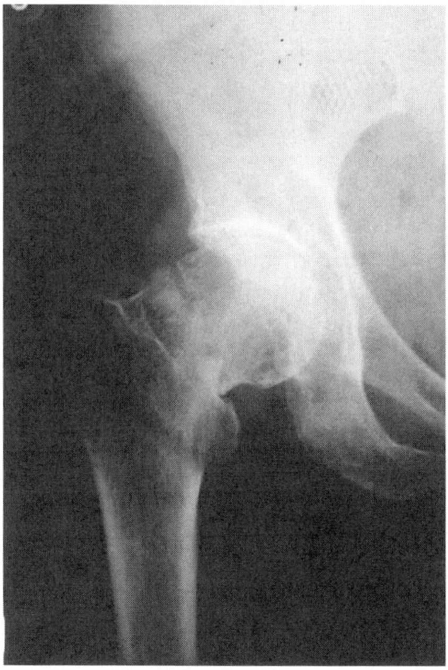

(A)

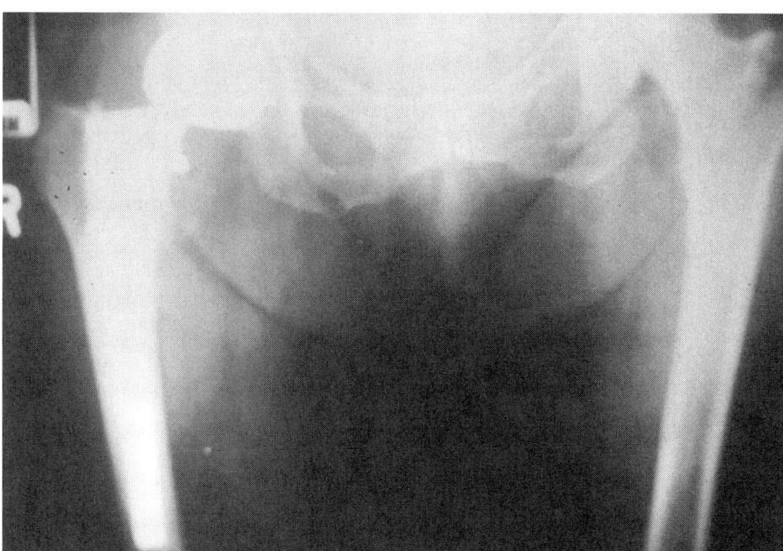

(B)

Figure 4 (A) Radiographs demonstrate osteopenia and a displaced subcapital femoral neck fracture. (B) Postoperative radiographs show a cemented right hemiarthroplasty.

isfactory results of hemiarthroplasty and reserve total hip replacement for patients who later become symptomatic. The preferred treatment of the displaced femoral neck fractures in the active patient will vary, depending on the training and experience of the surgeon.

2. Complications

The mortality after a hip fracture in persons 65 years and older is increased compared with the mortality of individuals, matched for age, who do not have a fracture. White and associates calculated the standard mortality ratio to be six times higher in hip fracture patients than in the general population (56). Surgical management has become the standard of care because prompt surgical treatment has been shown to be associated with the best chance of survival (57–60). Despite the improvements associated with surgical intervention, the reported mortality in high-risk groups remains high. An isolated fracture of the hip does not directly result in the death of a patient. Therefore, researchers have concentrated on the additional factors that contribute to mortality. Tierney and Goulet reported a mortality rate of 63% among patients with chronic renal disease, and Foster and coworkers reported a mortality rate of 70% in severely malnourished patients (61,62). In a prospective study of more than 400 patients, Wood and coworkers found the most significant predictors of 6-month mortality to be dementia, postoperative pneumonia, malignancy, advanced age, and deep wound infection (63). In that study, patients older than 85 years with dementia experienced 75% mortality. Davidson and Bodney noted a death rate of 80% among elderly patients with diabetes mellitus (64). These data suggest that high-risk individuals may be approaching the end of life at the time the hip fracture occurs, and the bone failure serves as a warning of impending failure of multiple organ systems.

Deep infection presents an immediate threat to the life and limb of the hip fracture patient. The incidence of postoperative wound infection after the internal fixation of hip fractures has been reported to range from 1% to 16% (65–66). The unstable infected fracture provides an environment that is unsuitable for fracture healing. Surgical debridement, local wound care, (gauze packing, antibiotic beads, or suction drains) and a 6-week course of parenteral antibiotics create conditions that are unfavorable to the offending bacteria. Internal fixation is retained if the implant provides adequate fracture stability. Internal fixation is removed if there has been loss of fixation, sepsis cannot be controlled, or the fracture has united. Prosthetic hip infections diagnosed within 2 to 4 weeks of surgery have been treated successfully with this same approach. However, late infections and virulent organisms will require removal of the prosthesis and all bone cement. The resulting resection arthroplasty leaves the patient without a functioning hip joint until reimplantation can be attempted at 6 weeks to 1 year, when clinical and diagnostic examinations show no evidence of infection (67,68).

Nonunion can occur in conjunction with infection or osteonecrosis. However, it is usually a separate event. Hip aspiration should be part of the diagnostic evaluation to exclude infection. Excessive motion at the fracture site can result from inadequate reduction, poor screw purchase in the femoral head, or excessive weight bearing. Metabolic changes may also contribute to the high incidence of nonunion in older patients with femoral neck fractures. Continued weight bearing on an ununited fracture will result in implant breakage, loss of fixation, and screw penetration through the femoral head.

The rate of avascular necrosis of the femoral head is related to the degree of displacement, the delay before fracture reduction, and the location of the fracture. The osteonecrotic femoral head will support viable articular cartilage because the articular cartilage is nourished by synovial fluid. The patient may remain asymptomatic until osteonecrosis is associated with femoral head collapse. Disabling symptoms are treated with total hip arthroplasty in the community ambulator and hemiarthroplasty in patients who are sedentary.

IV. FRACTURE PREVENTION IN OSTEOPOROSIS

Fracture prevention should start with education. Peak bone mass is achieved by the age of 35 years and appropriate diet, calcium intake, and exercise should be incorporated in childhood and early adult life. Patients at high risk for osteoporosis (i.e., family history, smokers, excessive alcohol intake, white, thin, fair-skinned females, women having early menopause or removal of ovaries) should be identified and educated before the onset of bone loss by their primary care providers or through other informative means. The judicious use of early estrogen replacement in patients at high risk for osteoporosis should be considered, providing no significant family history of uterine or breast cancer or history of these malignancies exists in the patient.

Early detection with bone densitometry (i.e., dual-energy x-ray absorptiometry) is also important so that medical management can be initiated to reduce the rapid bone resorption seen in type I or early-onset osteoporosis. Not only should estrogen replacement be considered in some patients but calcium replacement (1500 mg/day), vitamin D (400 IU/day), and third-generation bisphosphonates (i.e., Fosamax 10 mg/day) should also be considered. Calcitonin given subcutaneously or intranasally can also improve bone quality and has been effective in pain control, particularly in patients with compression fractures of the spine. These medications should be given in conjunction with an appropriate exercise program directed at weight-bearing activities. Senile or type II osteoporosis, which affects both men and women undergoing a slower bone resorption phase, can be treated with an exercise programs and medical management as needed.

REFERENCES

1. Tosi LL, Lane JM. Osteoporosis prevention and the orthopaedic surgeon. J Bone Joint Surg Am 1998; 80A:1567–1569.
2. Jette AM, Harris BA, Cleary PD, Campion EW. Functional recovery after hip fracture. Arch Phys Med Rehabil 1987; 68:735–740.
3. Kenzora JE, McCarthy RE, Lowell JD, Sledge CB. Hip fracture mortality, relation to age, treatment, preoperative illness, time to surgery, and complications. Clin Orthop Rel Res 1984; 186:45–56.
4. Koval KJ, Zuckerman JD. Hip fractures: I. Overview and evaluation and treatment of femoral neck fractures. Am Acad Orthop Surg 1994; 2:141–149.
5. Preamer A, Furner S, Rice DP. Musculoskeletal conditions in the United States. Park Ridge, IL: American Academy of Orthopaedic Surgeons, 1992.
6. Koval KJ, Aharonoff GB, Su ET, Zuckerman JD. Effect of acute inpatient rehabilitation on outcome after fracture of the femoral neck or intertrocanteric fracture. J Bone Joint Surg Am 1998; 80:357–364.
7. Zuckerman JD, Skovron ML, Koval KJ, Aharonoff G, Frankel VH. Postoperative complications and mortality associated with operative delay in older patients who have a fracture of the hip. J Bone Joint Surg Am 1995; 77:1551–1556.
8. Farmer ME, White LR, Brody JA, Bailey KR. Race and sex differences in hip fracture incidence. Am J Public Health 1984; 74:1374–1380.
9. Beck TJ, Ruff CB, Scott WW Jr, Plato CC, Tobin JD, Quan CA. Sex differences in geometry of the femoral neck with aging. Calcif Tissue Int 1992; 50:24–29.
10. Ruff CB, Hayes WC. Bone-mineral content in the lower limb. Relationship to cross-sectional geometry. J Bone Joint Surg Am 1984; 66A:1024–1031.
11. Melton LJ, Chrischilles EA, Cooper C, Lane AW, Riggs BL. Perspective. How many women have osteoporosis? Bone Miner Res 1992; 7:1005–1010.
12. Melton LJ. Epidemiology of osteoporosis. Baillieres Clin Obstet Gynaecol 1991; 5: 785–805.
13. Cummings SR. Epidemiologic studies of osteoporotic fractures. Methodologic issues. Calcif Tissue Int 1991; 49(suppl):S15–S20.
14. Fielding JW. Displaced femoral neck fractures. Orthop Rev 1973; 2:11–17.
15. Cleveland M, Bosworth DM, Thompson FR. Intertrocanteric fractures of the femur. J Bone Joint Surg 1947; 29:1049–1067.
16. Hayes WC. Biomechanics of cortical and trabecular bone. Implications for assessment of fracture risk. In: Moe VC, Hayes WC, eds. Basic orthopaedic biomechanics. New York: Raven Press, 1991. pp 93–142.
17. Alho A, Stomsoe K, Hoiseth A. Bone mineral related to mechanical strength of cancellous bone [abstract]. Trans Eur Orthop Res Soc 1992; 2:16.
18. Alho A, Husby T, Hoiseth A, Fonstelien E. Bone mineral content and mechanical strength of human femur. Finn J Orthop Traum 1985; 8:56–57.
19. Lane JM, Boskey AL, Li WKP. A temporal study of collagen, proteoglycan, lipid and mineral constitutents in a model of endochondral osseous repair. Metab Bone Dis 1979; 1:319–324.

20. Dalen N, Hellstrom LG, Jacobson B. Bone mineral content and mechanical strength of the femoral neck. Acta Orthop Scand 1976; 47(5):503–508.
21. Snyder SM, Schneider E. Estimation of mechanical properties of cortical bone by computed tomography. J Orthop Res 1991; 9(3):422–431.
22. Borrie MJ, Campbell AG, Caradoc-Davies TH. Osteomalacia in the elderly: investigation and diagnosis. N Z Med J 1985; 98:989–991.
23. Wilton TJ, Hosking DJ, Pawley E, Stevens A, Harvey L. Osteomalacia and femoral neck fractures in the elderly patient. J Bone Joint Surg Br 1987; 69:388–390.
24. Hinton RY, Smith GS. The association of age, race, and sex with the location of proximal femur fractures in the elderly. J Bone Joint Surg Am 1993; 75:752–759.
25. Aitken JM. Relavence of osteoporosis in women with fracture of the femoral neck. BMJ 1984; 288:597–601.
26. Long WT, Brien EW, Boucree JB Jr, Filler B, Stark HH, Dorr LD. Management of civilian gunshot injuries to the hip. Orthop Clin North Am 1995; 26:123–132.
27. Garden RS. Low angle fixation in fractures of the femoral neck. J Bone Joint Surg Br 1961; 43:647–663.
28. Evans EM. The treatment of trocanteric fractures of the femur. J Bone Joint Surg Br 1949; 31:190–203.
29. Jensen JS, Sonne-Holm S, Tondeuold E. Unstable trocanteric fractures: A comparative analysis of four methods of internal fixation. Acta Orthop Scand 1980; 51:949–962.
30. Quinn SF, McCarthy JL. Prospective evaluation of patients with suspected hip fracture and indeterminant radiographs: Use of T1 weighted MR images. Radiology 1993; 187:469–471.
31. Holder LE, Schwartz C, Werniche PG, Michael RH. Radionuclide bone imaging in the early detection of fractures of the proximal femur (hip): Multifactorial analysis. Radiology 1990; 174:509–515.
32. Macpherson DS. Preoperative laboratory testing: Should any test be ''routine'' before surgery? Med Clin North Am 1993; 77:289–308.
33. Karp AH, Koval KJ. Preoperative medical evaluation of the elderly patient. Arch Am Acad Orthop Surg 1998; 2:81–87.
34. Pemberton LB, Manax WG. Relationship of obesity to postoperative complications after cholecystectomy. Am J Surg 1971; 121:87–90.
35. Pitkin RM. Abdominal hysterectomy in obese women. Surg Gynecol Obstet 1976; 142:532–536.
36. Postlethwait RW, Johnson WD. Complications following surgery for duodenal ulcer in obese patients. Arch Surg 1972; 105:438–440.
37. Pasulka PS, Bistrian BR, Benotte PN, Blackburn GL. The risks of surgery in obese patients. Ann Intern Med 1986; 104:540–546.
38. Lehman DE, Capello WN, Feinberg JR. Total hip arthroplasty without cement in obese patients. A minimum two year clinical and radiographic follow-up study. J Bone Joint Surg Am 1994; 76:854–862.
39. Behr T, Dobozi WR, Badrinath K. The treatment of pathologic and impending pathologic fractures of the proximal femur in the elderly. Clin Orthop 1985; 198:173–178.

40. Paiement G, Wessinger SJ, Waltman AC, Harris WH. Low-dose warfarin versus external pneumatic compression for prophylaxis against venous thromboembolism following total hip replacement. J Arthroplasty 1987; 2:23–26.
41. Hull R, Raskob G, Pineo G, Rosenbloom D, Evans W, Mallory T, Anquist K, Smith F, Hughes G, Green D, Elliot CG, Panju A, Brant R. A comparison of subcutaneous low-molecular-weight heparin with warfarin sodium for prophylaxis against deep-vein thrombosis after hip or knee implantation. N Engl J Med 1993; 329:1370–1376.
42. Lieberman JR, Wollaeger J, Frederick D, Thomas BJ, Kilgus D, Grecula MJ, Finerman GA, Amstutz HC. The efficacy of prophylaxis with low-dose warfarin for prevention of pulmonary embolism following total hip arthroplasty. J Bone Joint Surg Am 1997; 79A:319–325.
43. Francis CW, Pellegrini VD, Totterman S, Boyd AD, Marder VJ, Liebert KM, Stulberg BN, Ayres DC, Rosenberg A, Kessler C, Johanson NA. Prevention of deep venous thrombosis after total hip arthroplasty. Comparison of warfarin and Dalteparin. J Bone Joint Surg Am 1997; 79:1365–1372.
44. Morris HD. Trocanteric fractures. South Med J 1941; 34:571–578.
45. Ganz R, Thomas RJ, Hammerle CP. Trocanteric fractures of the femur: treatment and results. Clin Orthop Rel Res 1979; 138:30–40.
46. Den Hartog BD, Bartal E, Cooke F. Treatment of the unstable intertrocanteric fracture: Effect of the placement of the screw, its angle of insertion, and osteotomy. J Bone Joint Surg Am 1991; 73:726–733.
47. Bridle SH, Patel AD, Bircher M, Calvert PT. Fixation of intertrocanteric fractures of the femur: A randomized prospective comparison of the gamma nail and the dynamic hip screw. J Bone Joint Surg Br 1991; 73:330–334.
48. Goldhagen PR, O'Connor DR, Schwarze E. A prospective comparative study of the compression hip screw and the gamma nail. J Orthop Trauma 1994; 5:367–372.
49. Hardy DCR, Descamps P, Krallis P, Laurent F, Smets P, Bertens CL, Philippe DE. Use of an intramedullary hip-screw compared with a compression hip-screw with a plate for intertrocanteric femoral fractures. J Bone Joint Surg Am 1998; 80:618–630.
50. Stern MB, Angerman A. Comminuted intertrocanteric fractures treated with a Leinbach Prosthesis. Clin Orthop 1987; 218:75–80.
51. Mehlhoff T, Landon GC, Tullos HS. Total hip arthroplasty following failed internal fixation of hip fractures. Clin Orthop 1991; 269:32–37.
52. Barnes R, Brown JT, Garden RS, Nicholl EA. Subcapital fractures of the femur. J Bone Joint Surg Br 1976; 58:2–24.
53. Bray TJ, Smith-Hoefer E, Hooper A, Timmerman L. The displaced femoral neck fracture: Internal fixation versus bipolar endoprosthesis: Results of a prospective, randomized comparison. Clin Orthop 1988; 230:127–140.
54. Greenough CG, Jones JR. Primary total hip replacement for displaced subcapital fracture of the femur. J Bone Joint Surg Br 1988; 70:639–643.
55. Delamarter R, Moreland JR. Treatment of acute femoral neck fractures with total hip arthroplasty. Clin Orthop 1987; 218:68–74.
56. White BL, Fisher WD, Laurin AC. Rate of mortality for elderly patients after fracture of the hip in the 1980's. J Bone Joint Surg Am 1987; 69:1335–1340.

57. Elmerson S, Zetterberg C, Andersson G. Ten-year survival after fractures of the proximal end of the femur. Gerontology 1988; 34:186–191.
58. Ions GK, Stevens J. Prediction of survival in patients with femoral neck fractures. J Bone Joint Surg Br 1987; 69:384–387.
59. Sexson S, Lehner J. Factors affecting hip fracture mortality. J Orthop Trauma 1988; 1:298–305.
60. Lee BPH, Berry DJ, Harmsen WS, Sim FH. Total hip arthroplasty for the treatment of an acute fracture of the femoral neck. J Bone Joint Surg Am 1998; 80:70–75.
61. Tierney GS, Goulet JA. Mortality after hip fracture in patients with chronic renal failure. Orthop Trans 1992; 16:332–339.
62. Foster MR, Heppenstall RB, Friedenberg ZB, Hozak WJ. A prospective assessment of nutritional status and complications in patients with fractures of the hip. J Orthop Trauma 1990; 4:49–57.
63. Wood DJ, Ions GK, Quimby JM, Gale DW, Stevens J. Factors that influence mortality after subcapital hip fracture. J Bone Joint Surg Br 1992; 74:199–202.
64. Davidson TI, Bodney WN. Factors influencing survival following fractures of the upper end of the femur. Injury 1986; 17:12–14.
65. Masterson EL, Masri BA, Duncan CP. Treatment of infection at the site of total hip replacement. J Bone Joint Surg Am 1997; 79:1740–1749.
66. Hanssen AD, Rand JA. Evaluation and treatment of infection at the site of a total hip or knee arthroplasty. J Bone Joint Surg Am 1998; 80:910–922.
67. Fitzgerald RH Jr, Nolan DR, Ilstrup DM, Scoy RE, Washington JA, Coventry MB. Deep wound infections following total hip arthroplasty. J Bone Joint Surg Am 1977; 59:847–855.
68. Fitzgerald RH, Jones DR. Hip implant infection: Treatment with resection arthroplasty and late total hip arthroplasty. Am J Med 1985; 78(6B):225–228.

9
Acute Conditions of the Abdomen

David Vo and Samuel Eric Wilson
UCI Medical Center, Orange, California

I. UNIQUE ASPECTS IN THE ELDERLY

The "acute abdomen" can be defined as abdominal pain that necessitates prompt assessment, diagnosis, and early treatment, often operative. This emergency is increasingly common in patients aged 65 and older. First, the elderly represent one of the fastest growing segments of the population in North America. Second, not only are people living longer because of advances in medicine, nutrition, and sanitation, but they are also enjoying relatively good health and remaining active. Not unexpectedly, the primary care physician will be confronted with an increasing number of elderly patients complaining of abdominal pain. Diagnosis of acute conditions of the abdomen in the geriatric patient is a major challenge because of its protean manifestations and diverse causes. This chapter will review the diagnosis and treatment of conditions specific to acute conditions of the abdomen in the older patient.

Delay in diagnosis may contribute to the significantly higher morbidity and mortality rates found in elderly patients with acute abdominal emergencies. From an analysis of three large series of patients, Telfer et al. confirmed that a higher mortality in older patients was associated with a lower diagnostic accuracy compared with that of younger patients (1). They also noted that the causes of acute abdominal diseases differed in older patients compared with younger age groups. Recognition of the different causes would likely expedite diagnosis of abdominal emergencies in elderly patients (Table 1). Patients older than 50 years of age with a chief complaint of abdominal pain most commonly had acute cholecystitis, whereas younger patients were more likely to have nonspecific abdominal pain or appendicitis. In addition, bowel obstruction and pancreatitis were about four times more common in older patients. Cancer, especially adenocarcinoma of the

Table 1 Rates of Disease in 2406 Patients >50 Years Old and 6317 Patients <50 Years Old Initially Seen with Acute Abdominal Pain from the OMGE[a] Series[b]

Disease	% younger than 50 (6317 total)	% older than 50 (2406 total)
Nonspecific abdominal pain	39.5	15.7
Appendicitis	32.0	15.2
Cholecystitis	6.3	20.9
Obstruction	2.5	12.3
Pancreatitis	1.6	7.3
Diverticular disease	<0.1	5.5
Cancer	<0.1	4.1
Hernia	<0.1	3.1
Vascular	<0.1	2.3

[a] World Organization of Gastroenterology (OMGE) Research Committee Multi-National Survey.
[b] From Ref. 1.

colon and rectum, mesenteric ischemia, and diverticular complications were more typical in the geriatric patient. Vascular causes initially seen as an upper abdominal pain syndrome included mesenteric arterial ischemia, embolus, myocardial infarction, and symptomatic abdominal aortic aneurysm.

Additional factors complicate the diagnosis of acute conditions of the abdomen in the elderly patient. The history may be inadequate because of mental confusion or underlying dementia, and co-existing illnesses can be distracting variables. Signs of peritonitis may be attenuated, with guarding being less pronounced because of a thinned abdominal musculature. Temperature elevation can be dampened to the point of hypothermia, and the white blood cell count tends to respond less vigorously. The use of nonsteroidal anti-inflammatory drugs (e.g., for arthritis) is more prevalent in the older patient and can mask abdominal pain. Seeking medical care may be delayed, leading to more advanced disease at presentation. Social factors such as living alone or fear of being institutionalized, losing one's independence, attributing symptoms to constipation and indigestion, or financial concerns may cause elderly people to avoid seeking medical attention early.

Elective surgery is generally well tolerated in the fit geriatric patient with minimal increase in morbidity and mortality compared with younger patients. However, in an emergency situation, the risks increase dramatically for older patients, in part because of a decrease in physiological reserves, an impaired immune response to infections, and a high incidence of chronic cardiopulmonary diseases associated with advancing age. Early surgery for most geriatric abdominal emergencies is the goal, but adequate time should be allowed for appropriate studies and preoperative preparation. (See Chapters 5 and 6.) Diagnostic exploratory laparoscopy has recently been suggested as having a potential role in the assessment of abdominal pain, thus abbreviating extensive preoperative studies (2). Important perioperative principles include optimization of associated medical conditions, timely but judicious replacement of fluids and electrolytes, aggressive respiratory care to prevent atelectasis and pneumonia, and early mobilization to avoid deep venous thrombosis and pulmonary embolism. The simplest operation that will do most to correct the immediate problem should be the goal when performing emergency abdominal surgery in the geriatric patient. One-stage definitive procedures should be attempted whenever safe and stomas avoided if feasible.

II. ACUTE CHOLECYSTITIS

A. Clinical Relevance

Acute cholecystitis is one of the most common abdominal illnesses that require surgical intervention in elderly people. The incidence of cholelithiasis increases with age in North Americans, ranging from 25% to 40% for those in their 60s to more than 50% in those 70 years of age and older (3). Biliary tract disease should be considered prominently in the differential diagnosis of acute upper abdominal pain in the geriatric population. In most cases, acute cholecystitis results from obstruction of the cystic duct by an impacted gallstone. Steady and persistent epigastric or right subcostal abdominal pain that may radiate to the back or to the tip of the right scapula is the most common complaint. Nausea, vomiting, fever, and chills may follow. A history of known gallstones, prior attacks of similar pain, or occasionally pancreatitis can be elicited in most cases. Physical findings are most remarkable for right upper quadrant abdominal tenderness with or without fever, jaundice, and a palpable right upper quadrant abdominal mass in about a third of the cases. Laboratory studies will reveal an elevated leukocyte count. Major complications are empyema, gangrene, and perforation of the gallbladder. A pericholecystic abscess should be suspected when the patient appears toxic with high fever and leukocyte count. Free perforation occurs infrequently and manifests as sudden spreading of previous localized pain and tenderness.

B. Immediate Diagnostic Approach

Acute cholecystitis should be strongly suspected if a tender, palpable gallbladder is present together with the preceding history. The first diagnostic study is abdominal ultrasonography, which is highly sensitive in showing gallstones in more than 95% of cases. Findings of gallstones, dilated and thickened gallbladder wall, pericholecystic fluid, and an ultrasonographic Murphy's sign are all suggestive of acute cholecystitis. If the ultrasonogram is equivocal, a technetium 99m-labeled derivative of iminodiacetic acid (e.g., HIDA) scan should be performed. After intravenous injection of the radionuclide, imaging of the bile ducts and gallbladder normally appears within 15 to 30 minutes and of the small intestine within 60 minutes. Failure to visualize the gallbladder while contrast appears in the common bile duct or duodenum indicates cystic duct obstruction.

Elderly patients differ in that they are initially seen with more advanced stages of biliary disease. Secondary complications such as jaundice caused by common bile duct (CBD) stones, cholangitis, empyema, gangrene, free perforation, and subphrenic or liver abscesses are all more common in the older age group (4). Clinical findings may be deceptively benign despite severe underlying pathological conditions, leading to a delay in diagnosis and poorer outcomes. Morrow et al. found that abdominal tenderness, peritoneal signs, temperature elevation, and leukocytosis can be absent in about 26%, 50%, 38%, and 35% of elderly patients with acute cholecystitis, respectively (5). In addition, the incidence of CBD stones increases with age and occurs in about 20% of patients 65 years and older with acute cholecystitis. CBD stones should be suspected in those with severe gallstone pancreatitis, a bilirubin value >3 mg/dL, a dilated CBD or stones seen in the CBD on ultrasonography.

Acute suppurative cholangitis is a serious complication of stones in the CBD. Right upper quadrant abdominal pain, jaundice, fever, and chills, known as Charcot's triad, may be absent in 30% of patients with cholangitis. Leukocyte count and alkaline phosphatase levels are usually elevated. Mental confusion and hypotension in the presence of Charcot's triad indicate sepsis from ascending cholangitis (Reynold's pentad) and may be the initial presenting symptoms in the older patient. Emergency decompression of the CBD and intravenous antibiotics are required. Endoscopic retrograde cholangiopancreatography (ERCP) with sphincterotomy has been reported to be successful in removing CBD stones over 90% of the time (6).

C. Therapeutic Intervention

Elective cholecystectomy should be strongly considered for symptomatic cholelithiasis before the development of complications. Elective biliary surgery in the elderly patient, including laparoscopic cholecystectomy, is safer and associated with reduced postoperative morbidity and mortality compared with emergency surgery. Most deaths from acute cholecystitis occur in patients older than 60 or those with diabetes mellitus. Emergency cholecystectomy in the elderly has a reported mortality rate of about 10%. The major causes of death postoperatively are due to sepsis and resultant multisystem organ failure, heart failure, pneumonia, and pulmonary embolus (7). Morrow et al. showed that medical therapy failed for most elderly patients with acute cholecystitis (5). Resuscitation consisting of hydration, nasogastric decompression, and intravenous antibiotics should be followed by prompt operation. Early cholecystectomy is the definitive treatment for acute cholecystitis in the elderly and is associated with decreased morbidity and mortality compared with medical management followed by elective cholecystectomy at a later date (8). In addition, early surgery will avoid overlooked diagnoses from other causes such as perforated duodenal ulcer or appendicitis and recurrent attacks of cholecystitis during a waiting period. Given the increased incidence of CBD stones in the older patient, the routine use of intraoperative cholangiography is encouraged. If stones are discovered, they may be removed intraoperatively or alternatively by ERCP with sphincterotomy postoperatively.

An initial approach with laparoscopic cholecystectomy is safe and effective in many young and elderly patients with acute cholecystitis. However, older patients have greater risk for conversion to open cholecystectomy than younger patients and the rate can be as high as 50% (9). The operative duration, analgesic requirement, recovery and hospitalization times, and postoperative complications were all increased in those requiring conversions to open surgery in the elderly group. A planned open cholecystectomy or early conversion from a laparoscopic cholecystectomy if severe adhesions are encountered should be considered in critically ill elderly patients (10).

When cholecystectomy is contraindicated because of the patient's critical condition or it is deemed technically dangerous, cholecystostomy should be considered as an alternative. A drainage tube is placed in the dome of the gallbladder through a limited incision performed with the patient under general or local anesthesia or by image-guided percutaneous cathether placement. It is important to ensure there is no co-existing cholangitis. After resolution of the crisis, an elective interval cholecystectomy should be performed if stones are present versus simple removal of the drainage tube if no stones are detected by cholangiogram (11).

III. ACUTE APPENDICITIS

A. Clinical Relevance

The diagnosis of acute appendicitis still rests primarily on clinical assessment. Acute appendicitis should not be disregarded as a possible cause of abdominal pain in patients older than 50 because appendicitis accounts for approximately 15% of all abdominal emergencies in this older age group (1). Advancing age is associated with increasing morbidity and mortality in patients with acute appendicitis. Although the elderly group accounts for only 5% to 10% of all cases of appendicitis, about half of the fatalities from appendicitis occur in this age group (12). The mortality rate of 0.8% to 1.6% in the general population contrasts sharply with that of approximately 10% and greater in those older than 70 (13, 14). These deaths are primarily related to the septic complications arising from perforated appendicitis. Prompt diagnosis followed by surgery, before the development of gangrene, perforation, or abscess formation, is crucial in reducing the increased morbidity and mortality observed in the older patient.

B. Immediate Diagnostic Approach

The clinical presentation of acute appendicitis is often thought to be atypical in the older person, but some recent studies suggest that the clinical features of appendicitis in the elderly are similar to those in the younger population (15, 16). Right lower quadrant abdominal pain and tenderness were the most common findings. Associated nausea, vomiting, fever, chills, anorexia, and leukocytosis with increased immature cells were not infrequent. Vague pain that moves from the periumbilical area to localize in the right lower quadrant, is exacerbated by movement, and occurs with focal right lower quadrant tenderness, guarding, and rebound should all favor acute appendicitis. However, the elderly patient will usually not have all these classical findings in a clear-cut fashion. In one series, only 20% of elderly patients with appendicitis had all the following findings: nausea or vomiting, fever, right lower quadrant tenderness, and an elevated white blood cell count (WBC) or left shift of the WBC (high percentage of neutrophils and band forms) (16). In addition, the symptoms and signs of appendicitis are often similar to other disease processes that are more common in the older age groups, leading to significantly higher errors in diagnosis. Common misdiagnoses in the older patient include diverticulitis, bowel obstruction, carcinoma, acute cholecystitis, or even ruptured abdominal aortic aneurysm. Diagnostic studies may often obscure the diagnosis, such as elevated bilirubin levels suggesting hepatobiliary disease, and roentgenograms showing ileus, bowel obstruction, or incidental nephrolithiasis or cholelithiasis.

The elderly patient is more likely to have complications. Franz et al. found that 91% of their patients older than 50 had either perforated appendicitis or an associated intra-abdominal abscess compared with only 25% in patients less than 50 years old (17). Those older than 70 carried the greatest risk of having perforated appendicitis associated with an intra-abdominal abscess. This is compatible with other studies, showing that the risk of gangrene and perforation are about two to four times more likely in patients older than 50 (4, 18, 19). The symptoms and signs in older patients may alert the clinician to the severity of the underlying pathological condition (Table 2). Franz et al. also found that prolonged duration of symptoms before presentation to the hospital correlated strongly with the incidence of complications and final outcome (17). Those with simple appendicitis

Table 2 Differences in Presentation of Acute Appendicitis in 366 Patients >50 Years Old and 1970 Patients <50 Years Old from the OMGE[a] Series[b]

Clinical feature	% of patients <50 yr old	% of patients >50 yr old
Generalized pain	2.2	13.1
Pain duration >24 hr	57.2	75.4
Previous surgery	3.2	21.0
Distention	6.2	23.8
Generalized tenderness	2.1	14.2
Rigidity	18.9	40.1
Decreased bowel sounds	19.0	38.0
Mass	4.0	12.1

[a] World Organization of Gastroenterology.
[b] From Ref. 1.

complained of symptoms lasting less than 24 hours, whereas those who had progressed to rupture or abscess experienced symptoms for more than 48 hours. In addition, Thorbjarnarson and Loehr postulated that anatomical changes in the appendix associated with aging could lead to earlier perforation (18). These changes include narrowing of the appendiceal lumen, thinning of its mucosa, and a decrease in the number of lymphocytes, all of which result in a structurally weakened appendix with decrease vascularity.

C. Therapeutic Intervention

Given all these factors, early diagnosis within 24 hours of symptom onset and prompt appendectomy before development of gangrene and perforation are crucial in reducing the morbidity and mortality of acute appendicitis in the older patient. A computer tomographic scan of the abdomen may be obtained to look for focal fat stranding, small bowel thickening, or abscess in the right lower quadrant. Diagnostic laparoscopy may be considered in very ill elderly patients with an unclear diagnosis to exclude acute appendicitis and other life-threatening conditions (20). This could avoid untimely delays from extensive diagnostic studies. If appendicitis is found, a laparoscopic appendectomy may be performed at the same time. (The cecum should be examined intraoperatively and the pathology reviewed to ensure that a primary appendiceal malignancy was not the cause of acute appendicitis.) The role of the surgeon in the management of the acute abdomen resulting from appendicitis in the elderly patient is to expedite diagnosis and proceed with appendectomy, while acknowledging a negative laparotomy rate in exchange for decreasing the rate of perforation and gangrene.

IV. INTESTINAL OBSTRUCTION

A. Clinical Relevance

Adhesions, malignant disease, and incarcerated hernias account for most intestinal obstruction in industrialized nations. The peak incidence for each occurs in the eighth decade of life. Obstruction caused by postoperative adhesions has become the most common cause, but strangulated hernias and intra-abdominal malignancies, particularly colorectal cancer, still account for 50% of all cases and deaths. Colon cancer may present with large bowel obstruction manifesting as early abdominal distention and constipation, followed by pain and vomiting at later stages. However, small bowel obstruction (SBO) can be more prominent if the ileocecal valve is incontinent.

B. Immediate Diagnostic Approach

Diagnosis of SBO is made on the basis of colicky abdominal pain, nausea, vomiting, diffuse abdominal tenderness, and distention. Although some controversy is acknowledged regarding the optimal timing of operation for small bowel obstruction, it is agreed that urgent surgery is required if peritoneal signs are present, indicating strangulation. The accepted criteria for strangulation may not be accurate in elderly patients (21). Approximately one-third of elderly patients with strangulation obstruction will display minimal symptoms or signs of ischemic bowel preoperatively. Leukocytosis and tachycardia are noted most consistently, whereas presence of an abdominal mass, change in the nature of pain from intermittent to constant, localized tenderness, fever, shock, and bloody diarrhea occurred less reliably. The use of computed tomography (CT) scans of the abdomen may increase the detection of strangulation obstruction. CT findings of poor enhancement of bowel wall, a serrated beak, ascites, and engorgement of mesenteric veins are suggestive of strangulated obstructions (22).

C. Therapeutic Intervention

It is recommended that elderly patients with complete SBO be operated on within 24 hours because delay carries a high risk of increased morbidity and mortality (23). Mortality rates escalate from 3% for simple obstructions to 30% when the bowel becomes necrotic or perforated (24). The presence of a malignancy is a significant risk factor for mortality in the elderly patient. The currently accepted indications for selective conservative management of SBO include carcinomatosis, Crohn's disease, early postoperative obstruction, and partial SBO. In the absence of these specific conditions, surgery should be performed expeditiously in elderly patients to avoid the sequelae of unrecognized strangulated obstruction. In addition, other studies have shown that a significant increase in the complication rate and mean length of hospital stay exists for those who received delayed operation versus early operation within 48 hours. Wound infection is the most common postoperative complication and has been shown to be related to the number of enterotomies made (21). Delayed wound closure should be considered in patients operated on for SBO after having an enterotomy because of the significant increased risk of wound infection despite appropriate prophylactic antibiotics.

D. Specific Causes of Intestinal Obstruction

1. Postoperative Adhesions

Postoperative adhesions are the leading cause of small intestinal obstruction, accounting for more than 40% of all cases and 60% to 70% of those involving the small bowel (25). Intestinal obstruction caused by adhesion is likely to increase as the numbers of major elective abdominal operations in the geriatric population increases. Laparoscopy does not seem to eliminate the risk of adhesions and obstruction. A high risk of recurrence is present after operative relief for obstructions caused by adhesions. Some patients who have had repeated operations for SBO may develop a ''frozen abdomen,'' in which adhesions are so dense that the bowel becomes fixed and is unable to achieve the degree of torsion necessary for strangulation. In these patients, a trial of nasogastric or small bowel decompression is warranted.

2. Strangulated Hernias

Elderly patients account for most of those presenting with obstruction caused by strangulated hernias, with the peak age occurring in the seventh and eighth decades. Abdominal wall hernias usually present little diagnostic challenge, but hernias are often neglected by the patient who views it as a nuisance and by the primary care physician who may erroneously consider the patient too frail to undergo an operation. The surgeon may also overlook the diagnosis of incarcerated hernia in an elderly patient by failing to examine the inguinal orifices. Elective hernia repair is well tolerated in the geriatric group, whereas emergency repair for incarceration is associated with excessive morbidity and mortality that can climb as high as 55% and 15%, respectively (26). Factors associated with increase risk of groin hernia incarceration include advanced age, femoral more than inguinal location, and recent appearance of the mass.

The obturator hernia is a rare and usually overlooked cause of intestinal obstruction in the older patient. There is a 7:1 ratio of women versus men affected. The classical patient is an elderly emaciated woman with chronic medical illnesses presenting with recurrent abdominal pain or partial intestinal obstruction and no history of previous abdominal operations. Most are residents of nursing homes or chronic care hospitals. A palpable groin mass is absent in most cases. Any patient with the aforementioned profile who is suspected of having a bowel obstruction should undergo a prompt CT scan to diagnose internal herniation. However, diagnosis continues to be delayed in these debilitated patients and often is made only at laparotomy, where bowel resection is required in about 75% of cases (27). This reflects the high morbidity and mortality rates of 65% and 25%, respectively.

3. Volvulus

Several other causes of intestinal obstruction are unique to the geriatric patient, including sigmoid and colonic volvulus. Sigmoid volvulus often occurs in elderly persons residing in institutions who have multiple co-existing diseases. Patients usually have abdominal pain, distention, and constipation, and it is correctly diagnosed only in about 60% of patients. A history of recurrent minor attacks may be present. Features suggestive of subclinical volvulus are recurrent abdominal pains, distention, and constipation relieved by a dramatic passage of flatus. Plain abdominal reoentgenograms characteristically display a dilated sigmoid loop with a ‘‘bird’s beak’’ narrowing. Conservative treatment with endoscopic decompression and rectal tube placement is indicated in the absence of peritoneal signs. Endoscopic treatment has a high success rate but is associated with frequent recurrences. Endoscopic decompression should be followed by elective sigmoid resection during the same hospital stay in otherwise healthy patients because the risk of recurrence is high with nonoperative treatment, and emergency surgery has a 30% mortality rate versus 5.6% for elective resection (28). Resection of redundant colon and creation of an end colostomy should be considered in patients with sigmoid volvulus who are bedridden or incontinent of stool and would not benefit from maintenance of bowel continuity.

4. Colonic Pseudo-Obstruction

Colonic pseudo-obstruction, also known as Ogilvie’s syndrome, occurs generally in elderly, bedridden patients with chronic disease who are receiving polypharmacy. Gangrene, infarction, and perforation may ensue as colon diameter increases and particularly if cecal distention reaches greater than 12 cm. Mortality approaches nearly 50% when perforation and gangrene occur. Colonoscopic decompression is the treatment of choice. If this fails, surgical decompression may take the form of cecostomy or may require exteriorization or resection of the colon if infarction has occurred (29).

5. Gallstone Ileus

Gallstone ileus is characterized by mechanical SBO caused by the passage of a large biliary calculus from the gallbladder to the duodenum through a fistula.

The insidious clinical presentation and the lack of specific signs of biliary disease are responsible for the delayed preoperative diagnosis that leads to an overall mortality rate of 15%. Signs of Rigler's triad: small bowel obstruction, ectopic gallstones, and air in the biliary tree are virtually diagnostic. Plain films, ultrasonography, or CT scan may help establish the diagnosis by detecting the obstruction. Operative intervention consists of simple enterolithotomy that is associated with an operative mortality of 12% and a recurrence of less than 5% (30). Others may advocate a one-stage procedure consisting of removal of the impacted gallstone, fistula repair, and cholecystectomy for low-risk patients despite a slightly higher operative mortality of about 17% (31).

V. ACUTE MESENTERIC INFARCTION

A. Clinical Relevance

The first description of acute intestinal infarction was reported by Antonio Benivene from Florence in the latter fifteenth century. Today, the exact incidence of intestinal ischemia is difficult to assess, but some studies estimate it to be 0.1% of all patients referred to a hospital and 1% of all patients initially seen with an acute condition of the abdomen. In the 1930s to 1960s, the reported mortality rates varied from 70% to 90%; this has changed little from recent rates of 45% to 90%. Reasons contributing to these high mortality rates may be late diagnosis leading to intestinal infarction and gangrene, continued unrecognized bowel ischemia even after correction of the underlying cause, and an increasing incidence of patients with nonocclusive mesenteric ischemia. The pathophysiological changes of intestinal ischemia range from reversible alterations to transmural hemorrhagic necrosis of all or part of the small intestine and right half of the colon. Segmental ischemic colitis of the sigmoid colon represents another variant of mesenteric ischemia.

Arterial causes of acute mesenteric ischemia include superior mesenteric artery (SMA) embolus or thrombosis and nonocclusive mesenteric ischemia. SMA embolus accounts for 40% to 50% of cases and is usually caused by embolization of a left atrial or ventricular mural thrombus after a period of cardiac dysrhythmia or infarction. A history of peripheral artery embolism and synchronous arterial emboli should be sought. SMA thrombosis contributes to $<25\%$ of cases. The acute thrombosis is usually due to progressive atherosclerotic stenosis at the origin of the SMA, until eventually complete occlusion occurs. Symptoms of chronic mesenteric ischemia can be ascertained in 20% to 50% of patients. Coronary artery, cerebrovascular, and peripheral vascular diseases are inevitably present. An aortogram will reveal occlusion of the superior mesenteric artery near its origin and usually a concomitant obstructive lesion of the celiac axis.

A venous cause represents the least common cause of acute mesenteric ischemia and is primarily due to mesenteric venous thrombosis. It is usually associated with a hypercoagulable state, abdominal trauma, portal hypertension, pancreatitis, viscus perforation, intra-abdominal sepsis, and cancer. Diagnosis is made with CT or MRI scan.

Nonocclusive mesenteric ischemia (NOMI) is a more common cause of acute mensenteric ischemia than previously recognized, although the true incidence remains unknown. Earlier studies suggested that it accounted for 20% to 30% of acute mesenteric ischemia cases. In a recent series, Newman et al. documented an increased incidence of 47%, and when SBO was excluded as a cause, this figure rose to 58% (32). This incidence compares similarly to that reported by Ottinger and Austen of 50% (33). Furthermore, patients diagnosed with NOMI carried the highest mortality rate compared with the other causes. NOMI is caused by prolonged splanchnic vasoconstriction occurring usually in the clinical setting of tissue hypoperfusion, decreased cardiac output, and hypotension. Precipitating factors include atrial fibrillation, myocardial infarction, congestive heart failure, aortic insufficiency, hypovolemia, sepsis, and cardiopulmonary bypass. Digoxin toxicity, vasopressors, and cocaine use may cause mesenteric vasoconstriction. Patients on high-flow hemodialysis have also developed this syndrome. Diagnosis is made on the basis of clinical suspicion and angiographic findings that consist of patent mesenteric vessels with segmental vascular spasms mimicking ''chain of sausages'' in the origins of multiple branches of the SMA, ''pinching off'' of the intestinal branches, spasm of the arcades, and impaired filling of intramural vessels. It is important to realize that intestinal ischemia may not manifest until hours or days after the precipitating event, and vasospasm may persist even after the initial cause is corrected (34).

B. Immediate Diagnostic Approach

The clinical characteristics of intestinal ischemia consist of acute onset of severe abdominal pain that is out of proportion to findings on physical examination, a forceful episode of bowel evacuation, and bloody diarrhea. Decompensation may occur acutely over hours or insidiously over days. Risk factors associated with acute intestinal ischemia include age >50 years, atherosclerotic cardiac and peripheral vascular diseases, history of intestinal angina, hypertension, critically ill postoperative patients, and the presence of multiple comorbidities. Newman et al. found that a high proportion of mesenteric infarction developed in patients who were already hospitalized and being treated for a different illness (32). This was particularly evidenced by patients with a prolonged intensive care course, those being treated with digoxin or vasopressors, and postoperative cardiovascular patients. Intestinal ischemia may manifest in these critically ill patients as systemic sepsis or multiple organ failure. A nonspecific abdominal examination is not uncommon early in course of ischemia. Unexplained abdominal distention, gastrointestinal bleeding, or mental confusion may be the only early signs of acute intestinal ischemia in the elderly patient. Increasing abdominal tenderness, rebound, guarding, distention, bloody diarrhea, and shock are highly suspicious for infarcted bowel. In addition, laboratory studies may reveal leukocytosis with a left shift, hemoconcentration, elevated alkaline phosphatase, metabolic acidosis with an increased base deficit, increased serum lactate level, hyperamylasemia, and hyperphosphatemia. Of these tests only an elevated serum lactate level may be a predictor of mortality. As with clinical findings, plain films of the abdomen are generally unremarkable in early ischemia. However, later in the course of the disease dilated and gasless loops of small intestine containing air-fluid levels, ''thumb printing'' of the bowel wall, intramural or portal venous gas, and free intraperitoneal air or fluid can be seen (35).

Early diagnosis of acute mesenteric ischemia is usually not apparent on the basis of clinical and biochemical assessments alone. The history is often incomplete as a result of the debilitated nature of these patients, and abdominal pain and tenderness may be absent in approximately 25% to 30% of cases. By the time findings become evident there has already been severe progression to nonviability of the involved bowel. CT of the abdomen and selective mesenteric angiography may assist in establishing a diagnosis earlier in the course of the disease, but so far these diagnostic studies have had little impact on the overall mortality. The main usefulness of CT lies in its ability to exclude other abdominal pathological conditions in a fast and noninvasive manner. Although CT is sensitive for the evaluation of intestinal ischemia, the findings are not specific (22). Bowel wall thickening is the most common CT finding that reflects submucosal edema and hemorrhage. Luminal dilation may be seen and reflects ileus in the ischemic segments. Fluid-filled bowel loops containing minimal intraluminal gas are due to exudation of blood and fluid into the lumen. The mesenteric fat may have increased attenuation because of edema. Intramural gas or ''pneumatosis intestinalis'' is observed in only 4% to 16% of proven bowel ischemia and is caused by dissection of luminal gas into the bowel wall across the compromised mucosa. Mesenteric or portal venous gas is even more infrequent and represents escape of intramural gas into the mesenteric venous system. Obviously, free intraperitoneal air and fluid indicate perforation and peritonitis. CT is the study of choice for evaluating mesenteric venous thrombosis and may also detect SMA thrombosis.

C. Therapeutic Intervention

An aggressive roentgenological and surgical approach to mesenteric ischemia proposed by Boley et al. has been reported to reduce mortality to 50% to 60% if delay is less than 12 hours (36). The premises are based on a high clinical suspicion in any atherosclerotic elderly patient with vague abdominal pain and early use of angiography. Initial treatment consists of resuscitation, restoration and monitoring of cardiac output with a pulmonary artery catheter, and discontinuation of digitalis or vasopressors. Broad-spectrum antibiotics are warranted as a result of intraluminal bacterial translocation across the ischemic wall. A mesenteric angiogram should be obtained expeditiously if the CT is unremarkable or shows signs of ischemia. Aggressive and early use of angiography will result in a large number of negative studies, but it is the most precise method for diagnosing both occlusive and nonocclusive intestinal ischemia (36). Mesenteric arterial vasospasm is often present and may continue for several days even after correction of the underlying cause. If mesenteric vasoconstriction is present on the angiogram, papaverine infusion through an SMA catheter may be tried.

Persistent peritoneal signs usually occur in the presence of infarcted bowel and are an indication to proceed with an explorative laparotomy. Goals would be to restore intestinal arterial flow, resect irreparably damaged bowel, or both. In some cases, revascularization should precede resection of questionable viable bowel segments because surprising recovery may occur after restoration of blood flow. Techniques for assessment of bowel viability include clinical criteria, Doppler ultrasonography, and fluorescein injection. Questionable segments of viable bowel can be left intact and reassessed at second exploration planned within 12 to 24 hours. Transarterial embolectomy can be performed for SMA embolus, and heparin may be instituted for prophylaxis against further emboli. SMA thrombosis may be revascularized by bypass or transaortic SMA endarterectomy. If gangrenous bowel is present as a result of NOMI, the surgeon may favor performing a delayed anastomosis with stoma until perfusion is adequate to maintain an anastomosis (37). Thrombolytic therapy has yet proven to have a significant role in this disease.

Recognition of chronic visceral ischemia may permit elective revascularization before the development of acute mesenteric infarction. Atherosclerotic narrowing of the mesenteric arteries accounts for about 95% of cases, and usually involvement of at least two major arteries is required to produce symptoms. Symptomatic patients usually have dull and gnawing periumbilcial or epigastric abdominal pain. Intestinal angina begins between 15 and 30 minutes after meals and may persist for several hours. As the occlusion worsens, the angina will be brought on by smaller amounts of food until the patient develops a fear of eating. This eventually leads to weight loss. The ratio of women to men is 3:1. A history of coronary artery, cerebrovascular, and peripheral vascular diseases is not uncommon, and an epigastric bruit may be heard on examination. Diagnosis depends on a high index of suspicion in any elderly patient with postprandial abdominal pain, food aversion, and weight loss (38). This should prompt an arteriogram followed by surgical revascularization if results are confirmatory.

VI. COLORECTAL CANCER

A. Clinical Relevance

Intra-abdominal cancer should be a consideration in every elderly patient with abdominal pain, particularly if the pain is nonspecific, associated with weight loss, and the diagnosis is not immediately obvious. Colorectal cancer accounts for most intra-abdominal cancers in North America, with the incidence estimated to be about 150,000 cases per year. It is the second leading cause of cancer deaths in Western countries. Adenocarcinomas account for 95% of the malignant tumors in the colon and rectum. The geriatric patient is primarily affected, with approximately two-thirds to three-quarters of the incident cases occurring in those 65 years of age or older. The age-adjusted colorectal cancer incidence rate for persons 65 years and older is 20 times greater than the rate for those younger. About 40% of these patients will initially be seen with advanced disease. Other known risk factors include a low-fiber, high-fat diet, hereditary polyposis syndromes, long-standing inflammatory bowel disease, adenomatous polyps, previous colorectal cancer, and a family history of colorectal cancer.

The pathogenesis of colorectal carcinoma represents a multistep process with a mean doubling time of 130 days. This translates to about 10 years of silent growth before a cancer reaches significant size to produce symptoms. During this asymptomatic period, screening is necessary to detect early curable lesions. Studies have suggested a reduced mortality from colorectal cancer by screening asymptomatic individuals over the age of 50 (39, 40). Patients with additional risk factors as previously mentioned should undergo earlier and more frequent screening examinations. Detection of cancers at earlier stages and removal of premalignant adenomatous polyps explain the basis for mortality reduction (41). Fecal occult blood tests or flexible sigmoidoscopy are currently recommended for the screening of asymptomatic elderly persons. Fecal occult blood testing has been shown to be effective in detecting cancers at earlier and more curable stages than unscreened groups, and mortality has been shown to be reduced in screened versus control populations. Screening sigmoidoscopy is also thought to reduce colorectal cancer mortality. If the fecal blood test is positive or adenomatous polyps are found on sigmoidoscopy, full colonoscopy is indicated. Nonspecific abdominal pain in the elderly patient should prompt an appropriate evaluation, such as barium enema, colonoscopy, or CT of the abdomen, to exclude cancer.

B. Immediate Diagnostic Approach

Colorectal cancer commonly presents in an insidious manner with an average delay between onset of symptoms and definitive treatment of 7 to 9 months. Any complaints of change in bowel function should raise suspicion for colorectal carcinoma. The elderly patient may be experiencing multiple chronic illnesses, which may cause the patient to attribute some disturbance of bowel function to these disorders. Symptoms and signs that are clues to the diagnosis of colorectal cancer include iron deficiency anemia, lower gastrointestinal bleeding, vague abdominal pain, tenesmus, mucous diarrhea, unexplained weight loss, fatigability, presence of an abdominal mass, and abdominal distention. Clinical findings usually correlate with the tumor's anatomical location. Right-sided lesions tend to grow as large polypoid fungating masses that produce minimal obstructive changes resulting from the fluid content of feces and large diameter of bowel wall in this location. Patients complain of fatigue and weakness because of iron deficiency anemia from occult blood loss in the stool, vague right lower abdominal discomfort, and, not infrequently, a palpable mass. Bowel obstruction caused by cecal carcinoma is uncommon, but it should be suspected in any elderly patient with distal small bowel obstruction because of its associated poor survival (42). In contrast, left-sided colon cancers grow in an annular fashion, producing a ''napkin-ring'' constriction. Alterations of bowel function are common and are attributed to the smaller caliber of the left colon and semisolid nature of feces. Gradual occlusion of the bowel occurs and is manifested by alternating constipation and diarrhea, narrowing of stools, and occasionally mild mucous bleeding mixed with stool. Cancer in the rectum produces bright red blood usually in association with defecation and tenesmus. Even in the presence of hemorrhoids, cancer must be excluded in the elderly patient with rectal bleeding.

Additional evaluation should include a complete blood count, liver enzymes, carcinoembryonic antigen level, and chest film. Colonoscopy aides in obtaining a pathological diagnosis, and CT will help evaluate for lymphadenopathy and metastatic disease. Endorectal ultrasonographic scanning should be obtained for local staging of rectal carcinomas.

C. Therapeutic Intervention

The only possible curative treatment for colorectal cancer is surgical resection. Various studies have shown that elective surgical resection is well tolerated in elderly patients (43, 44). This involves en bloc removal of the tumor with 10-cm proximal and 2-cm distal margins, along with complete resection of the involved lymphatic nodal basin. Resection of limited and accessible hepatic metastases has been shown to improve survival with minimal adverse effects. Cryosurgery and intraoperative ultrasonography show promise in this field. Solitary pulmonary metastases should also be considered for resection (45). Surgery is also indicated for palliation of large tumors that may obstruct, perforate, or bleed.

Colorectal cancers that present with obstruction or peritonitis caused by perforation require emergency surgery. Prognosis is poorest for this group of patients, with mortality rates ranging from 16% to 48%. Presence of multiple comorbidities increases the mortality. Long-term survival is decreased even after successful radical resection in the emergency versus elective groups. In addition, tumors tend to be more advanced and metastases more common in the emergency group (46). The minimal operation, such as bypass or diversion, should be strongly considered for the critically ill elderly patient with multiple cormorbidities presenting with an emergency complication. A staged resection can be attempted after recovery from the acute stress under optimized conditions (47).

VII. PEPTIC ULCER DISEASE

A. Clinical Relevance

The incidence and prevalence of peptic ulcer disease (PUD) have declined over the past several decades and may be related to the introduction of histamine H_2-receptor antagonists and proton pump inhibitors in the 1970s. This has correlated with a decline in elective surgical intervention for PUD. However, the number of emergency operations for complicated ulcer disease has remained relatively unchanged. In addition, the incidence and mortality of complicated PUD (i.e., hemorrhage and perforation) have been steadily rising in the elderly population, which constitutes most of those requiring emergency surgery for PUD. This trend is especially prominent in elderly women (48–51). The increased prevalence of nonsteroidal anti-inflammatory drug (NSAIDs) use among older people is believed to be a major incriminating factor. NSAIDs damage the gastric mucosa through the inhibition of prostaglandin synthesis and cytoprotective factors. The use of NSAIDs increases the risk of bleeding, perforation, and death from peptic ulcers (52–55).

B. Immediate Diagnostic Approach

Perforation of a peptic ulcer classically manifests as severe acute epigastric pain with radiation to one or both shoulders. The patient bends forward in agony and appears in distress. A lull period may follow as the initial chemical peritonitis becomes diluted from increased peritoneal secretions. The pain may shift to the right lower abdominal quadrant as the irritating fluid drains down the right paracolic gutter, but a generalized peritonitis is most common. Examination will reveal a thready pulse, labored respirations, diffuse abdominal tenderness, rigidity, and distention. Free air that appears on an acute abdominal radiographic series should confirm the diagnosis (56). However, this dramatic presentation is often subdued in the elderly patient (57, 58). It is not infrequent for perforation or bleeding to occur without any prior history or symptoms of PUD. Typical ulcer pain is less likely to be present in elderly patients, and the analgesic properties of NSAIDs may mask the severity of pain. Peritoneal signs may be lacking, and mental confusion can be the initial presentation. Distinguishing findings between

Table 3 Clinical Differences Between Perforated Peptic Ulcer and Colonic Perforation[a]

Feature	Favors perforated peptic ulcer	Favors colonic perforation
Age (yr)	<50	>60
Location of pain at onset	Upper half	Lower half
Duration of pain (h)	<12	>24
Severity	Dramatic	Less severe
Bowel habit	Normal	Abnormal
Previous indigestion	Present	Absent

[a] From Ref. 1.

peptic ulcer perforation and colonic perforation are displayed in Table 3. Acute myocardial infarction should be excluded in elderly patients with substernal or high epigastric pain. Abdominal radiographs may not show subdiaphragmatic free air in 25% of cases. Upper gastrointestinal endoscopy or barium series can aid in the diagnosis.

C. Therapeutic Intervention

The morbidity and mortality of complicated PUD are high, especially in elderly patients taking anti-inflammatory drugs and with multiple medical problems. Morbidity occurs in about 65% of patients and consists of pneumonia, cardiac dysrhythmia, wound infection, urinary tract infection, and sepsis. Overall mortality for emergency peptic ulcer surgery consisting of perforations, hemorrhage, and penetration is about 30% (59). Sepsis and multiple organ failure are the leading causes of death. Boey et al. found that a treatment delay of more than 24 hours, concurrent medical diseases, and preoperative shock all increased the mortality in patients with perforated peptic ulcers. The presence of one, two, or three of these factors was associated with a mortality of 10%, 46%, and 100%, respectively (60). Svanes et al. also found that a delay of more than 24 hours increased mortality, morbidity, and length of hospital stay (61). Elderly patients should undergo the simplest surgical treatment consisting of explorative laparotomy or laparoscopy and suture closure of the perforation. The rate of recurrence with this is low (59).

Elderly patients with peptic ulcer bleeding are more likely to rebleed, require an operation, and die compared with their younger counterparts, especially if they require more than 5 units of blood transfusion (62, 63). (See also Chapter 19.) The risk of rebleeding is higher, about 70%, for patients admitted in shock.

Resuscitation needs to be performed adequately but cautiously because elderly patients will not tolerate hypotension as well and are at risk for cardiac failure with overhydration. Treatment requires communication between the surgery team and gastrointestinal endoscopist for initial attempts at hemostasis. Endoscopic stigmata of a visible vessel or sentinel clot in the ulcer base indicates a high risk of rebleeding. The surgical procedure depends on the condition of the patient, age, location of the ulcer, and the treatment preference and training of the individual surgeon. These can include simple closure with or without omental patch, vagotomy and drainage, pyloroplasty or gastrojejunostomy, or resection. Endoscopically or radiographically documented peptic ulcer should be followed until healing occurs. Cancer or Zollinger-Ellison syndrome should be suspected if healing has not occurred within 8 weeks.

VIII. COMPLICATED DIVERTICULAR DISEASE

A. Clinical Relevance

Most colonic diverticula are acquired and considered ''false'' because they consist of only herniated mucosa and submucosa. A low-fiber diet is believed to play a causative role. The prevalence of colonic diverticula in Western countries is significantly higher and increases with age. Only about 10% to 20% of persons with documented colonic diverticulosis will have symptomatic disease develop (i.e., acute diverticulitis or hemorrhage) (64). Complicated diverticular disease occurs primarily in the middle-aged and elderly populations, with about three-quarters of all patients hospitalized for acute diverticulitis being older than 60. Acute diverticulitis is the most common complication and occurs when a divertculum becomes inflamed and perforates. The sigmoid colon is invariably involved in more than 90% of all cases. Contained perforation may result in abscess formation, fistulization, small bowel obstruction from adhesions, and large bowel obstruction from fibrotic luminal narrowing after repeated episodes. Free perforation may lead to generalized peritonitis.

B. Immediate Diagnostic Approach

Acute diverticulitis resembles acute appendicitis in pathophysiology and presentation except the pain is situated in the left lower quadrant. The attack occurs suddenly, and the pain can be steady or colicky in nature. The location of the pain may be variable because of the redundancy of the sigmoid colon and occasionally can be felt in the suprapubic area, right lower quadrant, or throughout the lower abdomen. When located in the right lower quadrant, it can easily be mistaken for acute appendicitis. Passage of flatus or stool may alleviate the pain. Alteration in bowel habits, nausea, and vomiting are not uncommon. Urinary symptoms may occur when adjacent bladder irritation is present. Physical findings consist of low-grade fever, mild abdominal distention, left lower quadrant tenderness and or mass, and leukocytosis. Caution must be taken to not underestimate the extent of disease in the elderly because their symptoms may be insidious and attenuated (65). Plain abdominal films may show nonspecific findings of ileus or obstruction, free air in the bladder indicating a colovesical fistula, or a pneumoperitoneum suggesting free perforation of a diverticulum. Abdominal CT scan with water-soluble contrast enema is the initial study of choice and affords the option of percutaneous drainage of any abscesses identified. Barium enema and lower endoscopy should be avoided during the acute attack because of possible leakage of barium into the peritoneal cavity and the risk of perforation from high pressure.

C. Therapeutic Intervention

Most patients with acute diverticulitis will have their disease resolve with medical treatment consisting of bowel rest, hydration, and antibiotics. Oral feeding is slowly advanced as the inflammation subsides and a stool-bulking agent started. The patient should be evaluated with colonoscopy or barium enema several weeks after resolution of the initial attack. The risk of another attack is 25%, usually occurring within the first 5 years, for those whose disease resolves with medical therapy (66).

Approximately 25% of patients hospitalized with acute diverticulitis will require surgical treatment. Surgery is indicated for cases refractory to medical treatment, recurrent diverticulitis that is associated with increased rate of complications, and age younger than 50. Patients experiencing their first episode of acute diverticulitis before the age of 50 are at high risk for recurrent diverticular disease requiring urgent operation and thus should undergo elective resection after resolution of their initial episode (67). Recurrent diverticulitis after resection is infrequent, occurring in 3% to 7% of cases. In cases of free perforation with peritonitis, abscess formation, obstruction, or fistula formation, surgery is mandatory. The operative mortality rate is about 5% in recent reports.

The type of operation is determined mainly by the surgeon's experience and preference. Efforts should be made to convert an emergency operation into an urgent or elective one. The use of intravenous antibiotics and CT-guided percutaneous catheter drainage of well-localized paracolic abscesses have played a large role in promoting successful one-stage operative procedures when peritoneal contamination is slight and contained and the patient is in good health (68). This consists of resection of diseased colon with anastomosis during the same operation. In the emergency setting, especially with elderly patients, a two-stage procedure is preferable (69). This consists of primary resection with the proximal end of colon brought out as temporary colostomy and the distal end closed into a Hartmann's pouch or exteriorized as a mucous fistula. Reanastomosis is performed at a second operation after the infection subsides. Three-stage procedures are not performed commonly today but may retain a role in colonic obstruction resulting from diverticulitis.

IX. CONCLUSION

Improving the outcome of acute abdominal disease in the elderly patient requires action on three fronts. Patients must be educated to seek medical attention early in the course of symptoms. The primary care physician should evaluate nonspecific abdominal complaints in the elderly and seek surgical referral for elective conditions before development of complications necessitates urgent operation. Last, the surgeon must recognize the variable presentations and higher morbidity and mortality associated with advanced age and therefore not delay treatment while awaiting a definitive diagnosis.

REFERENCES

1. Telfer S, Fenyo G, Holt PR, de Dombal FT. Acute abdominal pain in patients over 50 years of age. Scand J Gastroenterol 1988; 23(suppl 144):47–50.
2. Geis WP, Kim HC. Use of laparoscopy in the diagnosis and treatment of patients with surgical abdominal sepsis. Surg Endoscopy 1995; 9:178–182.
3. Crump C. The incidence of gallstones and gallbladder disease. Surg Gynecol Obstet 1981; 53:447–455.
4. Reiss R, Deutsch AA. Emergency abdominal procedures in patients over 70. J Gerontology 1985; 40:154–158.
5. Morrow DJ, Thompson J, Wilson SE. Acute cholecystitis in the elderly. Arch Surg 1978; 113:1149–1152.
6. Chock E, Wolfe BM, Matolo NM. Acute suppurative cholangitis. Surg Clin North Am 1981; 61:885–892.
7. Harness JK, Strodel WE, Talsma SE. Symptomatic bilieary tract disease in the elderly patient. Am Surgeon 1986; 52:442–445.
8. Edlund G, Ljungdahl M. Acute cholecystitis in the elderly. Am J Surg 1990; 59(3): 414–416.
9. Magnuson TH, Ratner LE, Zenilman ME, Bender JS. Laparoscopic cholecystectomy: applicability in the geriatric population. Am Surgeon 1997; 63:91–96.
10. Le CM, Fan ST, Liu CL, Lai EC, Wong J. Early decision for conversion of laparoscopic to open cholecystectomy for treatment of acute cholecystitis. Am J Surg 1997; 173:513–517.
11. Sugiyama M, Tokuhara M, Atomi Y. Is percutaneous cholecystostomy the optimal

treatment for acute cholecystitis in the very elderly? World J Surg 1998; 22:459–463.
12. Andersson A, Bergdahl L. Acute appendicitis in patients over sixty. Am Surgeon 1978; 44:445–447.
13. Owens BJ, Hamit HF. Appendicitis in the elderly. Ann Surg 1978; 187:392–396.
14. Addiss DG, Shaffer N, Fowler BS, Trauxe RV. The epidemiology of appendicitis and appendectomy in the United States. Am J Epidemiol 1990; 132:910–925.
15. McCallion J, Canning G, Knight PV, McCallion JS. Acute appendicitis in the elderly: a 5 year retrospective study. Age Ageing 1987; 16:256–260.
16. Horattas M, Guyton DP, Wu D. A reappraisal of appendicitis in the elderly. Am J Surg 1990; 160:291–293.
17. Franz MG, Norman J, Fabri PJ. Increased morbidity of appendicitis with advancing age. Am Surgeon 1995; 61:40–43.
18. Thorbjarnarson B, Loehr WJ. Acute appendicitis in patients over the age of 60. Surg Gynecol Obstet 1967; 125:1277–1280.
19. Hubbell DS, Barton WK, Solomin OD. Appendicitis in older people. Surg Gynecol Obstet 1960; 110:289–292.
20. Kuster GGR, Gilroy SBC. The role of laparoscopy in the diagnosis of acute appendicitis. Am Surgeon 1992; 58:627–629.
21. Zadeh BJ, Davis JM, Canizaro PC. Small bowel obstruction in the elderly. Am Surgeon 1985; 51:470–473.
22. Bartnicke B, Balfe D. CT appearance of intestinal ischemia and intramural hemorrhage. Imaging Acute Abdomen 1994; 32:845–859.
23. Playforth RH, Holloway JB, Griffen WO. Mechanical small bowel obstruction: a plea for earlier operative therapy. Ann Surg 1970; 171:783–788.
24. Green WW. Bowel obstruction in the aged patient. Am J Surg 1966; 118:542–545.
25. McEntee G, Pender D, Mulvin D, McCullough M, Naeeder S, Farah S. Current spectrum of intestinal obstruction. Br J Surg 1987; 74:976–980.
26. Bender JS, Busuito MJ, Graham C, Allaben RD. Small bowel obstruction in the elderly. Am Surgeon 1989; 55:385–388.
27. Lo CY, Lorentz TG, Lau PWK. Obturator hernia presenting as small bowel obstruction. Am J Surg 1994; 167:396–398.
28. Ballantyne GH, Brandner MD, Beart RW, Ilstrup DM. Volvulus of the colon. Ann Surg 1985; 202:83–91.
29. Geelhoed GW. Colonic pseudo-obstruction in surgical patients. Am J Surg 1985; 149:258–265.
30. Reisner RM, Cohen JR. Gallstone ileus: a review of 1001 reported cases. Am Surgeon 1994; 60:441–445.
31. Berliner SD, Burson LC. One stage repair for chlecystduodenal fistula and gallstone ileus. Arch Surg 1965; 90:313–316.
32. Newman TS, Magnuson TH, Ahrendt SA, Smith-Meed MA, Bender JS. The changing face of mesenteric infarction. Am Surgeon 1998; 64:611–616.
33. Ottinger LW, Austen WG. A study of 136 patients with mesenteric infarction. Surg Gynecol Obstet 1967; 124:251–261.
34. Wilcox MG, Howard TJ, Plaskon LA, Unthank JL, Madura JA. Current theories of

pathogenesis and treatment of nonocclusive mesenteric ischemia. Dig Dis Sci 1995; 40:709–716.
35. Klein HM, Lensing R, Klosterhalfen B, Tonc C, Gunther RW. Diagnostic imaging of mesenteric infarction. Radiology 1995; 197:79–82.
36. Boley SJ, Sprayregan S, Siegelman SS, Veith FJ. Initial results from an aggressive roentgenological and surgical approach to acute mesenteric ischemia. Surgery 1977; 82:848–855.
37. Ward D, Vernava AM, Kaminski DL, Ure T, Peterson G, Garvin G, Arends TW, Longo TW. Improved outcome by identification of high risk nonocclusive mesenteric ischemia, aggressive reexploration, and delayed anastomosis. Am J Surg 1995; 170:577–581.
38. Mikkelsen WP. Intestinal angina: its surgical significance. Am J Surg 1957; 94:262–266.
39. Morris JB, Stellato TA, Guy BB, Gordon NH, Berger NA. A critical analysis of the largest reported mass fecal occult blood screening program in the United States. Am J Surg 1991; 161:101–105.
40. Selby JV, Friedman GD, Quesenberry CP, Weiss NS. A case control study of screening sigmoidoscopy and mortality from colorectal cancer. N Engl J Med 1992; 326: 653–657.
41. Winawer SJ, Zauber AG, Ho MN, O'Brien MJ, Gottlieb LS, Sternberg SS, Waye JD, Schapiro M, Bond JH, Panish JF. Prevention of colorectal cancer by colonoscopic polypectomy. N Engl J Med 1993; 329:1977–1981.
42. Rovito PR, Verazin G, Prorok JJ. Obstructing carcinoma of the cecum. J Surg Oncol 1990; 45:177–179.
43. Vivi AA, Lopes A, Cavalcanti S, Rossi BM, Marques LA. Surgical treatment of colon and rectal carcinomas in elderly patients. J Surg Oncol 1992; 51:203–206.
44. Payne JE, Chapuis PH, Pheils MT. Surgery for large bowel cancer in people aged 75 years and older. Dis Colon Rectum 1986; 29:733–737.
45. Asbun HJ, Hughes KS. Management of recurrent and metastatic colorectal carcinoma. Surg Clin North Am 1993; 1:145–166.
46. Kyllonen, L. Obstruction and perforation complicating colorectal carcinoma. Acta Chir Scand 1987; 153:607–614.
47. Fitzgerald SD, Longo WE, Daniel GL, Vernava AM. Advanced colorectal neoplasia in the high risk elderly patient: is surgical resection justified? Dis Colon Rectum 1993; 36:161–166.
48. Coggan D, Lambert P, Langman MJS. Twenty years of hospital admissions for peptic ulcer in England and Wales. Lancet 1981; 1:1302–1304.
49. Paimela H, Joutsi T, Kiviluoto T, Kivilaakso E. Recent trends in mortality from peptic ulcer disease in Finland. Dig Dis Sci 1995; 40:631–635.
50. Fineberg HV, Pearlman LA. Surgical treatment of peptic ulcer in the United States. Trends before and after the introduction of cimetidine. Lancet 1981; 1:1305–1307.
51. Scheeres DE, DeKryger LL, Dean RE. Surgical treatment of peptic ulcer disease before and after introduction for H2 blockers. Am Surgeon 1987; 53:392.
52. Jick SS, Perera DR, Walker AM, Jick H. Non-steroidal anti-inflammatory drugs and hospital admission for perforated peptic ulcer. Lancet 1987; 2:380–381.

53. Armstrong CP, Blower AL. Nonsteroidal anti-inflammatory drugs and life threatening complications of peptic ulceration. Gut 1987; 28:527–532.
54. Collier DSJ, Pain JA. Non-steroidal anti-inflammatory drugs and peptic ulcer perforation. Gut 1985; 26:359–363.
55. Griffin MR, Ray WA, Schaffner W. Non-steroidal anti-inflammatory drug use and death from peptic ulcer in elderly patients. Ann Intern Med 1988; 109:359–363.
56. Cope, Zachery, Sir. Early diagnosis of the acute abdomen. 18th ed. In: Silen W, ed. New York: Oxford University Press, 1991, pp 109–110.
57. Clinch D, Banerjee AK, Ostick G. Absence of abdominal pain in elderly patients with peptic ulcer. Age Ageing 1984; 13:120–123.
58. Coleman JA, Denham MJ. Perforation of peptic ulcer in the elderly. Age Ageing 1980; 9:257–261.
59. Bulut O, Rasmussen C, Fischer A. Acute surgical treatment of complicated peptic ulcers with special reference to the elderly. World J Surg 1996; 20:574–577.
60. Boey J, Choi SKY, Alagaratnam TT, Poon A. Risk stratification in perforated duodenal ulcers: a prospective validation of predictive factors. Ann Surg 1987; 205:22–26.
61. Svanes C, Lie RT, Svanes K. Adverse effects of delayed treatment for perforated peptic ulcer. Ann Surg 1994; 220:168–175.
62. Larson G, Schmidt T, Gott J, Bond S, O'Connor CA, Richardson JD. Upper gastrointestinal bleeding: predictors of outcome. Surgery 1986; 100:765–773.
63. Booker JA, Johnston M, Booker CI, Tydd T, Mitchell R. Prognostic factors for continued or rebleeding and death from gastrointestinal hemorrhage in the elderly. Age Ageing 1987; 16:208–214.
64. Parks TG. Natural history of diverticular disease of the colon. Clin Gastroenterol 1975; 4:53–69.
65. Cheskin LJ, Bohlman M, Schuster M. Diverticular disease in the elderly. Gastroenterol Clin North Am 1990; 19:391–401.
66. Larson DM, Masters SS, Spiro HM. Medical and surgical therapy in diverticular disease. Gastroenterology 1976; 71:734–737.
67. Eusebio EB, Eisenberg MM. Natural history of diverticular disease of the colon in young patients. Am J Surg 1973; 125:308–311.
68. Wedell J, Banzhaf G, Chaoui R, Reichmann J. Surgical management of complicated colonic diverticulitis. Br J Surg 1997; 84:380–383.
69. Konsten J, Gouma DJ, Soeters PB. Effect of preoperative risk factors and the outcome after surgery for complicated diverticular disease. Netherlands J Surg 1990; 42:101–104.

10
Acute Vascular Emergencies

J. Dennis Baker
UCLA School of Medicine, Los Angeles, California

Atherosclerosis and other degenerative conditions affecting the arterial wall are rarely seen in younger patients and most frequently become clinically significant in the older population. Consequently, the most important arterial vascular emergencies are found predominantly in this age group, and physicians caring for these people need to consider the possibility of vascular problems higher on the list of differential diagnoses of acute symptoms than might be customary in the average population.

I. RUPTURED ABDOMINAL AORTIC ANEURYSM

A. Clinical Relevance

The abdominal aortic aneurysm (AAA) is primarily a disease of the aging population. Contemporary screening studies have found an incidence in the range of 3% in males ages 65 to 74, with the rate increasing to the range of 11% in elderly subjects with hypertension (1,2). The most serious complication of an AAA is rupture. The risk of rupture increases with maximum diameter, because the larger the aneurysm the more attenuated the vessel wall thickness and the greater the tension on the wall. Although small aneurysms (<4 cm) can rupture, this is a rare occurrence. However, the 5-year risk of rupture of a 6-cm diameter AAA is in the range of 50%. Aortic aneurysm rupture carries a high mortality and is within the top 15 most frequent causes of death in the United States (3). Over the past three decades a progressive decrease in the mortality has been associated with the elective repair of AAA; however, little improvement exists in the salvage of patients in whom a rupture has occurred. The major factor accounting for the persistent high mortality is that many patients die before reaching medical care. A study from the United Kingdom reported that only 38% of patients reached the hospital alive and only half of these survived operation, for an overall mortality of 80% (4). Even in communities with rapid access to hospital care, the mortality rate is in the 70% range (5).

Most commonly the infrarenal aorta ruptures into the retroperitoneum (Figure 1). This location of the bleeding allows for initial limitation of the blood loss by tamponade. If untreated, essentially all of these contained ruptures will break through the posterior peritoneum with uncontrolled bleeding into the abdominal cavity, usually leading to rapid death. Most patients who survive have ruptured into a retroperitoneal site, allowing them to reach the hospital and undergo emergency operation. Primary rupture into the peritoneal cavity results in a larger and more rapid hemorrhage, and few of these patients are saved. In rare cases the aneurysm may rupture into the inferior vena cava. Although the patient does not lose blood from the circulation, the high flow arteriovenous fistula causes severe heart failure and often acute onset of renal failure occurs, resulting from the high venous pressure at the level of the renal veins. In addition, these patients rapidly have massive leg edema develop from the venous hypertension. A loud, harsh bruit heard over the abdomen is diagnostic for the aortocaval fistula.

B. Immediate Diagnostic Approach

The classic presentation of a ruptured AAA includes severe pain in the back or the abdomen, a palpable pulsatile abdominal mass, and hypotension. The pain is usually on the left side and is described as ''knifelike'' and severe. The pain may radiate to the hip, the thigh, or the genitalia. This pattern and severity often suggests to the physician that the patient has ureteral colic, leading to a less rushed work-up with time taken to obtain an intravenous pyelogram and to call a urology consultant. This delay in identification of the true cause of the pain may result in death in the emergency department. Because of the urgency in diagnosing and treating a ruptured AAA, any patient older than 60 who is seen with acute onset of severe back or flank pain should be considered to have this condition as the top item on the list of differential diagnoses. A high level of suspicion will help save patient lives.

Only about half of patients are seen with all three findings that are clearly detected. In some cases a large, easily palpable mass is present. Often what is felt is a pulsatile hematoma rather than a large AAA. Alternatively, no palpable mass may be detected, especially in obese patients. Hypotension may not be a dominant finding, especially if retroperitoneal tamponade has limited blood loss to a few hundred milliliters. Another source for error can be found in the patient with undocumented hypertension, who may be hypotensive relative to his or her baseline pressure but not in absolute terms. In most of these cases an elevated

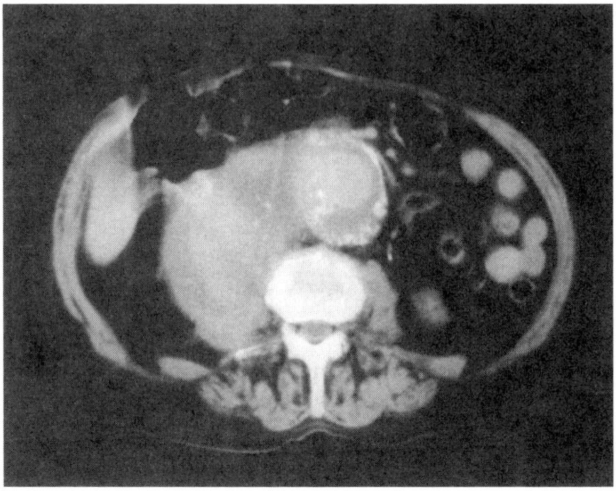

(A)

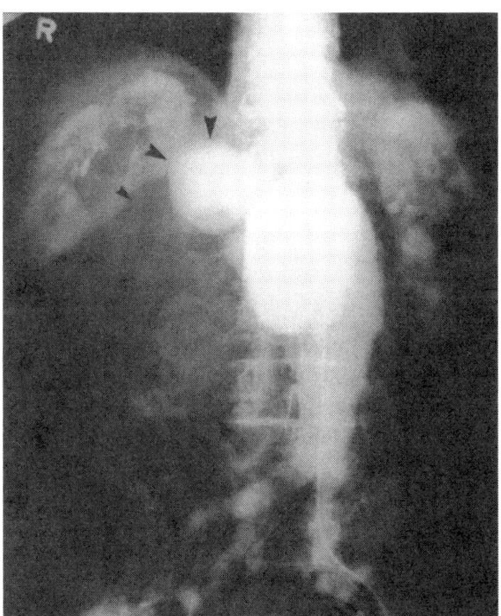

(B)

Figure 1 Large retroperitoneal rupture of abdominal aortic aneurysm. (A) CT scan at level of rupture. (B) Aortogram shows persisting flow into upper end of retroperitoneal hematoma. Note large volume of thrombus to right of aorta, with upward displacement of right kidney.

pulse rate or a low hematocrit point toward significant blood loss. An occasional person will be seen with symptoms dating back several days, and the presence of periumbilical or flank ecchymosis points to a significant retroperitoneal hematoma.

As soon as the condition is suspected, vascular surgery consultation should be obtained. In many patients, the initial findings are sufficient for a decision to be made for immediate operation. (Other conditions such as viscus perforation or acute visceral ischemia may mimic the severe pain and hypotension of a ruptured AAA, but most of these diagnoses also require emergency surgery.) The patient must be taken directly to the operating room. Unlike most other conditions, the clinician should not try to resuscitate the patient before going to surgery. Transfusing up to a reasonable hematocrit or trying to get blood pressure back to a normal level may actually be harmful in that a higher systemic pressure may increase the risk of secondary rupture of the tamponading posterior peritoneum and massive hemorrhage. Most surgeons do not want the systolic pressure greater than 80 to 90 mm Hg. The key to improving the chances of survival is to operate as soon as possible; anything that adds to delay increases mortality.

In some cases of ruptured aneurysm, the amount of blood loss may be limited and the patient may be stable. In this situation the diagnosis of AAA that is rupturing may be uncertain, and additional evaluation is needed. A computed tomographic (CT) scan with intravenous contrast is the preferred examination (6). An initial screening study with wide cuts should be carried out, and if this does not show a significant abnormality, a more complete study can be done. When ongoing bleeding is occurring, extravasation of the contrast is seen, but in many cases the key finding is a unilateral hematoma, often with displacement of the kidney (Figure 1, B). The sensitivity of the CT scan has been shown to be in the range of 75%, with specificity of 90% to 100%; however, Adam and his associates have reported a specificity of 77% (7). This incidence of false-positive findings emphasizes the importance of relying on clinical presentation and maintaining a high index of suspicion if the scan shows an aneurysm, especially a large one. In some cases, the pain that led to the patient seeking medical help may result from an acute expansion of the aneurysm as a prelude to rupture. Some centers use abdominal ultrasonography as the initial diagnostic test, but it is less accurate than the CT scan and often an inadequate examination is obtained because of bowel gas. Insistence on an initial ultrasonogram often just adds to a delay in the diagnostic pathway. In general the ultrasonogram should not be ordered unless a CT scan is not available.

C. Therapeutic Intervention

The initial treatment of a ruptured aneurysm is the application of a vascular clamp proximal to the site of leak to control bleeding; therefore, as soon as the diagnosis is made the patient should be taken to the operating room without delay. The initial preparation and preliminary resuscitation is best done in that setting. Large-bore intravenous lines are placed and crystalloid infusion is started. Operation is not delayed for the usual preoperative preliminaries such as obtaining a full electrocardiogram, chest x-ray film, and full blood cross match. The operation consists of replacing the aneurysmal portion of the aorta by a prosthetic graft. In many cases, a simple tube graft is inserted in the infrarenal aorta, but if the aneurysmal disease extends to the bifurcation or into the iliac branches, a bifurcation graft is required, extending to either the iliac or the femoral arteries.

Intraoperative management is often complicated by hypothermia and coagulopathies. The latter should be anticipated, and early use of platelets and fresh frozen plasma is an important adjunct. Major postoperative complications are frequent and when they occur, the mortality is increased. A Mayo Clinic study of patients with ruptured aneurysms reported respiratory failure in 48%, renal failure in 29%, sepsis in 25%, and myocardial infarction or congestive heart failure in 24% (8). Seventy-six percent of patients who had renal failure developed died. An uncommon but catastrophic complication is paraplegia or paraparesis, occurring in about 2%, which is about 10 times the incidence occurring with elective aneurysm repair (8,9). Patients who survive operation usually have a longer postoperative course than those who have had an elective aneurysm repair. Intensive care unit stays and total hospitalizations are longer.

D. Follow-up Management

Physicians caring for these patients after discharge shold be aware of the marked stress of this type of surgery and the resulting convalescence. A gradual recovery should be anticipated. The typical person finds that return to preoperative status often takes 3 months. Once this period has passed, return to preoperatvie level of activity is the norm. Rohrer et al., used a questionnnaire to determine quality of life for survivors of ruptured aneurysm repair and found the parameters to be similar to patients who had undergone elective aneurysm repair (10).

Patients with aortic aneurysms have an increased incidence of aneurysms at other sites. The most common are femoral and popliteal arteries. Because the typical patient with a ruptured aneurysm does not receive a careful preoperative evaluation, it is important to check for the additional aneurysmal disease, especially in the popliteal arteries.

II. ACUTE AORTIC DISSECTION

A. Clinical Relevance

Acute aortic dissection occurs more frequently than rupture of the abdominal aortic aneurysm but is probably undiagnosed in a higher proportion of patients.

(The condition was formerly labeled ''dissecting aneurysm,'' but the initial dissection very rarely involves an existing aneurysm.) In a review of autopsy series Hirst and colleagues found one dissection per 363 autopsies (11). An untreated dissection is a highly lethal condition, with a mortality of 1% per hour in the first day and a cumulative mortality of 37% at 2 days (11). The initiating process is an intimal tear with secondary dissection through the media. A dissection rarely occurs in a healthy aorta, and degenerative changes in the media are a prerequisite. Most of the younger patients with dissection have a genetic connective tissue abnormality, such as Marfan's or Ehlers-Danlos syndrome, which results in degeneration of elastic tissue in the media. In the older age group, hypertension is common and is thought to cause the medial smooth muscle degeneration usually found in the involved segments of aorta (12). Once the initial tear occurs, there is rapid extension of pulsating blood through the weakened media. The partial thickness of media and the adventitia form the new outer wall of the aorta. The length of dissection depends on a variety of factors, including the severity of medial degeneration and the presence and extent of atherosclerotic plaque formation in the aortic wall. Likewise, the extent of circumferential separation varies, but it is common to see about half of the circumference involved. In many patients a second tear of the intima occurs some distance from the initial entry point forming a re-entry site, providing two parallel flow channels—a true and a false lumen. It is typical for some of the aortic branches to remain in continuity with the true lumen, whereas others are supplied by the false channel (Figure 2).

A variety of schemes have been used to describe aortic dissections, but the simplest and most practical is the Stanford classification. Type A includes any dissection with involvement of the ascending aorta, whereas type B includes only the dissections of the descending aorta, distal to the origin of the left subclavian artery. Table 1 lists typical characteristics of the two types of dissections. The potential complications and the therapeutic approaches are quite different for the two types. The most common complications occur from rupture of the thin residual wall of the false lumen with bleeding outside the aorta. Hirst and colleagues found that 70% of deaths in acute dissection resulted from hemopericardium and the resulting tamponade (11). Most of these patients were found to have a type A dissection. The rupture can also occur into the pleural cavity (usually the left).

Figure 2 Descending aortic dissection. (A) Lateral aortogram shows filling primarily of true lumen anterior to larger false lumen. (B) Aortogram of abdominal aorta shows only filling of the superior mesenteric artery from the true lumen. (Renal and iliac arteries being perfused from the false lumen.) (C) MRI scan at level of superior mesenteric artery origin. Single arrowhead points to true lumen; double arrowhead, points to false lumen. Superior mesenteric artery comes off true lumen. Note the larger size of the false lumen and the thin membrane separating lumens.

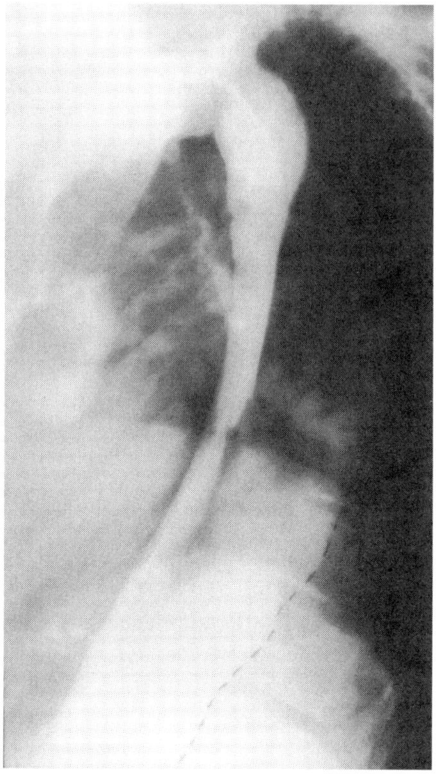

(A)

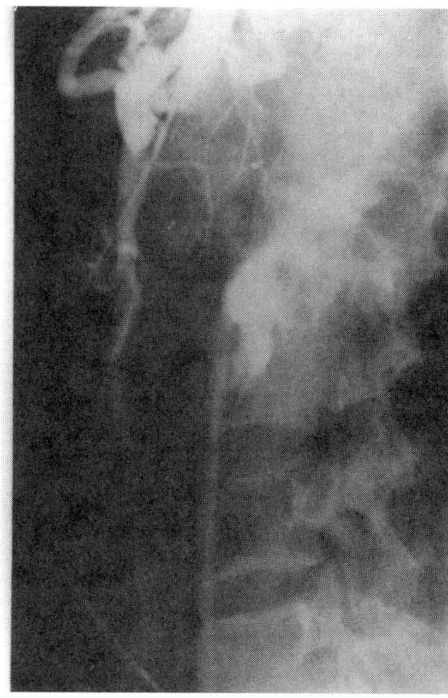

(B)

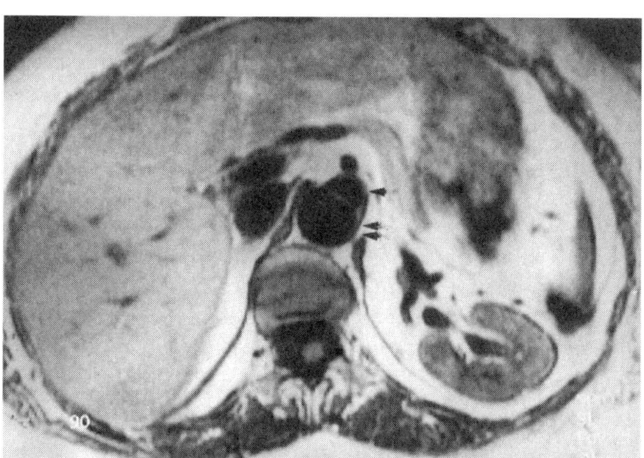

(C)

Table 1 Characteristics of Aortic Dissection by Type

	Ascending	Descending
Stanford classification	Type A	Type B
Relative frequency	70%	30%
Age group	Younger	Older
Associated factors	Connective tissue disorder	Hypertension
Degeneration involves	Elastic tissue	Medial smooth muscle
Main complications	Intrapericardial rupture, intrapleural rupture, coronary artery occlusion, aortic valve regurgitation	Intrapleural rupture, organ ischemia, extremity ischemia
Treatment	Immediate surgery	Possible medical management

Unusual complications of aortic valve regurgitation and pulmonary artery narrowing can be produced by retrograde dissection into the root of the aorta. Most of the other acute complications result from damage to arterial branches. In some cases, the branch may be sheared off the true lumen and remain open with perfusion from the false lumen. Another alternative is compression of the orifice of the branch vessel by the false lumen, with decrease or cessation of flow, usually followed by thrombosis. The presenting clinical manifestations are determined by the involved ischemic organs and can include myocardial ischemia, stroke, paraplegia (spinal cord ischemia), renal failure, visceral insufficiency, and acute leg symptoms. A review of the Stanford University experience in 1990 found that 31% of patients with aortic dissections had one or more peripheral arterial complications (13). The incidences were 38% in type A and 20% in type B dissections.

B. Immediate Diagnostic Approach

The patient typically is seen with severe pain of sudden onset, variously described as tearing, ripping, or knifelike. The most common location of the pain is the chest, but other sites include the neck, the abdomen, and the lower back. Type A dissections typically present with pain in the anterior chest, whereas type B dissections produce pain predominantly in the intrascapular region. Other presenting symptoms are determined by the ischemic complications discussed earlier. The decrease or loss of one or more peripheral pulses points to the occlusive effects of the dissection. The femoral is the most common pulse to be missing as the result of the frequent extension of dissections down to the common iliac branches (11). Pulse loss can also be found in the carotid or subclavian branches. Measurement of blood pressures in both arms may help to document an asymmetry. Most patients are admitted with hypertension; however, 25% of patients have shock, resulting either from tamponade or hemorrhage. Auscultation of the heart is important in establishing the presence of aortic regurgitation. Whenever dissection is suspected, the physical examination must include neurological assessment and a search for signs of visceral or extremity ischemia. Even if this part of the examination is initially negative, the findings may change at a later time.

Acute aortic dissection carries such a high early mortality that physicians must be alert to any patient who has a suggestion of this diagnosis. The confirmatory tests must be carried out rapidly. Transesophageal echocardiography (TEE) has become the initial examination in most medical centers. It can be completed quickly at the bedside with appropriate sedation. The technique can image the flow in the false lumen and often the proximal extent can be detected, which will define the type of dissection—a critical consideration in treatment. In addition, TEE can document aortic valve regurgitation. If a strong suspicion of a dissection exists and the initial examination is negative, additional tests should be carried out to try to exclude a false-negative result. Further definition of the anatomy is obtained with a CT scan, usually performed with intravenous contrast. In some patients contrast angiography is obtained to refine the anatomical information, especially when planning an operation. The arteriogram is especially valuable when dissection is complicated by associated occlusions of major branch vessels.

C. Therapeutic Intervention

1. Initial Management

All patients suspected of acute dissection should be admitted immediately to an intensive care unit and started on antihypertensive treatment. This treatment was originally advocated in the 1960s by Wheat, who postulated that reduction of pulsatility and of mean blood pressure would limit the extent of dissection and reduce complications (14,15). Animal experiments demonstrated that trimethaphan (Arfonad) reduced both myocardial contractility and mean pressure. Wheat's clinical protocol used an initial intravenous drip to lower systolic pressure to the range of 100 mm Hg and because most patients become refractory to trimethaphan within 48 hours, reserpine or guanethidine was started to provide longer term hypotensive control. Various series reported in the 1970s and 1980s showed a benefit of medical therapy in the management of type B dissections (20% mortality) but not the type A ones (69% mortality) (14).

Current protocols usually start with intravenous nitroprusside for the treatment of hypertension, with the drip titrated to keep the systolic pressure between 100 and 120 mm Hg. An intravenous beta-adrenergic blocker such as propranolol or esmolol is given concurrently to counteract the increase in cardiac contractility that can occur with nitroprusside. Repeat doses are given until the heart rate is in the range of 70 beats per minute. An alternative treatment is the use of calcium channel blockers such as diltiazem or nifedipine. These agents have the advantage of lowering both contractility and blood pressure.

2. Type A Dissections

Patients with type A dissections have a high early mortality and poor results with medical therapy. Surgery should be carried out immediately except for patients with severe strokes or advanced systemic disease without significant survival potential. The damaged part of the ascending aorta and the arch are replaced with a prosthetic graft. In many cases of aortic valve regurgitation, it is possible to repair the annulus and avoid the use of a prosthetic valve with its attendant complications and need for anticoagulation. Some patients require reimplantation of the coronary arteries. The 30-day mortality after ascending aortic replacement for acute dissection ranges from 5% to 27% (16). The mortality is greater in more complicated reconstructions, and Crawford and colleagues reported a 3% rate for ascending aorta replacement in contrast to 16% for resection of both the ascending aorta and the arch (17). Factors associated with operative mortality include older age, hypertension, coronary artery disease, preoperative congestive heart failure, diabetes mellitus, postoperative renal failure, visceral ischemia, or reoperation for control of bleeding. Overall, surgical repair provides survival benefit. Of those patients discharged, 91% are alive at 1 year and 76% to 82% at 5 years (16).

3. Type B Dissections

Patients with uncomplicated descending aortic dissections are treated with the medical hypotensive protocol just described. Close observation and monitoring are required in the early phase of medical management. Frequent physical examination must include attention to status of peripheral pulses, heart auscultation, and neurological assessment. Daily chest films are indicated. Patients who remain stable with resolution of the presenting pain are weaned off intravenous drugs and given oral medications. Ongoing oral medical treatment has the same goals as were sought initially: reduction of cardiac contractility and control of blood pressure. Ideally, the systolic pressure should be kept below 120 mm Hg, but some elderly patients will not tolerate this level. It may be necessary to compromise and aim for between 130 and 140 mm Hg. The first line of treatment is the beta-adrenergic blockers, including atenolol, labetalol, metoprolol, and propranolol. A common alternative is to combine calcium channel blockers (diltiazem, nifedipine, verapamil) with one of the major antihypertensives (captopril, clonidine, lisinopril, methyldopa). (Hydralazine should be avoided because of concerns that its incorporation into the mucopolysaccharide of the aortic wall may produce further weakening.)

The patient should remain hospitalized until appropriate control with oral medications is confirmed. Before discharge, a repeat CT or magnetic resonsnce imaging (MRI) scan should be done to verify that no early progression of the dissection has occurred. In a combined series from Stanford and Duke Universities, Glower and colleagues found similar early outcomes resulted with medical or surgical treatment of patients with uncomplicated type B aortic dissections (18).

The medical management is abandoned in favor of operation for patients who have uncontrolled hypertension, especially if severe pain continues. Patients who have complications of aortic branch ischemia, including involvement of the brain, kidneys, intestines, or extremities, also need to be considered as surgical candidates. In this group early replacement of the descending aorta can eliminate the false lumen and re-establish perfusion, but some patients require adjunctive procedures including fenestration (removal of part of the septum separating the true and false lumens creating a common channel) and bypass grafting. Reported surgical mortality for repair of type B lesions ranges from 6% to 50%; however, reports with high fatalities include patients with complicated dissections (16).

Many centers with experience in surgery for this condition choose to perform early elective repairs on young, good-risk patients with type B dissections. This group commonly has Marfan's or Ehlers-Danlos syndrome as the cause and is considered to be at a higher risk for late complications developing, especially in view of greater projected longevity and lower incidence of other risk factors. An early elective operation offers a better risk/benefit ratio compared with a delayed urgent or emergency one.

D. Follow-up Management

A patient treated for any aortic dissection should never be considered cured. Close follow-up is needed initially to check on satisfactory control of blood pressure. A CT or MRI scan should be obtained at 3 and 6 months after the acute episode. If these remain unchanged, annual follow-up is appropriate. Because the entire aorta is at risk for further deterioration, the imaging studies should not be limited to the region of initial injury. An important warning sign is aneurysmal dilation, particularly of the weakened wall of the false channel. Aortic dilation greater than 6 cm in diameter is an indication for elective repair. A relative indication for late operation is loss of control of blood pressure either because of medical factors or patient noncompliance.

III. ARTERIAL EMBOLUS

A. Clinical Relevance

Embolization occurs when a piece of thrombus or atheromatous plaque breaks off and is carried distally in the arterial circulation until it becomes lodged, usually at a bifurcation. This condition is an important cause of mortality and morbidity, especially in the older population. A long-term study from the Massachusetts General Hospital reported a mean age of patients with emboli of 52 years in the period 1937 to 1953 and of 70 years between 1964 and 1980 (19). The source of emboli is the heart in 75% of cases: two-thirds of cardiac thrombi are associated with atrial fibrillation and one-third with acute myocardial infarction (20). Other sources of emboli include arterial aneurysms and plaques; the source is undetermined in 5% to 10% of patients. The size of the embolus determines the site of occlusion, but the extent of ischemia is affected as well by the extent of thrombosis, resulting not only in the main artery but also in the branch vessels. Most series report the site of embolic occlusion in the terminal aorta or below in 70% to 75% of cases. Incidence of emboli to other sites is approximately 10% each for the carotid arteries and upper extremities and 5% to visceral branches. (See Chapter 9 for a discussion of visceral emboli.)

B. Immediate Diagnostic Approach

Typically, the patient has a sudden onset of symptoms of acute ischemia, usually including most or all of the ''5 Ps'': pulselessness, pain, pallor, paresthesias, and paralysis. Presence of paralysis is an ominous sign, because it indicates a profound degree of ischemia. The diagnosis is made easier if the patient has had prior examinations documenting the presence of peripheral pulses. In carrying out the physical assessment, it is important to remember that a transmitted pulse may be palpated at the proximal limit of the thrombosis, especially in the first hours. The highest risk case is the saddle embolus, in which a large thrombus occludes the aortic bifurcation. The serious impact of this embolus is related to the simultaneous involvement of the pelvis and both legs. The critical part of both initial and follow-up examinations is the assessment of severity of ischemia. Pulse loss, an abnormal temperature gradient, distal pallor, and some element of pain or paresthesias are common to most patients, even when limb-threatening ischemia is not present. The pain is typically described as a steady, severe ache predominantly in the distal muscles. Preservation of light touch is a good index of viability. Alternatively, anesthesia and motor weakness indicate advanced ischemia; paralysis signals impending gangrene. The signs of irreversible injury include anesthesia, loss of voluntary contraction, muscle rigor, and absent capillary filling of the skin.

A competing differential diagnosis in the setting of acute ischemia is acute arterial thrombosis. This condition usually occurs in areas of pre-existing advanced atherosclerotic disease, and the patient has evidence of chronic arterial insufficiency (Table 2). The absence of trophic changes such as skin atrophy, loss of sweating, and nail deformity points to a lack of antecedent arterial insufficiency and favors the diagnosis of an embolus. Another differential diagnosis is aortic dissection, but this condition is usually accompanied by impressive chest or back pain, as discussed previously.

Initial confirmation of the level and extent of the thrombosis can be obtained noninvasively with a duplex scan; however, evaluation and initial treatment should not be delayed while the examination is obtained. A contrast angiogram can provide a clear picture of the anatomy proximal to the occlusion, but it may not be possible to define the distal vessels because of inadequate perfusion by way of the collateral vessels. Angiograms are not always obtained in the initial treatment of peripheral emboli. (See below)

C. Therapeutic Intervention

The first step in treatment is an intravenous bolus of heparin as soon as the diagnosis is considered. A common regimen is an initial dose of 10,000 units and a continuous infusion of 1000 to 1500 units per hour. Blaisdell and colleagues have recommended a higher dose of 20,000 units with a drip at 2000 to 4000 units per hour (21). The purpose of immediate heparin is to arrest the progression of thrombosis not only in the axial but also in the branch vessels. The protection of the branch vessels is essential to a good outcome because it is difficult to clear thrombus from these. Even though some patients with atrial fibrillation may be on a coumarin regimen, they should be given the same treatment with heparin. The further treatment of the embolic occlusion depends on the status of the extremity and the patient's overall condition. An important decision to be made is whether revascularization aimed at limb salvage should be attempted. A patient with a foot or leg that is clearly not viable should not be put through the added risks with hopeless attempts but should have a primary amputation.

Table 2 Differential Diagnosis of Acute Ischemia

	Embolus	Thrombosis
History of claudication	Rare	Usual
Atrial fibrillation	Usual	Less common
Contralateral pulses	Normal	Decreased or absent
Lower leg skin	Normal	Trophic changes

1. Surgical Embolectomy

The standard approach is the operative removal of the embolus and the resulting thrombus. In many cases, the surgeon may elect to proceed directly to the operating room without obtaining an arteriogram, because the study often adds little information to the obvious clinical manifestation. In some cases, the operation can be done with local anesthesia. Usually either the common femoral or the popliteal artery is exposed and a balloon catheter is used to extract the thromboembolus. In the case of aortic saddle embolus or an embolus to the iliac artery, the femoral artery approach can still be used. Once the thrombectomy is completed, the success of the procedure is assessed with an intraoperative angiogram. This allows confirmation that all the thrombus has been removed. If residual thrombus is demonstrated, repeated passes are made with the catheter with angiography for re-evaluation. One of the limitations of catheter embolectomy is that thrombosed side branches cannot be reopened. In some cases, in which treatment, has been delayed the large side branches or the runoff vessels in the calf remain occluded after optimal balloon thrombectomy. In such cases, intraoperative thrombolytic therapy can be attempted as an adjunct and often succeeds in opening the runoff vessels, allowing perfusion to the lower leg. Surgical treatment has the advantage of being completed rapidly with early restoration of flow. Recent studies have reported limb salvage rates in the order of 90% with a mortality of 10% (20).

Patients are at high risk of major complications in the early period after re-establishing perfusion. Many patients have had a recent myocardial infarction and are at risk from the related instabilities. Intraoperatively, cardiac problems may be aggravated by the potassium and acid load resulting from flushing stagnant blood out of a severely ischemic leg. This problem is reduced by establishing reperfusion slowly, but the risk of dysrhythmias and cardiac depression still exists. Two major problems must be anticipated in the early postoperative course: myoglobinemia and acute compartment syndrome. Patients with prolonged muscle ischemia will have cell necrosis with release of myoglobin. This complication must be anticipated, and urine must be frequently monitored for myoglobin. Prophylactic treatment includes inducing high diuresis (increased intravenous fluids together with diuretic administration) and alkalinization of urine to reduce the precipitation of myoglobin in the renal tubules. Compartment syndrome occurs most frequently in the lower leg and results from increased capillary leak caused by the ischemia injury. The external muscle fascia forms a unyielding envelope so that small increases in volume within the compartments cause considerable increase in pressure. This abnormal pressure can cause nerve damage and new episode of ischemia by interfering with arterial flow within the compartment. In some cases, a prophylactic fasciotomy is performed at the end of the thrombectomy. If this has not been done, careful, frequent examination of the lower leg is necessary. If a question of onset of abnormal pressure, exists, the pressure within the compartment should be measured. Any significant increase in pressure must be treated with immediate fasciotomy in an attempt to limit further injury.

2. Thrombolytic Therapy

In recent years, the use of urokinase or tissue plasminogen activator for the primary treatment of acute emboli has a greatly increased. The most effective method is to use a high dose of the drug infused directly through a multihole catheter embedded into the thrombus (22). A critical limitation is that thrombolytic (lytic) therapy requires considerably more time that operative thrombectomy. It is common to take 12 to 48 hours to re-establish direct flow in the axial artery. Consequently, this approach is contraindicated for patients with severe ischemia, as indicated by advanced neurological loss or motor weakness. It is necessary for the patient to be able to tolerate the prolonged treatment without risk of additional injury. Thrombolytic therapy carries additional complications of its own. One of the major concerns is bleeding from remote sites as a result of the systemic effect of the drug. Therefore, this mode of therapy is contraindicated for patients who have had a recent operation or have other sources of potential bleeding. An additional problem is that during therapy partial clot lysis may be achieved, permitting distal embolization of fragment. Although the complication can usually be treated by continued infusion, it may result in a longer period of treatment. Contraindications to lytic therapy include a history of gastrointestinal bleeding, intracardiac thrombus, recent myocardial infarction, recent stroke or neurosurgical operation, coagulation disorder, and severe hypertension. Overall, recent series have demonstrated limb salvage rates of the order of 80% with mortality around 5% (20).

The reperfusion that occurs with thrombolysis is more gradual, so that one does not usually encounter the acute problems of dysrhythmias or cardiac depression. Myoglobin problems and compartment syndrome are not as common with lytic therapy as after surgical thrombectomy, partly because patients with more severe symptoms do not undergo this treatment. Alternatively, either of these complications may develop in the patient undergoing lysis, and ongoing monitoring is important.

D. Follow-up Management

All patients are kept on heparin in the early postoperative period. Although there is a moderate increase in postoperative or post procedure hematoma, the practice has led to lower mortality and higher limb salvage (23). As a general rule, all patients who have sustained an arterial embolus should be started on coumarin and kept on chronic anticoagulation to reduce the risk of recurrence. A study from Henry Ford Hospital reported a 22% incidence of recurrent embolus at 5 years in patients on chronic anticoagulation compared with 38% for those not treated (24). In each patient, the risks and benefits of anticoagulation must be judged in deciding on long-term management.

In many patients, atrial fibrillation is the cause of the embolus. In the patient with regular rhythm and no evidence of recent myocardial infarction, it is still necessary to exclude the heart as a source of embolus. In the past, this was problematic because of inaccuracies of transthoracic echocardiography; however, TEE offers a better diagnostic tool. If the heart has been excluded as a likely source, it is necessary to seek aneurysms or atherosclerotic plaques as culprits. Screening can be carried out with CT or MRI scans, reserving contrast angiography to further examine abnormalities found on the former.

These three conditions, i.e., AAA, acute aortic dissection, and arterial embolus attack, the elderly patient at a higher rate than the balance of the population. Vascular disease is one area in which accurate assessment and early treatment are critical. The physician caring for the geriatric patient must alter the usual or ordinary order of differential diagnoses and the evaluation priorities if morbidity and mortality are to be reduced to a minimum.

REFERENCES

1. Bengtsson H, Bergqvist D, Ekberg O, Janzon L. A population based screening of abdominal aortic aneurysms (AAA). Europ J Vasc Surg 1991; 5:53–57.
2. Scott RAP, Ashton HA, Kay DN. Abdominal aortic aneurysm in 4237 screened patients: Prevalence, development and management over 6 years. Br J Surg 1991; 78:1122–1125.
3. Ernst CB. Abdominal aortic aneurysm. N Engl J Med 1993; 328:1167–1172.
4. Ingolby CJH, Wujanto R, Mitchell JE. Impact of vascular surgery on community mortality from ruptured aortic aneurysm. Br J Surg 1986; 73:551–553.
5. Johansen K, Kohler TR, Nicholls SC, Zierler RE, Clowes AW, Kazmers A. Ruptured abdominal aortic aneurysm: The Harborview experience. J Vasc Surg 1991; 13:240–247.
6. Weinbaum FI, Dubner S, Turner J, Pardes JG. The accuracy of computed tomography in the diagnosis of retroperitoneal blood in the presence of abdominal aortic aneurysm. J Vasc Surg 1987; 6:11–16.
7. Adam DJ, Bradbury AW, Stuart WP, Woodburn KR, Murie JA, Jenkins AM, Ruckley CV. The value of computed tomography in the assessment of suspected ruptured abdominal aortic aneurysm. J Vasc Surg 1998; 27:431–437.
8. Gloviczki P, Pairolero PC, Mucha P, Farnell MB, Hallett JW, Ilstrup DM, Toomey BJ, Weaver AL, Bower TC, Bouchier RG, et al. Ruptured abdominal aortic aneurysms: Repair should not be delayed. J Vasc Surg 1992; 15:851–859.

9. Szilagyi DE, Hageman JH, Smith RF, Elliott JP. Spinal cord damage in surgery of the abdominal aorta. Surgery 1978; 83:38–56.
10. Rohrer MJ, Cutler BS, Wheeler HB. Long-term survival and quality of life following ruptured abdominal aortic aneurysm. Arch Surg 1988; 123:1213–1217.
11. Hirst AE, Johns VJ, Kime SW. Dissecting aneurysm of the aorta: A review of 505 cases. Medicine 1958; 37:217–279.
12. Roberts WC. Aortic dissection: Anatomy, consequences and causes. Am Heart J 1981; 101:195–214.
13. Fann JI, Sarris GE, Mitchell RS, Shumway NE, Stinson EB, Oyer PE, Miller DC. Treatment of patients with aortic dissection presenting with peripheral vascular problems. Ann Surg 1990; 212:705–713.
14. Wheat MW. Intensive medical therapy. In: Doroghazi RM, Slater EE, eds. Aortic Dissection. New York: McGraw-Hill, 1983, pp 165–191.
15. Wheat MW, Palmer RF, Bartley TD, Seelman RC. Treatment of dissecting aneurysms of the aorta without surgery. J Thorac Cardiovasc Surg 1965; 50:364–373.
16. Fann JI, Miller DC. Aortic dissection. Ann Vasc Surg 1995; 9:311–323.
17. Crawford SE, Kirklin JW, Naftel DC, Svensson LG, Coselli JS, Safi HJ. Surgery for acute dissection of ascending aorta—Should the arch be included? J Thorac Cardiovasc Surg 1992; 104:46–59.
18. Glower DD, Fann JL, Speier RH, Morrison L, White WD, Smith LR, Rankin JS, Miller DC, Wolfe WG. Comparison of medical and surgical therapy for uncomplicated descending aortic dissection. Circulation 1990; 82 (suppl IV):IV-39–IV-46.
19. Abbott WM, Maloney RD, McCabe CC, Lee CE, Wirthlin LS. Arterial embolism: A 44 year perspective. Am J Surg 1982; 143:460–464.
20. Mills JL, Porter JM. Basic data related to clinical decision-making in acute limb ischemia. Ann Vasc Surg 1991; 5:96–98.
21. Blaisdell FW, Steele M, Allen RE. Management of acute lower extremity arterial ischemia due to embolism and thrombosis. Surgery 1978; 84:822–834.
22. McNamara TO, Bomberger RA, Merchant RF. Intra-arterial urokinase as the initial therapy for acutely ischemic lower limbs. Circulation 1991; 83 (suppl I):I-106–I-119.
23. Tawes RL, Beare JP, Scribner RG, Sydorak GR, Brown WH, Harris EJ. Value of postoperative heparin therapy in peripheral thromboembolism. Am J Surg 1983; 146: 213–215.
24. Elliott JP, Hageman JH, Szilagyi DE, Ramakrishnan V, Bravo JJ, Smith RF. Arterial embolization: Problems of source, multiplicity, recurrence and delayed treatment. Surgery 1980; 88:833–845.

11
Management of Shock

Merlyn M. Asuncion and Vidya S. Kaushik
Charles R. Drew University of Medicine and Science, and Martin Luther King, Jr.–Charles R. Drew Medical Center, Los Angeles, California

I. CLINICAL RELEVANCE

Although the elderly make up only 12% of the general population, approximately 50% of patients admitted to critical care units are patients aged 65 or older (1,2). Because of age-related diseases and certain biological changes that occur with aging, the elderly are at a higher risk for complications, mortality, and morbidity from shock. Table 1 lists many of the reported age-associated biological changes in the cardiovascular, pulmonary, and renal systems and their potential physiological and clinical impact. During periods of hypoperfusion, these age-associated changes will greatly influence the entire response, compensatory mechanisms, and recovery from a state of shock. With these pre-existing changes, the heart, lungs, kidneys, and other organs need only small changes in the perfusion pressure to adversely affect them. Thus, even minor and short duration of hypoperfusion and hypoxemia can precipitate hepatic or renal failure and cardiac or cerebral ischemia. With timely and vigorous institution of treatment, shock may be reversible. The elderly who have diminished cardiac, pulmonary, or renal reserves do not tolerate prolonged states of shock. Even when their vital signs are eventually restored, they can continue to have cellular decompensation (3). In one study 100% of traumatized elderly patients, who were hypotensive (systolic blood pressure <80 mm Hg) for just 15 minutes, died (3). To date, few studies and observations of outcomes of elderly patients admitted with shock have been reported.

Table 1 Organ Changes Caused by the Aging Process

Organ changes	Physiological or clinical effects
Cardiovascular system	
Atherosclerosis	Decreased compliance
Amyloid/collagen deposition	Decreased compliance
Left ventricular hypertrophy	Decreased compliance
Decreased heart rate	Limited compensatory reserve
Decreased beta-adrenergic receptor responsiveness	Limited compensatory reserve
Altered catecholamine response	Hypertension
Kidneys	
Decreased renal mass	
Sclerotic renal arteries	
Decreased glomerular filtration rate	Reduced clearance of drugs
Pulmonary system	
Stiff chest wall and lungs	Decreased vital capacity, increased FRC
Decreased FVC and FEV_1	Decreased Po_2

FVC, Forced vital capacity; FEV_1, forced expiratory volume in 1 minute; FRC, functional residual capacity; Po_2, partial pressure of oxygen.

II. IMMEDIATE DIAGNOSTIC APPROACH AND CLINICAL MANIFESTATIONS

Shock is present when the circulatory system fails to maintain adequate cellular perfusion and function because of significant impairment of blood flow to vital organs and tissues, leading to microcirculatory insufficiency (4). Shock is most often clinically evident when the systolic blood pressure is less than 90 mm Hg (or mean arterial pressure is <60 mm Hg), vasopressors are required to maintain systolic blood pressure >90 mm Hg, or evidence of end organ hypoperfusion (low urine output, altered mental status, cold/diaphoretic extremities) exists (5). The clinical manifestations of shock depend on its cause. Four varieties of shock exist: cardiogenic, distributive, obstructive, and hypovolemic (Table 2). Several symptoms and signs of shock in the elderly may differ from those in younger adults, depending on the presence or absence of underlying age-related organ changes (Table 3).

A. Cardiogenic Shock

From 1975 to 1988, the incidence and mortality of cardiogenic shock associated with acute myocardial infarction remained unchanged at 7.5% and 80%, respec-

Table 2 Types of Shock

Cardiogenic shock		
	Acute myocardial infarction	
	Ventricular tachycardia/fibrillation	
Distributive shock		
	Sepsis	
	Anaphylaxis	
	Neurogenic	
Obstructive shock		
	Cardiac tamponade	
	Pulmonary embolism	
	Aortic stenosis	
Hypovolemic shock		
	Hemorrhagic	
		Trauma
		Gastrointestinal bleeding
	Dehydration	
	Severe diarrhea/vomiting	
	Polyuria	
	Burns	

tively (6). In a recent trend analysis from the same community, it was noted that although the incidence of shock complicating myocardial infarction remained unchanged, a significant trend toward an increase in in-hospital survival in mid-to-late 1990s was seen (7). The most common presentation of cardiogenic shock is in the setting of an acute myocardial infarction with loss of 35% to 40% of functioning left ventricular myocardium (8). Reduced cardiac output and hypotension associated with loss of a large amount of functioning myocardium further aggravate ischemia and cell death and a vicious circle of events begins, resulting in a state of shock. Lactic acidosis induced by tissue hypoxia, which is more

Table 3 Atypical Manifestations of Shock in the Elderly

Altered mental status
Delirium
Bradycardia
Hypothermia
Tachypnea

manifest in the elderly, also depresses myocardial contractility. The location of the infarction, in most analysis, is not an independent predictor of the development of cardiogenic shock. Cardiogenic shock is seen more commonly with anterior infarctions because the amount of myocardium at risk is greater in occlusions of the left anterior descending artery. It occurs in inferior and right ventricular infarction because of insufficient left ventricular filling pressure (9). Cardiogenic shock resulting from myocardial infarction can also develop because of mechanical complications, such as ventricular septal defect, mitral regurgitation, and rupture of the free wall of the left ventricle. Mitral regurgitation occurs more frequently in inferoposterior infarctions, whereas ventricular septal defect develops with equal frequency in anterior and inferior infarctions. Rupture of the left ventricular free wall is found in 10% of fatal myocardial infarctions. It is more often observed in older hypertensive women, >60 years old, sustaining a first myocardial infarction and commonly occurs within 1 to 10 days after the acute event. Patients with dilated congestive cardiomyopathy may also terminally be seen in cardiogenic shock resulting from severe biventricular dysfunction. These patients have a history of chronic heart failure with four chamber dilation, S_3 and S_4 gallops, murmurs of mitral and tricuspid insufficiency, and signs of increased right and left ventricular filling pressures.

B. Distributive Shock

Sepsis associated with hypotension is the classical example of distributive shock. It is the most common cause of death in the intensive care unit, with an annual estimate of 200,000 cases (4). The most common sources of infection in community-dwelling older patients are the lungs and urinary tract. Septic shock is most commonly due to gram-negative bacteremia in 50% of cases, whereas gram-positive bacteremia causes shock in 25% of cases. Shock resulting from sepsis or endotoxemia is a syndrome of vascular collapse and multiple organ failure in response to bacterial products. It is characterized by the presence of hypotension (systolic blood pressure <90 mm Hg), low systemic vascular resistance, fever or hypothermia (>101°F or <97°F), tachycardia, tachypnea, positive blood culture or an obvious source of infection, leukocytosis, or ''left shift'' (high percentage of neutrophils and band neutrophils). The hypotension persists despite administration of adequate fluids and catecholamines to maintain systolic blood pressure to >90 mm Hg. The hypotension caused by sepsis is produced by the release of potent vasodilator agents in response to mediators of sepsis such as lipopolysaccharides, tumor necrosis factor, and other mediators. One such vasodilator substance is an endothelial-derived relaxing factor recently identified as nitric oxide. Other mediators such as anaphylatoxins C3a and C5a cause vasodilation, increased vascular permeability, and platelet and neutrophil aggregation.

Septic shock should be suspected in the elderly, manifesting with hypotension and symptoms and signs of decreased tissue perfusion in the absence of other causes of shock, with or without overt evidence of infection. The patient may have symptoms from the primary source of infection such as pneumonia, pyelonephritis, cellulitis, or intra-abdominal infections. Alternatively, elderly, debilitated, and immunocompromised patients may not show localizing signs. A careful history and physical examination and directed laboratory tests are the most important tools to investigate the source of infection. (See also Chapter 18.) The elderly may have respiratory alkalosis develop caused by tachypnea or lactic acidosis; thus, serum electrolytes and arterial blood gas determination should be done. Blood cultures confirm the presence of sepsis when invading pathogens are isolated; however, positive blood cultures are seen in less than 50% of cases. The elderly who are initially seen with sepsis must be aggressively treated for the infection before the onset of septic shock.

C. Obstructive Shock

Hypotension and circulatory insufficiency caused by vascular obstruction, such as cardiac tamponade, aortic stenosis, and pulmonary embolism, belong in this category of shock and must be suspected in the setting of cardiogenic shock. The most common form of obstructive shock is acute cardiac tamponade. Massive pulmonary embolism is also quite common in the hospitalized elderly patient. As in younger patients, the clinical manifestations of pulmonary embolism are varied and nonspecific. When the index of clinical suspicion for the presence of pulmonary embolism is high, it should be investigated. It must be considered in patients who are immobilized or bed-bound; have underlying malignancy, congestive heart failure, or hypercoagulable states; or have shortness of breath, nonspecific chest pains, agitation, tachycardia, or hypoxemia develop postoperatively, especially after hip and knee surgeries. The clinical manifestations, course, outcome, and treatment have not been extensively reported in the elderly. Siddique et al. conducted an extensive analysis of elderly patients with a primary or secondary discharge diagnosis of pulmonary embolism from 1984 to 1991 (10). The median age of this population was 73 years for men and 76 years for women. The case fatality rate of primary pulmonary embolism was higher in men (13.7%) than women (12.8%), and among blacks (16%) compared with whites (12.9%). Secondary pulmonary embolism had a similar case-fatality rate in both gender and race. The mortality significantly increased with advancing age, with higher rates in the older elderly (i.e., those older than 85).

Shock resulting from massive pulmonary embolism in the elderly is difficult to diagnose. Rapid assessments include acid-base and arterial oxygenation status, chest radiography (mainly to exclude parenchymal or alveolar lung abnormality), and electrocardiogram (primarily to exclude massive acute myocardial infarction because the changes caused by pulmonary embolism are nonspecific tachycardia or may be more characteristic of sudden right axis deviation). Ventilation-perfusion scan and, lately, spiral computed tomographic (CT) studies can be done after stabilizing the patient's hemodynamic status. In the unstable patient, a bedside transesophageal echocardiogram can be done. Some studies have reported a high specificity of transesophageal echocardiogram in determining the presence of massive pulmonary embolus or right ventricular dysfunction (11). The inclusion of massive pulmonary embolism as the cause of shock is of paramount importance because emergency institution of surgical embolectomy or thrombolytic treatment must be quickly decided.

Aortic stenosis has a chronic progressive natural course in which the patient has a history of angina, syncopal attacks, or congestive heart failure. It is recognized by its characteristic physical findings of carotid shudder, delayed and low volume pulse (pulsus parvus et tardus), and systolic ejection murmur at the apex and second right intercostal space with radiation to the carotid vessels. Systolic click, best heard at the apex, is rare in elderly patients with valvular aortic stenosis. Even the pathognomonic slowly rising carotid pulse may be masked by the sclerosed inelastic carotid vessels in the elderly. Systolic murmurs along the parasternal area caused by aortic sclerosis are far more common in the elderly and must be differentiated from hemodynamically significant aortic stenosis. Echo-Doppler study is helpful in the diagnosis and assessment of severity of stenosis. Shock caused by aortic stenosis is rare. It may follow the injudicious use of diuretics or aggressive vasodilators to treat the congestive heart failure. When recognized early, critical aortic stenosis should be managed surgically in all otherwise functional elderly patients.

Shock resulting from acute cardiac tamponade is caused by sudden impairment of diastolic ventricular filling from pericardial compression. Slow accumulation of large pericardial effusions caused by malignancies can cause clinical findings of cardiac tamponade but rarely shock, whereas rapid accumulation of small amounts of pericardial fluid can cause hemodynamic collapse and shock. Patients complain of shortness of breath, may have altered level of consciousness, and have distended jugular veins, hypotension, and pulsus paradoxus. Electrocardiograms may show electrical alternans and low QRS voltage. Chest radiographic studies may demonstrate enlarged cardiac silhouette with a "bottle-neck" sign when the effusion is large, but this is not observed with small pericardial effusions. When cardiac tamponade is suspected, a transthoracic echocardiogram should be done immediately to measure the amount of effusion and observe tamponade changes such as collapse of the right ventricle during diastole.

D. Hypovolemic Shock

Sudden reduction in the circulating blood volume by about 20% will result in decreased cardiac output and hypotension. Loss of more than 40% of the circulating blood volume will result in profound hypotension. The elderly, because of physiological changes as a result of the aging process, may respond differently. The expected tachycardia caused by reflex sympathetic stimulation is abrogated. Thus, the tachycardia seen in younger patients as a result of loss of blood or circulating blood volume may not be observed in the elderly. This inability to hemodynamically compensate for the loss of plasma volume leads to decreased blood pressure and cardiac output. The ischemia from an underlying coronary disease may be aggravated by the reduced blood volume and coronary perfusion. Common causes of sudden loss of volume in older persons are gastrointestinal bleeding, severe diarrhea and vomiting, external losses caused by burns, or redistribution of body fluids. Thirty percent of intensive care unit admissions are elderly patients with acute gastrointestinal bleeding. (See also Chapter 19.) They are at an increased risk for mortality and morbidity. Patients with hypovolemic shock may have dizziness, body weakness, syncope, falls, angina, shortness of breath, altered consciousness, delirium, or cognitive impairment.

III. THERAPEUTIC INTERVENTION

A. General Management of Shock

In general, managing patients in shock state requires quick assessment of vital signs and the possible cause of the shock. Initial and serial measurements of blood pressure, heart rate, respiratory rate, gas exchange, tissue perfusion, and end-organ functions must be done. Laboratory determination for complete blood count, serum electrolytes, renal function, liver function, and random blood sugar, as well as an electrocardiogram, arterial blood gas tests, and a chest radiograph should be done initially. Assessment of airways and oxygenation can be quickly undertaken to determine the need for endotracheal intubation. If active bleeding from the gastrointestinal tract is present, a blood sample for typing and cross-matching must be quickly sent to the laboratory. While assessment and procedures are being undertaken, the circulating plasma volume should be maintained. Fluid resuscitation can be initiated with either colloid or crystalloids to maintain euvolemia. In the absence of invasive hemodynamic monitoring, such as Swan-Ganz (pulmonary artery) catheter monitoring, the patient's response to initial fluid resuscitation can be assessed by vital signs; bedside parameters such as level of sensorium, urinary output, and skin temperature; and acid-base status. Intravenous fluids are infused generously but cautiously to raise the systolic blood pressure to about 90 to 100 mm Hg. The development of shortness of breath, rales, or distended neck veins can give bedside clues to overhydration. If blood pressure fails to rise after infusion of approximately 2 L of intravenous fluids, vasopressors should be started, either dopamine, levophed, or phenyleprine. Additional interventions then will depend on the cause of the shock. Further diagnostic and therapeutic interventions are best continued in the intensive care unit.

Intra-arterial pressure monitoring for continuous blood pressure determination is ideal. Patients in shock unresponsive to initial fluid resuscitation, especially with alteration of mental status, should be considered for endotracheal intubation and ventilation support. Those with massive upper gastrointestinal bleeding must be considered, likewise, for intubation to protect the airways. Because of their unpredictable response to the shocked state, fluid replacement, vasopressors, and inotropic agents, it is conceivable that hemodynamic monitoring would be most valuable, both for diagnostic and therapeutic maneuvers, in the elderly. However, routine use of pulmonary artery balloon flotation catheters for hemodynamic monitoring has been challenged by several reports recently. Prospective, randomized study or even observational studies on the outcome of using hemodynamic monitoring in the management of these patients is lacking. Concern exists about the cost-effective use of medical resources and the increasingly widespread use of the pulmonary catheter (12,13).

B. Specific Shock Management

1. Cardiogenic Shock

The presence of hypovolemia must be considered when hypotension and evidence of diminished perfusion are noted in a patient with acute myocardial infarction. (See also Chapter 12.) It is easily treatable and carries a much better prognosis than other varieties of cardiogenic shock. If no clinical evidence of congestive heart failure such as distended neck veins, S_3 gallop, or pulmonary rales is present, judicious infusion of intravenous fluid (crystalloids or colloids) should be tried. The older patient responds differently to volume replacement and may not tolerate rapid infusion of intravenous fluids. Despite the controversy (as stated earlier), hemodynamic monitoring with the pulmonary artery balloon flotation catheter may assist in guiding the clinicians toward achieving adequate plasma volume and minimize the risk of iatrogenic pulmonary edema. Typically patients in hypovolemic shock have low cardiac output and low pulmonary capillary wedge pressure. Intravenous fluid administration should aim to maintain the left ventricular filling pressure in the range of 15 to 18 mm Hg and a cardiac index >2.2 L/min/m^2 (14). If the blood pressure remains low despite adequate hydration, vasopressor or inotropic agents should be started. In the patients who have cardiogenic shock develop as a result of a large infarct, therapy is directed to salvage the viable but nonfunctioning myocardium (stunned myocardium). Early reperfusion with primary angioplasty of the infarct-related coronary artery is probably the best approach at this time (5,15–17). A few large multicenter randomized controlled studies are in progress, which should yield definitive answers to the validity of interventional strategies. Noninterventional therapy includes thrombolytic therapy, low-dose dopamine drip to maintain adequate perfusion pressure, and, if feasible, vasodilator therapy with nitroprusside infusion to reduce preload and afterload. Intraaortic balloon counterpulsation (IABP) is an effective short-term stabilization treatment and, if needed, can be combined with vasopressor or vasodilator therapy. Use of floppy, flexible guide wires and newer smaller diameter catheters facilitates successful insertion of the balloon in elderly patients with highly tortuous vessels. With IABP, deflation of balloon in systole reduces the impedance to left ventricular emptying (afterload), and balloon inflation in diastole increases central aortic diastolic pressure, which augments coronary perfusion. Thus, IABP provides both systolic and diastolic advantages to the supply-demand discrepancy in the ischemic myocardium. It is particularly useful in cardiogenic shock resulting from potentially reversible mechanical complications such as ruptured ventricular septum or acute mitral regurgitation. In a study of 20 patients with acute myocardial infarction and cardiogenic shock with a mean age of 62 years, the use of IABP showed favorable initial clinical and hemodynamic response. It stabilized the patients enough to safely perform angiography and undertake percutaneous transluminal coronary angioplasty (PTCA), coronary artery bypass graft (CABG), or surgical correction of the mechanical complication of the infarction (18). Four of the five patients with mechanical complications had long-term survival (18).

Earlier reports on victims of acute myocardial infarction in shock showed lower mortality in patients after surgical revascularization compared with those who did not have surgery. More recent reports showed lower mortality rates among patients with myocardial infarction in shock who underwent early PTCA or CABG surgery (11,16). The practice trend in the management of elderly patients with acute myocardial infarction complicated by cardiogenic shock appears to be changing. In the Canadian retrospective study of both older and younger victims of acute myocardial infarction from 1989 to 1995, the use of cardiac catheterization, interventional procedures, and IABP was significantly increased in all age groups. The in-hospital survival of these patients was also significantly increased (17).

2. Distributive Shock

Treatment of septic shock is directed toward the eradication of the offending organism with appropriate antimicrobials or surgical drainage of abscesses or necrotizing tissues. Because the mortality of sepsis and septic shock in the elderly is >50%, it must be treated aggressively. After obtaining blood and other body fluid cultures, broad-spectrum antibiotics should be started immediately. Effective circulating plasma volume should be maintained with intravenous fluids, blood products, and vasopressor agents as needed. Adequate oxygenation with supplemental oxygen or ventilator support is essential. Careful monitoring of all system functions is mandatory because multiorgan system failure portends a poor prognosis. The onset of adult respiratory distress syndrome as a component of the sepsis further increases mortality. Sepsis is commonly associated with cardiovascular dysfunction despite initial elevated cardiac output and systemic vascular resistance. Because of these changes in the cardiovascular system, the elderly may benefit from the use of pulmonary balloon catheters for measurement of hemodynamic parameters and as a guide in titrating fluid replacement and use of vasopressor and inotropic agents.

Treatment emphasis must be on restoring mean blood pressure to greater than 65 mm Hg. Aggressive administration of volume should be followed by vasopressor agents such as dopamine if no improvement of blood pressure occurred with volume replacement alone. If the systolic pressure remains low with dopamine, norepinephrine should be added. Because of the association of myocardial depression with sepsis, some clinicians prefer to use inotropic agents such as dobutamine to maintain a cardiac index of greater than 4 L/min/m^2. Large, controlled trials on the use of polyclonal antisera and monoclonal antibody against endotoxins reveal improved survival in some subgroups. The role of this treatment in the elderly is not known. A recent study of patients with septic shock showed an inappropriately low level of plasma vasopressin in patients with advanced disease. A dose of exogenous vasopressin resulted in marked pressor response in these patients, which may indicate that low levels of the hormone contributes to vasodilation in sepsis (19).

3. Obstructive Shock

When symptoms and signs of cardiac tamponade are evident and the presence of significant pericardial fluid or blood is shown on echocardiographic studies, immediate pericardiocentesis must be performed.

Shock caused by pulmonary embolism usually occurs when a massive embolism is present. Hypotension should be managed first with intravenous fluid resuscitation followed by vasopressors as needed. As mentioned earlier, the presence of massive embolism must be confirmed with spiral CT scanning or transesophageal echocardiogram (20,21). Once pulmonary embolism is clinically suspected, heparin therapy should be started if no contraindications exist. Dalen et al. reviewed several studies on pulmonary embolism and compared the results of heparin or thrombolysis use. They found that the resolution of the embolus within 24 hours was more rapid with recombinant tissue plasminogen activator (r-TPA) than heparin. However, the clot resolution after 1 month was the same with heparin and r-TPA (22). Because of the bleeding risk associated with thrombolysis, it is recommended that thrombolytic therapy be given only to patients in shock with massive pulmonary embolism (23). Standard treatment for massive pulmonary embolism has been surgical embolectomy and lately it has been thrombolytic therapy, if there are no contraindications. Mikkola et al. reviewed

312 cases of pulmonary embolism and compared the complications of therapy between the older and younger patients. There was a fourfold increase in bleeding among older patients (70 years old and older) compared with younger patients (mean age of 62 years) (23). In a smaller study of 26 elderly patients (75 years old and older) and 28 younger patients with massive pulmonary embolism treated with thrombolytic therapy, Gisselbrecht et al. found no difference in the clinical presentation and tolerance between the two groups and suggested that provided there are no contraindications, old age should not preclude the use of thrombolytic therapy (24). Ohteki et al. reported prompt, noninvasive diagnosis in three cases of massive pulmonary embolism with transesophageal echocardiography. All three patients underwent successful emergency embolectomy under support of percutaneous cardiopulmonary bypass (25).

4. Hypovolemic Shock

The treatment of hypovolemic shock depends on the cause. As stated earlier, paramount to the treatment is volume resuscitation. Blood transfusion should be given for hypovolemia resulting from blood loss. As is true in the other states of shock, metabolic acidosis caused by lactic acidemia should be corrected accordingly.

IV. FOLLOW-UP MANAGEMENT

Once the vital signs are stabilized, further diagnostic special studies or therapeutic interventions can be undertaken.

A. Adequate Oxygenation

In shocked state, peripheral oxygen delivery is impaired. In nonintubated patients, Venturi masks provide sufficient oxygenation to achieve oxygen saturation equal to or greater than 90%. In cardiogenic, septic, or obstructive shock, the older patient may not be able to obtain adequate oxygenation or protect the airways, thus endotracheal intubation is indicated. Monitoring of adequate oxygenation can be followed by the use of transcutaneous pulse oximetry, but it is recommended that arterial blood gas analysis be done intermittently because peripheral vasoconstriction may not reflect the true status of oxygen delivery.

B. Acid-Base Status

Shock causes decreased blood flow to vital tissues, leading to abnormal cellular metabolism and cell death. Irreversible shock results in multiorgan system failure.

Decreased perfusion to the kidneys leads to acute tubular necrosis. As peripheral organs fail, cellular metabolism is altered, leading to metabolic acidosis. This poses more problems to the elderly person who has already diminished reserves because of aging and more so in those elderly with existing cardiovascular diseases.

C. Cardiac Dysrhythmias

All forms of supraventricular and ventricular dysrhythmias can occur as a result of hypoxia, ischemia/infarction, and acid-base abnormalities. Management of these dysrhythmias is the same as in younger patients, except that lower doses of drugs are usually indicated. Type 1 antiarrhythmic agents, which prolong QT interval, are not as well tolerated by older patients (26). Life-threatening dysrhythmias, such as ventricular tachycardias with hemodynamic compromise or ventricular fibrillation, must be treated promptly with cardioversion or defibrillation. Atrioventricular (AV) conduction abnormalities are not uncommon in the elderly. Additional ischemic insults can precipitate advanced AV blocks and may require temporary or permanent pacing. Depending on the extent of infarction, such as extensive anterior wall infarction, conduction abnormalities can progress to complete heart block and thus will need ventricular pacemaker insertion.

D. Pulmonary Artery Balloon Flotation

The use of the pulmonary artery balloon flotation for hemodynamic monitoring has been challenged for the past 12 years. Also a substantial concern exists about the widespread use of this monitoring procedure and its cost-effectiveness (27). Some concerned investigators have commented that no evidence of benefit to the patient exists with regard to mortality or morbidity. Other concerns are the complications (though rare), such as dysrhythmias, infections, or rupture of the pulmonary artery. Concerns about the lack of understanding of the physicians and nurses regarding measurements and interpretation of hemodynamic parameters exist. The controversy continues. However, until a less invasive technique for differentiating cardiogenic from noncardiogenic pulmonary edema or measuring parameters such as the pulmonary capillary wedge pressure to guide the clinician in balancing fluid infusion and use of drugs, hemodynamic monitoring should be used if deemed necessary for clinical management decisions (13). As previously mentioned, in the elderly, with limited cardiopulmonary reserves, and probably with underlying occult coronary artery disease or left ventricular dysfunction, pulmonary artery pressure monitoring will be beneficial in selected critically ill nonterminal cases.

E. Miscellaneous

The elderly patient in shock who is intubated will not be able to complain of pain. Pain is common in these patients. Narcotic medications for pain should be given cautiously in the elderly because they are more sensitive to their side effects. The metabolic requirement of the patient in shock should be met with adequate provision of nutrition. The intubated patient or patient with gastrointestinal hemorrhage should not have food withheld for longer than 72 hours. If enteral feeding is not possible, the nutritional needs can be met with parenteral hyperalimentation. Nutritional support is often overlooked in these patients and can be a source of problems for wound healing, tissue repair, and adequate muscle strength for weaning from ventilators.

REFERENCES

1. Campion EW, Mulley AG, Goldstein RL, Barnett OG, Thibault, GE. Medical intensive care for the elderly: A study of current use, costs and outcomes. JAMA 1981; 246:2052–2056.
2. Fedullo AJ, Swinburne AJ. Relationship of patient age to cost and survival in a medical ICU. Crit Care Med 1983; 11(3):155–159.
3. Oreskovich MR, Howard JD, Copass MK, Carrico CJ. Geriatric trauma injury patterns and outcomes. J Trauma 1984; 24:565–572.
4. Matthay M. Principles of managing the patient with hemodynamic insufficiency and shock. Chest Med 1995; 616:625–626.
5. Hockman JS, Boland J, Sleeper LA, Porway M, Brinker J, Col J, Jacobs A, Slater J, Miller D, Wasserman H, Menegus MA, Talley JD, McKinlay S, Sanborn T, LeJemtel T, The SHOCK Registry Investigators. Current spectrum of cardiogenic shock and effect of early revascularization on mortality: Results of an international registry. Circulation 1995; 91:873–881.
6. Goldberg RJ, Gore JM, Alpert JS, Osganian V, De Groot J, Bade J, Chen Z, Frid D, Dalen JE. Cardiogenic shock after acute myocardial infarction: incidence and mortality from a community-wide perspective, 1975 to 1988. N Engl J Med 1991; 325:1117–1122.
7. Goldberg RJ, Samad NA, Yarzebski J, Gurwitz J, Bigelow C, Gore JM. Temporal trends in cardiogenic shock complicating acute myocardial iinfarction. N Engl J Med 1999; 340:1162–1168.
8. Alonso DR, Scheidt S, Post M, Killip T. Pathophysiology of cardiogenic shock: Quantification of myocardial necrosis, clinical, pathologic and electrocardiographic correlations. Circulation 1973; 48:588–596.
9. Shah PK, Maddahi J, Berman DS, Pichler M, Swan HJ. Scintigraphically detected predominantly right ventricular dysfunction in acute myocardial infarction: Clinical, hemodynamic correlates and implications for therapy and prognosis. J Am Coll Cardiol 1985; 6:1264–1272.

10. Siddique RM, Siddique MI, Connors AF, Rim AA. Thirty-day case-fatality rates for pulmonary embolism in the elderly. Arch Intern Med 1996; 156:2343–2347.
11. Lee L, Erbel R, Brown TM, Laufer N, Meyer J, O'Neil WW. Multicenter registry of angioplasty therapy of cardiogenic shock: initial and long-term survival. J Am Coll Cardiol 1991; 17:599–603.
12. Naylor CD, Sibbald WJ, Sprung CL, Pinfold SP, Calvin JE, Cerra FB. Pulmonary artery catheterization: can there be an integrated strategy for guideline development and research promotion? JAMA 1993; 269:2407–2411.
13. Weil MH. The assault on the Swan-Ganz catheter: A case history of constrained technology, constrained bedside clinicians, and constrained monetary expenditures. Chest 1998; 113:1379–1386.
14. Forrester JS, Diamond G, Chatterjee K, Swan HJ. Medical therapy of acute myocardial infarction by application of hemodynamic subsets (Two parts). N Engl J Med 1976; 295:1356–1362; 1404–1413.
15. Emmerich K, Ulbricht LJ, Probst H, Krakau I, Hoffmeister T, Thale J, Gulker H. Cardiogenic shock in acute myocardial infarction. Improving survival rates by primary angioplasty. Zeitschrift fur Kardiologie 1995; 2:25–42.
16. Hibbard MD, Holmes DR, Bailey KR. Percutaneous transluminal coronary angioplasty in patients with cardiogenic shock. J Am Coll Cardiol 1992; 19:639–646.
17. Dzavik V, Burton JR, Kee C, Teo KK, Ignazewski A, Lucas AR, Tymchak WJ. Changing practice patterns in the management of acute myocardial infarction complicated by cardiogenic shock: elderly compared with younger patients. Can J Cardiol 1998; 14(7):923–930.
18. Fornaro G, Prando MD, Parodi F, Cordero G, Sansa M, Bongo AS, Campi A, Aralda D, Dellavesa P, Aina F, Lazzero M, Cernigliaro C. Short and intermediate term clinical outcome in patients with cardiogenic shock treated with aortic counterpulsation. Giornale Italiano di Cardiologia. 1996; 26(12):1385–1399.
19. Landry DW, Levin HR, Gallant EM, Ashton RC Jr, Seo S, D'Alessandro D, Oz MC, Oliver JA. Vasopressin deficiency contributes to the vasodilation of septic shock. Circulation 1997; 95:1122–1125.
20. Garg K, Welsh CH, Feyerabend AJ, Subber SW, Russ PD, Johnston RJ, Durham JD, Lynch DA. Pulmonary embolism: diagnosis with spiral CT and ventilation-perfusion scanning—correlation with pulmonary angiographic results or clinical outcome. Radiology 1998; 208(1):201–208.
21. Goldhaber SZ. Contemporary pulmonary embolism thrombolysis. Inter J Cardiol 1998; 65 (Suppl 1):S91–S93.
22. Dalen JE, Alpert JS, Hirsh J. Thrombolytic therapy for pulmonary embolism: Is it effective? Is it safe? When is it indicated? Arch Intern Med 1997; 157:2550–2556.
23. Mikkola KM, Patel SR, Parker JA, Grodstein F, Goldhaber SZ. Increasing age is a major risk factor for hemorrhagic complications after pulmonary embolism thrombolysis. Am Heart J 1997; 134(1):69–72.
24. Gisselbrecht M, Diehl JL, Meyer G, Sors H. Comparison of efficacy and tolerability of a thrombolytic treatment with r-TPA in acute massive pulmonary embolism in the elderly patients and patients under 75 years of age. Revue de Medecine Interne 1997; 18(7):521–527.

25. Ohteki H, Norita H, Sakai M, Narita Y. Emergency pulmonary embolectomy with percutaneous cardiopulmonary bypass. Ann Thorac Surg 1997; 63(6):1584–1586.
26. Aronow WS, Mercando AD, Epstein S, Kronzon I. Effect of quinidine or procainamide versus no antiarrhythmic drug on sudden death, total cardiac death and total death in elderly patients with heart disease and complex ventricular arrhythmias. Am J Cardiol 1990; 66:423–428.
27. Naylor CD, Sibbald WJ, Sprung CL, Pinfold SP, Calvin JE, Cerra FB. Pulmonary artery catheterization: can there be an integrated strategy for guideline development and research promotion? JAMA 1993; 269:2407–2411.

12
Cardiac Emergencies

Donald D. Tresch and Indu Poornima
Medical College of Wisconsin, Milwaukee, Wisconsin

Cardiovascular emergencies are common in elderly patients, which relates to the high prevalence of underlying cardiac disease in this age group. Not only are cardiovascular emergencies common, but associated morbidity and mortality are also high in these patients. A rapid and accurate diagnosis plus correct therapy are mandatory. The diagnosis, however, may be more challenging in older patients because of atypical presentations and the presence of concomitant diseases and aging changes that often mask the usual clinical findings. Emergency management will also be challenging in these elderly patients because of the presence and complexity of multiple disorders and aging changes that influence therapy.

Two common cardiac emergencies that are frequently encountered in elderly patients will be discussed: acute myocardial infarction (AMI) and acute cardiogenic pulmonary edema. Emphasis will be on the atypical presentations of these disorders in elderly patients and a practical approach to managing elderly patients with these cardiovascular emergencies will be presented.

I. ACUTE MYOCARDIAL INFARCTION

The incidence of AMI increases with age, as does associated morbidity and mortality (1–4). More than half of all AMIs occur in persons 65 or older, and one-third occur in persons older than 75. In-hospital mortality in AMI patients 70 or older is at least three times that of younger AMI patients, and 1-year and 2-year probability of survival has been reported to be as low as 60% and 50%, respectively, in patients 70 or older. In addition, such complications as heart failure, shock, and ventricular rupture are more common in elderly patients.

The reason for the high mortality and morbidity in elderly patients with AMI is multifactorial, with the increased prevalence of long-standing underlying cardiac disorders and left ventricular dysfunction being major factors. A difference in therapy between age groups, however, needs to be emphasized. Numerous studies have found that the therapeutic approach in elderly AMI patients is different than that in younger patients (5,6). Elderly AMI patients are less likely to receive interventional diagnostic procedures and therapies. In addition, beneficial drugs have been shown to be underused in this age group. Such underuse of therapy commonly occurs during the first few hours of hospitalization when therapies are so important in preventing myocardial damage and catastrophic complications, including death.

A. Clinical Manifestations

A quick correct diagnosis is mandatory when evaluating elderly patients who are suspected of having an AMI. The initial evaluation of an elderly AMI patient should be accomplished within 10 minutes of the patient's presentation. Evaluation should include a history, physical examination, and an electrocardiogram, which can be performed concurrently during the history taking. The clinical presentation of AMI, however, may be different and atypical in elderly patients compared with younger patients, and, too frequently, the diagnosis is delayed in elderly patients, which may significantly influence emergency therapy. In some elderly AMI patients the diagnosis will be completely overlooked. Studies have demonstrated that at least 25% of all AMIs are unrecognized (7,8). Either the patient may be without symptoms or the symptoms are unrecognized as an AMI by the patient or the patient's physician. The incidence of unrecognized MI increases with age, and as many as 60% of MIs may be unrecognized or silent in the very elderly.

In regard to history and risk factors, elderly AMI patients are more likely to be female and have a history of heart failure but are less likely than younger patients to have a family history of MI, elevated cholesterol, or smoking tobacco (9). Some studies have also found that a history of angina pectoris, previous MI, diabetes mellitus, and hypertension are more common in elderly AMI patients (10).

When present, symptoms in elderly AMI patients may be extremely vague. Numerous studies (11–15) have demonstrated the atypical presentation and wide variability of symptoms in elderly AMI patients (15) (Figure 1). These studies emphasize the importance of suspecting an AMI in elderly persons who experience unexplained behavior changes, acute signs of cerebral insufficiency, or dyspnea.

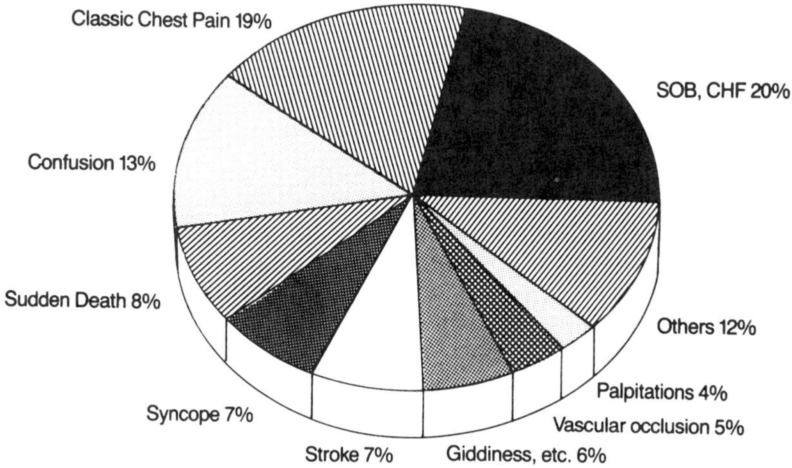

Figure 1 Chart illustrating the wide variability of symptoms in elderly AMI patients. SOB, shortness of breath; CHF, congestive heart failure. (From Ref. 15.)

Some studies have suggested that chest pain as the presenting symptom of an AMI decreases with age, whereas shortness of breath as the presenting symptoms increases with age (16–18). Paul and associates (16), in a study of 561 patients enrolled in the Myocardial Infarction Registry at Massachusetts General Hospital, found 80% of patients 65 or younger with AMI had chest pain compared with only 49% of patients 75 years or older. Bayer and associates (17) reported similar findings in a study of 777 patients 65 or older, who were hospitalized for an AMI in Cardiff, Wales. Chest pain was the presenting symptom of an AMI in 76% of the patients younger than age 70 but occurred in only 51% of the patients aged 80 to 84. Of the patients 85 or older, only 38% complained of chest pain as the presenting symptom of an AMI. Shortness of breath as presenting symptom, however, increased with age; only 37% of the patients younger than age 70 complained of shortness of breath compared with approximately 50% of patients between 80 and 84 years of age. In a prospective study of 145 older patients (mean age, 83 years) hospitalized during a 3-year period in a Geriatric University Hospital in Sweden, Wroblewski and associates (18) found only 20% of patients who had an AMI, diagnosed by autopsy findings, demonstrated chest pain at the onset of the acute infarction, whereas 70% complained of dyspnea.

The initial physical examination should be targeted to exclude disorders that can mimic AMI, including aortic dissection, acute pericarditis, spontaneous pneumothorax, acute pulmonary embolus, and peptic ulcer disease. In addition, the physical examination should assess for AMI complications, such as heart failure, ventricular rupture, hypotension, dyshythmias, and valvular insufficiency.

B. Immediate Diagnostic Evaluation

1. Electrocardiogram

As with the clinical presentation and physical examination, interpretation of the electrocardiogram (ECG) in elderly AMI patients may be more difficult than in younger AMI patients. Because of the high prevalence of underlying cardiac disorders, along with the presence of aging changes, the ECG in older AMI patients may demonstrate numerous abnormal findings such as left bundle branch block or ST-T wave changes, which will make the diagnosis of an AMI difficult. However, in most elderly AMI patients ECG findings will not only diagnose the AMI but will be helpful in assessing the size and extent of the AMI. Such an assessment is important in stratifying elderly AMI patients into low-risk and high-risk groups and in choosing appropriate therapy, such as thrombolysis or emergency percutaneous transluminal coronary angioplasty (PTCA). The amount of ST segment elevation, ST depression, and the number of leads in which these changes are present are all proportionate to infarct size: the higher the ST segment elevation, the deeper the ST depression, and the more leads involved, the larger the infarction (19). The presence of new bundle branch block and hemiblock are other electrocardiographic findings that are associated with increased complications, including high-grade atrioventricular (AV) block, heart failure, and increased mortality (20). Electrocardiographic findings of Q waves should not be used to exclude AMI patients from receiving thrombolytic therapy. It has been shown that Q waves do not reflect irreversible myocardial change, and significant myocardial salvage by thrombolysis or PTCA can occur in AMI patients with new pathological Q waves.

Interpretation of ECG V4R lead may be beneficial in recognizing high-risk elderly patients with acute inferior wall MI (21). ST segment elevation of 1 mm or more in lead V4R has a high sensitivity and specificity for detecting right ventricular infarction and identifies patients at high risk for AV block developing (21,22). The ST segment elevation in lead V4R usually disappears within 10 hours after the onset of AMI pain; therefore, it is important to assess the lead early during the elderly patient's evaluation.

2. Cardiac Enzymes

Typically, the biochemical markers of AMI, creatine kinase (CK-MB) isoenzymes, lactate dehydrogenase (LD-1) isoenzyme, and troponin T and I, are measured initially in all patients suspected of having an AMI and usually repeated at 3-hour intervals. Creatine kinase mass assay (isoform) is a sensitive and early direct marker of myocardial damage. Structural proteins, such as troponin T and troponin I, also detect early minimal myocardial damage and not only diagnose AMI but also enable risk stratification in patients with unstable angina. Myoglo-

Table 1 Biochemical Markers for Diagnosing Acute Myocardial Infarction

	Time to above URL (h)	Time to peak (h)	Time to normal	Sensitivity (%)	Specificity (%)
CK-MB	3–8	9–30	48–72	17–62	92–100
LD-1	10	24–48	10–14 days	—	—
Troponin T	2–6	10–24	10–15 days	50–59	74–96
Troponin I	2–6	12–24	7–10 days	6–44	93–99
Myoglobin	1–3	6–10	24–36	50–100	77–95

CK-MB, Creatine kinase, myocardial band; LD, lactate dehydrogenase; URL, upper reference limit.

bin is another sensitive, although nonspecific, early marker of myocardial injury. All these markers, with the exception of LD-1, will detect myocardial damage within 1 to 3 hours of onset of AMI (Table 1). LD-1 is a late marker of AMI and may not be elevated until later in the AMI patient's hospitalization. Creatine kinase isoform appears to have the best sensitivity, and its use in combination with the other markers provides the physician with a means for early detection of AMI; it is also helpful in estimating infarction size. However, none of the markers are 100% sensitive, and biochemical markers should not influence the initial therapeutic decision in elderly patients suspected of having an AMI.

C. Therapeutic Intervention

1. General Management

Initial general management of the elderly AMI patient should be to relieve discomfort and to treat complications, including hypotension, dysrhythmias, and heart failure. *Supplemental oxygen* is usually administered, although oxygen delivery will not be improved unless baseline oxygen saturation is less than 95%. *Intravenous morphine sulfate*, starting at 2 mg and titrating to higher dose, will usually relieve or reduce chest pain and decrease anxiety. *Nitroglycerin* will also be beneficial in reducing chest pain and can be administered sublingually, transdermally, or intravenously. In addition, myocardial oxygen demands are reduced with nitroglycerin, and some studies (23) have demonstrated survival improvement with the use of the drug. Nitroglycerin, however, may cause hypotension in elderly patients, especially in those who are hypovolemic or have a right ventricular infarction. Usually in these patients the hypotension is corrected quickly with the discontinuation of the drug or with increasing intravenous fluid.

Aspirin improves survival in AMI patients independent of other drugs (24), and, unless contraindicated, should be administered in all elderly patients who are suspected of having an AMI. A dose of 160 mg is recommended because higher dosage of 325 mg has not been shown to be more effective and may be associated with more complications. A nonenteric-coated preparation should be used, and the first dose should be chewed instead of swallowed to enhance rapid absorption.

2. Thrombolytic Therapy

Thrombolytic therapy with early perfusion of the acute myocardial infarcted area within 6 to 12 hours of infarction onset has been shown by all studies to reduce infarction size and improve survival (25–29). As in younger AMI patients, elderly AMI patients benefit from thrombolysis, and, from the standpoint of the number of lives saved, elderly patients may have the most to gain from the therapy (29,30). Pooled data from five major thrombolytic trials demonstrated an absolute reduction in mortality of 3.5% in the elderly (age 65 and older) compared with a 2.2% reduction in younger patients (Table 2) (30). Severe bleeding and strokes related to thrombolytic therapy have been reported to increase with age, although the absolute risk for both stroke and other major bleeding is less than 1% in elderly AMI patients (26,31,32). Therefore, on the basis of these favorable results immediate thrombolytic therapy should be considered in every elderly AMI patient unless contraindicated (Table 3). Minimizing delay of initiating thrombolytic therapy is paramount, and as soon as the ECG diagnosis is established,

Table 2 Mortality in Pooled Trials of Beta-Blocker[a] and Thrombolytic Therapy Use in AMI

		Mortality (%)				
	No. of patients	Therapy	Control	Difference	% Change	*P* Value
BB Therapy						
Younger	4687	2.5	2.6	−0.1	−5.0	NS
Older	8513	6.9	8.9	−2.1	−23.2	.0005
TT (early mortality)						
Younger	26,941	6.2	8.4	−2.2	−25.7	<.0001
Older	9984	17.2	20.7	−3.5	−16.9	<.0001
TT (late mortality)						
Younger	11,706	9.1	11.2	−2.0	−18.1	.0003
Older	6278	25.6	28.6	−3.0	−10.3	.009

AMI, Acute myocardial infarction; BB, beta-blocker; NS, not significant; TT, thrombolytic therapy.
[a] Pooled data from major trials. Younger age limit varied from ≤65 to <60 years old; older age range varied from ≥60 to 70, 66 to 75, and >75.
Source: Ref. 30.

Table 3 Contraindications to Use of Thrombolytic Therapy

Absolute	
	Active internal bleeding
	Recent head trauma
	Trauma or major surgery within 2 wk, especially head trauma
	Pregnancy
	Known bleeding disorder
	Severe persistent hypertension >200/120 mm Hg
	Aortic dissection
	CNS malignancy or AV malformation
	Previous hemorrhagic CVA
Relative	
	Altered consciousness
	Active peptic disease
	History of ischemia or embolic CVA
	Prolonged CPR

AV, Arteriovenous; CNS, central nervous system; CVA, cerebrovascular accident; CPR, cardiopulmonary resuscitation.

recombinant tissue plasminogen activator (r-TPA) should be administered by use of an accentuated weight-adjusted regimen consisting of an initial bolus of 15 mg, followed by 0.75 mg/kg over 30 minutes (not to exceed 50 mg) and 0.5 mg/kg over the next 60 minutes (not to exceed 35mg). *Intravenous heparin* should be given in conjunction with r-TPA to maintain the partial thromboplastin time (PTT) in range of 50 to 70 seconds for the first 6 to 8 hours. As previously mentioned, all AMI patients should receive aspirin regardless of thrombolytic therapy.

Despite the favorable results with thrombolytic therapy, it should be emphasized that elderly AMI patients are less likely to receive thrombolytic therapy than younger AMI patients. The decreased use of thrombolytic therapy is related to factors that need to be considered when managing elderly AMI patients, including (1) delay in seeking medical assistance, (2) atypical symptoms, (3) nondiagnostic ECG findings, (4) increased likelihood of contraindications to thrombolytic therapy, (5) high incidence of non-Q-wave MI, and (6) increased concerns about adverse side effects (bleeding and stroke).

3. Percutaneous Transluminal Coronary Angioplasty

The use of primary PTCA versus thrombolytic therapy is an important issue when managing elderly AMI patients. Most studies demonstrate that emergency PTCA can be performed successfully and safely in elderly AMI patients, including the very old (33,34), and is associated with better left ventricular function and fewer hemorrhagic strokes than thrombolysis (33–36). Some studies have reported emergency PTCA to be particularly beneficial in a high-risk subgroup of AMI patients, including the elderly and patients with large infarctions. Stone and associates (35) analyzed data from the Primary Angioplasty in Myocardial Infarction trial and found that in patients 65 or older, hospital mortality was reduced more with emergency PTCA than thrombolytic therapy (5.7% vs 1.5%, $P = .066$), and PTCA was associated with less intracranial hemorrhages and recurrent ischemic events. In a study of very elderly AMI patients (55 octogenarians), Laster and associates (36) reported an initial PTCA success of 96% and hospital mortality of 16% associated with emergency PTCA; no strokes occurred in these elderly patients. Other recent studies (37) have demonstrated emergency PTCA to be beneficial in elderly AMI patients with cardiogenic shock. The largest study (1138 patients) that compared emergent PTCA and thrombolysis in patients with AMI was the GUSTO IIB Trial (Global Use of Strategies to Open Occluded Coronary Arteries), which found no difference in mortality between the PTCA-treated or thrombolysis-treated groups (38). Although no difference in mortality was found between PTCA or thrombolysis in this study, the composite outcome of death, nonfatal reinfarction, and disabling stroke at 30 days was significantly reduced with primary PTCA compared with thrombolysis. In the 300 patients older than 70, mortality tended to be lower with PTCA, although the difference was not significant. The linear relationship between age and outcome was the same irrespective of whether the patient was treated with emergency PTCA or thrombolytic therapy.

The role of intracoronary stents in the managemnet of elderly AMI patients is uncertain. Studies have demonstrated that coronary stenting can be performed safely in elderly patients; however, further studies are necessary to assess the benefits in elderly AMI patients.

On the basis of this information it appears that primary PTCA can be beneficial in elderly AMI patients. In elderly AMI patients in whom thrombolysis is contraindicated and in high-risk elderly AMI patients with heart failure or shock, primary PTCA may be the best therapy. At this time, routine use of primary PTCA in elderly AMI patients needs to be individualized with consideration of the patient's risks and the experience and expertise of the physician and institution in performing emergency PTCA.

4. Beta-Blockers

Beta-blocker therapy has been shown to improve survival if administered early in the course of an AMI, and this benefit is more impressive in elderly AMI patients than younger AMI patients (Table 2) (30,39–41). Therefore, unless contraindicated, an intravenous beta-blocker should be administered emergently in all elderly AMI patients. Intravenous atenolol or metoprolol preparations are the two beta-blockers usually recommended for AMI patients. Ten milligrams of atenolol is given initially in two divided doses at 10-minute intervals, and 10 minutes after the last dose, 50 mg oral atenolol should be administered every 12 hours if no side effects occur. The recommended initial dose of intravenous metoprolol is 15 mg given in 5-mg increments at 2 minute intervals. Fifteen minutes after the last intravenous dose, 50 mg of oral metoprolol should be administered every 12 hours.

Contraindications to the use of intravenous beta-blockers are more common in elderly patients and include a history of asthma or of bronchospasm, moderate to severe heart failure, marked sinus bradycardia, prolong first-degree AV block (P-R interval $\geq$ 0.24 s) or higher level of AV block, or hypotension. Diabetes mellitus, peripheral vascular disease, chronic pulmonary disease without bronchospasm, or mild heart failure should not be considered a specific contraindication to use of beta-blocker therapy.

5. Angiotensin Converting Enzyme Inhibitors

Angiotensin converting enzyme (ACE) inhibitors administered within 24 hours of symptoms have been shown to be beneficial in certain AMI patients (42,43), and in some studies the benefits have been especially impressive in older AMI patients (43). The Survival of Myocardial Infarction Long-Term Evaluation study demonstrated a 34% reduction in the incidence of death or severe heart failure in AMI patients randomized to receive zofepril within the first 24 hours after onset of symptoms compared with patients given placebo; the benefits were approximately three times greater in patients aged 65 and older (43). In contrast to these favorable results, in one early study, the Cooperative New Scandinavian European Survival Study (44), a higher frequency of adverse outcomes was found in AMI patients receiving intravenous enalapril within 24 hours of hospital admission compared with AMI patients treated with placebo. Numerous other studies (45–47), however, have demonstrated the value of ACE inhibitors in MI patients with significant left ventricular dysfunction as determined by left ventricular ejection fraction (LVEF < 40% or heart failure), although in these studies the drug was usually given 3 to 16 days after onset of AMI.

On the basis of the findings of numerous studies assessing benefits of ACE inhibitors in a setting of AMI, early administration of an ACE inhibitor is recommended in hemodynamically stable elderly patients with a clinical large anterior wall MI and elderly AMI patients with heart failure or with LVEF of <40% regardless of the location of the AMI (48).

6. Heparin

Intravenous heparin is recommended in elderly patients who are suspected to have acute non-Q-wave MI or high-risk unstable angina. The drug is also recommended in conjunction with r-TPA. The recommended initial dose is a bolus of 80 units/kg (body weight) titrated to an activated PTT of two to three times control. Risk factors for bleeding resulting from heparin therapy include advanced age, female sex, hypertension with systolic blood pressure greater than 180 mm Hg, and patients with lower body weight.

7. Calcium Channel Blockers

Calcium channel blockers, in general, have not been shown to be beneficial in patients with AMI, and some studies have shown the drugs to be detrimental (49,50). In one small study 60 to 90 mg diltiazem administered 24 to 72 hours after admission was found to reduce reinfarction rate in patients with non-Q-wave MI, although the drug had no effect on mortality (51). In a study of Q-wave MI, diltiazem had no significant effect on mortality or recurrent MI; however, in patients with pulmonary congestion or a LVEF <40%, diltiazem caused an increase in new cardiac events (52). The American College of Cardiology/American Heart Association guidelines state that no Class I indications exist for the use of calcium channel blockers after MI (48).

8. Magnesium

Intravenous magnesium has been considered by certain studies to be an effective therapy in AMI patients (53). The International Study of Infarct Survival (ISIS-4 Study) (54), however, failed to show any benefit with magnesium other than to replete a demonstrated deficiency. Therefore, the routine use of intravenous magnesium in elderly AMI patients is not recommended (48).

9. Non-Q-Wave Myocardial Infarction

Non-Q-wave MI increases with age and accounts for greater than 40% to 50% of all MI in the elderly (55,56). Although in-hospital mortality and complications are less in non-Q-wave MI patients than in patients with Q-wave MI, morbidity and mortality rates in elderly patients with non-Q-wave MI are still high. And, as in Q-wave MI, mortality is significantly higher in non-Q-wave elderly patients compared with younger patients. Chung and associates (57) reported a 10% hospital mortality in patients older than 70 years of age with non-Q-wave MI compared with 3% in younger patients; the 1-year mortality was 36% in the older patients versus 16% in younger patients. Elderly patients with non-Q-wave MI also had significant ischemic events and reinfarctions during the first and second year after the AMI, and 1-year mortality was similar between elderly patients with non-Q-wave and Q-wave infarctions.

In reference to management of elderly patients with non-Q-wave MI, diltiazem has been shown to reduce early reinfarction rate, although the drug is contraindicated in patients with poor left ventricular function (51). Beta-blockers are also beneficial, as are aspirin and heparin. Recently, studies of the new platelet GP11b/111a blockage drugs have demonstrated impressive benefits in reduction of recurrent coronary events, including death, in patients with non-Q-wave MI, and these benefits have been as impressive in elderly patients as in younger patients (58,59).

Thrombolytic therapy is not recommended in non-Q-wave MI patients because studies have failed to demonstrate any reduction of reinfarction or death with use of this therapy in this setting (60,61). Similarly, routine emergency coronary angiography and interventional therapy (i.e., PTCA or CABG have not been shown to be beneficial in non-Q-wave MI patients) (62). Therefore, emergency coronary angiography and interventional therapy should be performed only in elderly non-Q-wave MI patients whose chest pain cannot be controlled with medical therapy or who are hemodynamically unstable.

10. Complications

(a). Ventricular Dysrhythmias. Cardiac dysrhythmias are common in elderly patients with AMI. Most elderly AMI patients will demonstrate a cardiac rhythm abnormality within the first 24 hours of onset of AMI, including tachyarrhythmias and conduction disturbances (63). The incidence (4.5%) of serious dysrhythmias such as ventricular fibrillation (VF) is greatest in the first hour of an AMI and declines rapidly thereafter (62). Elderly AMI patients are especially at increased risk for supraventricular tachycardia, including atrial fibrillation, and for conduction disturbances, such as bundle branch block and high-grade AV block. The incidence of ventricular tachycardia (VT), however, is similar in elderly and younger AMI patients, and primary VF is considered to occur less frequently in elderly AMI patients.

In the past, ventricular ectopy (more than 5 premature ventricular contractions [PVC], multiform PVCs, repetitive patterns in the form of couplets or salvos, and nonsustained ventricular tachycardia [NSVT]) was considered a predictor of VF, and intravenous lidocaine was recommended. It has now been shown that ventricular ectopy is not a reliable predictor of VF and suppression of PVCs with lidocaine does not improve survival (64); some studies have even reported an increased incidence of fatal bradycardia or asystole with the use of the drug (65,66). Therefore, prophylactic use of lidocaine is not recommended in elderly AMI patients. Instead, therapy should be directed at correcting metabolic and electrolyte abnormalities and suppression of ongoing myocardial ischemia.

Sustained VT is defined as consecutive PVCs at a rate greater than 110 beats/min and lasting longer than 30 seconds or causing hemodynamic compromise. Sustained VT associated with an AMI is a predictor of high hospital mortality and requires antiarrhythmic drug therapy (67). If sustained VT is associated with sustained hemodynamic effects, emergency direct-current (DC) cardioversion is necessary. If the dysrhythmia is hemodynamically well tolerated by the patient, antiarrhythmic drug therapy may be attempted. Usually, intravenous lidocaine is the first antiarrhythmic drug used; if lidocaine is ineffective, intravenous procainamide or amiodarone can be used (Table 4).

Primary VF occurs early in the setting of AMI, with 60% of episodes occuring within 4 hours of onset (68). Secondary VF occurs later, usually 48 hours after onset of AMI, and often occurs in conjunction with pump failure or cardiogenic shock (69,70). In this setting, secondary VF has been associated with an in-hospital mortality of 40% to 60% (70).

Treatment of VF is emergency unsynchronized electrical cardioversion with at least 200 to 300 J. Successful conversion of VF and patient survival are time dependent; the likelihood for survival decreases 10% for each minute of time after onset of uncorrected VF (71). If DC shock is unsuccessful in converting

Table 4 Drug Therapy for Ventricular Tachycardia in Acute Myocardial Infarction

Agent	Dose	Comments
Lidocaine (IV)	Initial IV bolus of 1.5 mg/kg (75–100 mg), followed by repeat dose every 5–10 min to maximum dose of 3 mg/kg. Maintenance dose of 4 mg/min	CNS side effects more common in elderly patients; reduction of dose necessary in patients with liver dysfucntion and in patients with heart failure
Procainamide (IV)	Loading dose of 12–17 mg/kg over 20–30 min, followed by maintenance dose of 1–4 mg/min. Alternative: 100 mg q 10 min to dose of 1.0 g, followed by maintenance dose of 1–4 mg/min	Monitor closely for hypotension and prolonged Q-T interval
Amiodarone (IV)	Loading dose of 150 mg in 10 min followed by perfusion of 1.0 mg/min up to 6.0 h, then maintenance dose of 0.5 mg/h	Monitor closely for bradycardia and AV block, hypotension, CNS effects, and liver abnormalities; increases digoxin, quinidine, and PT level

IV, intravenous; CNS, central nervous system; PT, prothrombin time; AV, atrioventricular.

VF, or if VF recurs after successful conversion, administration of lidocaine will be necessary.

Ventricular dysrhythmias, including PVC's and ventricular tachycardia, may occur after thrombolytic therapy in elderly AMI patients. Initially, these dysrhythmias were thought to be a reliable marker of successful myocardial reperfusion, although their specificity is low and it has now been shown that clinical findings, including dysrhythmias, are not reliably predictive of angiographically coronary artery patency (72). Ventricular dysrhythmias associated with thrombolytic therapy do not usually portend poor prognosis and should be managed as other ventricular dysrhythmias that occur in the setting of AMI.

(b). Supraventricular Dysrhythmias. Paroxysmal supraventricular tachycardia is an uncommon dysrhythmia in elderly AMI patients, although when present the rapid ventricular heart rate may produce increasing myocardial ischemia, and rapid correction of the dysrhythmia is necessary. Intravenous adenosine is the drug of choice for restoration of sinus rhythm in patients with paroxysmal supraventricular tachycardia because most of these tachyarrhythmias are related to AV nodal re-entry mechanism, which is abolished by AV node blockage with adenosine. Adenosine is also a drug with a very short half-life; therefore, any side effects quickly dissipate after a few seconds (73). The drug can be used safely in the setting of AMI if hypotension is not present. A dose of 6 mg given as a rapid intravenous injection should be initially administered and increased to 12 mg if there is no success with a 6-mg dose. If the patient is symptomatic or hypotensive, synchronized DC shock with an initial dose of 50 J should be performed after sedation of the patient. Intravenous beta-blockers or diltiazem are drugs that will slow ventricular heart rate and are acceptable alternative drugs if adenosine is not effective and if heart failure or hypotension is not present. The intravenous beta-blocker, esmolol, a drug with very short half-life, may be especially advantageous as the initial drug in that effects of the drug are quickly dissipated after discontinuing the drug. Digitalis may be beneficial in converting the supraventricular tachycardia and slowing the heart rate, although the drug is not recommended in the acute setting because of its delayed onset of action.

Atrial fibrillation occurs in approximately 10% to 15% of AMI patients and may occur in the first few hours of the onset of the AMI. The dyshythmia may be related to atrial infarction, pericarditis, electrolyte imbalance, drugs, or more commonly atrial enlargement caused by elevated ventricular diastolic pressure. In the setting of an AMI, atrial fibrillation is associated with increased mortality and stroke, particularly in elderly patients with anterior wall infarction (74).

Atrial fibrillation with rapid ventricular heart rate will increase myocardial oxygen demand and myocardial ischemia and impair left ventricular function. Therefore, early conversion of the dysrhythmia or rapid slowing of the heart rate is necessary in elderly AMI patients. If the elderly patient is experiencing new or increasing chest pain or is hypotensive or in heart failure, synchronized electrical conversion will be required. Electrical conversion voltage should be 100 J after the elderly patient is sedated, and the voltage should be gradually increased if the initial shock is unsuccessful. If conversion is not successful or not considered necessary, slowing of the heart rate will be essential. For elderly AMI patients who are not hemodynamically compromised, an intravenous beta-blocker that reduces sympathetic activity and relieves myocardial ischemia is the drug of choice. Intravenous esmolol should be used if any concern exists about the patient's ability to tolerate beta-blockade. Intravenous diltiazem or verapamil are effective alternatives that rapidly slow the ventricular rate in patients with atrial fibrillation; however, both drugs, because of their negative inotropic effect, should be used with caution in patients with heart failure or in patients with poor left ventricular function. Because of the increased risk of stroke with atrial fibrillation, intravenous heparin should be administered and later changed to warfarin, unless contraindicated. If warfarin is contraindicated, daily aspirin should be used.

(c). Bradycardias. Sinus bradycardia is the most common dysrhythmia associated with AMI. The dysrhythmia usually occurs early after onset of AMI and is particularly common in patients with acute inferior or posterior wall infarctions (75). Usually the dysrhythmia is benign, and specific therapy is not indicated unless symptoms or signs of cerebral hypoperfusion occur or if the patient is hemodynamically unstable. The dysrhythmia is commonly related to increased vagal tone and is easily corrected with intravenous atropine at doses of 0.5 to 1.0 mg. However, in elderly patients, repeated doses of atropine are often associated with serious side effects, including delirium; occasionally, atropine may aggravate sinus node slowing or produce tachycardia. Therefore, prophylactic atropine is not indicated in elderly AMI patients. If atropine is ineffective and the patient is hemodynamically unstable because of the bradycardia, temporary pacing is indicated.

Atrioventricular block is divided into first-, second-, and third-degree types. Electrocardiographic findings of first-degree AV block are a prolonged P-R interval with all P waves conducted; second-degree block has intermittent P waves not conducted to the ventricle and is divided into type I (Mobitz I or AV Wenckebach) and type II (Mobitz II). In third-degree AV block no conduction occurs between the atrium and the ventricle. First-degree AV block occurs in approximately 15% of AMI patients and, as with sinus bradycardia, is more common in inferior infarction (76). In general, the block is benign and no specific therapy is indicated.

In type I second-degree AV block (Wenckebach), the conduction is usually at the level of the AV node, and the nonconducted beat follows progressive lengthening of P-R interval, and the P-R interval before the nonconducted beat is longer than the P-R interval of the sinus impulse that follows the pause. Type I second-degree AV block occurs in 10% of patients with AMI and accounts for approximately 80% to 90% of all second-degree AV block associated with AMI. It usually occurs in inferior AMI, is usually transient, rarely progresses to third-degree AV block, and does not affect prognosis. Thus, type I second-degree AV block does not require treatment unless associated heart failure or hypotension is present. If treatment is necessary, intravenous atropine will usually be successful in resolving the block. Only in a few cases will the heart block persist and be associated with heart failure or hypotension, in which case temporary pacing will be necessary.

In contrast to type I second-degree AV block, in type II (Mobitz II) the block is located below the AV node and is characterized on electrocardiogram by a wide QRS with fixed P-R intervals before and after the nonconducted atrial beat. It is uncommon in association with AMI. When present, it occurs almost always with anterior MI, often progresses to third-degree AV block, and is associated with poor prognosis (77). The presence of type II second-degree AV block associated with AMI is an indication for immediate temporary pacing.

Third-degree AV block occurs in 5% to 15% of patients with AMI and is more common in patients with inferior AMI than in patients with anterior AMI. The significance and prognosis of the block depends on the location of the block and the size of the infarction. Third-degree AV block in patients with inferior AMI is usually located at or above the bundle of His, and the escape rhythm is stable with a heart rate usually exceeding 40 beats/min. The block usually responds to pharmacological intervention (atropine) and will resolve quickly, although in certain patients it may last for a few days (78). Associated mortality is significantly increased in the presence of co-existing right ventricular infarction. Temporary pacing will be necessary in hemodynamically unstable elderly AMI patients and in those elderly patients in whom the block persists for a prolonged period.

In elderly patients with anterior AMI, third-degree AV block usually denotes significant myocardial damage, and the block will be below the bundle of His, resulting in escape rhythms with rates less than 40 beats/min. The block may progress suddenly to asystole and is associated with high mortality rates (79). Immediate temporary pacing is required in elderly patients who demonstrate third-degree AV block associated with anterior wall MI. Besides second- and third-degree AV block, other indications for temporary pacing in the setting of AMI include certain intraventricular conduction disturbances (Table 5).

(d). Cardiac Arrest. The benefit of cardiopulmonary resuscitation (CPR) in elderly patients sustaining cardiac arrest is controversial. Some studies have reported poor outcomes in elderly patients, whereas other studies have found no significant difference in outcomes between age groups (80–84). Many studies

Table 5 Guidelines for Temporary Pacing in Acute Myocardial Infarction

ECG abnormality	Indication (yes or no)
First-degree AV block	No
Marked sinus bradycardia with unstable hemodynamics	Yes
Second-degree AV block	
Type I, asymptomatic	No
Type I, persistent, unstable hemodynamics	Yes
Type II, anterior wall MI	Yes
Alternating bundle branch block	Yes
RBBB with anterior or posterior hemiblock	Yes
LBBB with first-degree AV block or hemiblock	Yes
New RBBB with anterior MI	Yes[a]
Third-degree AV block	
Inferior wall, asymptomatic	No
Inferior wall, unstable hemodynamics	Yes
Anterior wall MI	Yes

AV, atrioventricular; LBBB, left bundle branch block; RBBB, right bundle branch block; ECG, electrocardiogram; MI, myocardial infarction.
[a] Relative indication.

have demonstrated that age alone is not the main determinant of CPR success. More important are the patient's prearrest comorbidity, the specific initial dysrhythmia, and the underlying cardiac disorder. Elderly patients who are functionally independent without multiple chronic illnesses are good candidates for CPR compared with frail nursing home residents; clinically, patients with VF as the initial dysrhythmia have the best chance of survival with CPR compared with patients with asystole or electrical mechanical dissociation. Elderly patients with an acute coronary disorder are more likely to benefit from CPR than elderly patients with such disorders as sepsis, renal disease, or cancer. Tresch and associates (85) recently reported a survival to hospital discharge rate of 39% in hospitalized patients 70 or older who received CPR and demonstrated VF as the initial documented dysrhythmia. Most of these patients were hospitalized for acute coronary artery syndromes, including AMI and unstable angina, and had their cardiac rhythm monitored at the time of their arrest. Functional status was excellent in the elderly survivors as was long-term survival, which was not significantly different from younger survivors.

On the basis of the findings of numerous studies that have shown patient's age alone is not the main determinant of success of CPR, it is recommended that all elderly AMI patients who have a cardiac arrest receive CPR with advanced cardiac life support (ACLS) guidelines unless a clear advance directive specifies that the patient does not want CPR institued.

(e). Right Ventricular Infarction. Approximately 25% to 30% of patients with acute inferior wall myocardial infarction (AIMI) will have right ventricular infarction (RVI) (86,87), and RVI is one of the strongest predictors of in-hospital complications and deaths in patients with AIMI. In a recent study of patients with AIMI, Bueno and associates (88) compared AIMI patients with and without RVI and found major complications including complete AV block and cardiogenic shock to be more common in patients with RVI (45% versus 19%, $P <$ .001) as was in-hospital mortality rate (22% vs 6%, $P < .001$). The incidence of RVI increased with age, and increasing age was directly associated with the in-hospital incidences of major complications and death. Because of this poor prognosis, elderly patients with AIMI and RVI are considered a high-risk group; it has been suggested that this is the group of AMI patients that would probably benefit most from reperfusion therapy.

Early diagnosis of RVI in elderly patients with AIMI is mandatory. Often RVI may be clinically silent, although a V4R electrocardiography lead is highly sensitive and specific for RVI. Therefore, interpretation of V4R lead is necessary in all elderly AIMI patients during their initial evaluation. The presence of ST-segment elevation in V4R not only makes the diagnosis of RVI but is also a powerful predictor of in-hospital death.

Elderly patients with AIMI and RVI may initially be seen with hypotension, and the physical examination will demonstrate right-sided heart failure, including elevated jugular venous pulsations with a positive Kussmaul's sign and right-sided cardiac gallop with clear lung fields. Associated complete AV block may be present. Echocardiography typically confirms the diagnosis with right ventricular dilation and related wall motion abnormalities. The diagnosis can be further confirmed with catheterization of the right side of the heart (Swan-Ganz monitoring) that demonstrates elevated right atrial and ventricular end-diastolic pressures with a normal or low pulmonary capillary wedge pressure and normal or low pulmonary artery pressures. On occasion, usually with an extensive RVI, the right-sided catheterization pressures may be confused with pericardial tamponade or constrictive pericarditis with equalization of diastolic filling pressures. An echocardiogram will quickly resolve the confusion.

Management of elderly AIMI patients with RVI and hemodynamic compromise consists of vigorous fluid administration to increase right ventricular output and maintain systemic blood pressure. Elderly patients who do not promptly respond to fluid therapy should undergo hemodynamic monitoring (Swan-Ganz). If systemic blood pressure and cardiac output do not improve after maximal volume infusion (pulmonary capillary wedge pressure between 15 and 20 mm Hg), inotropic support with dobutamine and dopamine should be initiated.

If complete AV block is present, temporary pacing will be necessary, preferably atriventricular sequential pacing.

(f). Myocardial Rupture. Three types of myocardial rupture are associated with AMI: (1) papillary muscle with acute mitral valvular regurgitation, (2) interventricular septum perforation (ventricular septal defect; VSD), and (3) ventricular free wall rupture. Although myocardial rupture is not a common complication in patients with AMI, the incidence increases with age and is associated with extremely high morbidity and mortality in this age group (89). Mortality rates as high as 50% to 80% are reported in cases of acute papillary muscle or interventricular septal ruptures, and in cases of free wall ventricular rupture the mortality rate is almost 100%. Myocardial rupture usually occurs within 7 to 10 days of the onset of AMI but may occur within hours of the onset of the AMI and be present when the elderly AMI patient initially seeks medical assistance. Acute papillary muscle rupture with acute mitral regurgitation and VSD both typically produce holosystolic murmurs, which may be preceded by severe chest pain and are associated with hemodynamic deterioration including heart failure, shock, or cardiac arrest. The bedside differentiation between these two catastrophic complications may be difficult, although emergency bedside echocardiography with Doppler ultrasonography will usually make the definitive diagnosis. Bedside right-sided cardiac catheterization (Swan-Ganz monitoring) will confirm the diagnosis by measuring a step-up of oxygen saturation from the right atrium to right ventricle (usually >8%–10%) in cases of VSD rupture, whereas a large V wave in the pulmonary capillary wedge pressure suggests mitral regurgitation. A large V wave, however, is not specific for mitral regurgitation, and large V waves have been reported in cases of acute VSD. Initial management of acute mitral regurgitation or VSD should include hemodynamic monitoring and use of nitroglycerin or nitroprusside to reduce afterload and ''unload'' the left ventricle. The use of intra-aortic balloon counter pulsation, and positive inotropic agents, such as dobutamine and dopamine, may be necessary in patients who are hypotensive or have low cardiac output. Subsequent cardiac catheterization and surgery are necessary in these patients, with most surgeons recommending early surgical correction because without surgery the course is one of progressive hemodynamic deterioration and death. Perioperative mortality is high, especially in elderly patients (90). Surgical success, however, depends more on the severity of left ventricular dysfunction and the patient's hemodynamic deterioration than age. Long-term prognosis after successful surgery of VSD and papillary muscle rupture is good.

Rupture of the ventricular free wall is almost alwys catastrophic, associated with pericardial tamponade and sudden death. Occasionally, the rupture will be locally contained because of pericardial adhesions, and there may be time for emergency surgical interviention. In some instances of ventricular rupture, the rupture may be preceded by pericardial pain resulting from the accumulation of blood in the pericardial space with or without signs of pericardial tamponade. Prompt recognition of this stage may allow for successful surgical intervention.

(g). Acute Pericarditis. Pericarditis is common in the early stage of AMI and occurs in 10% to 15% of cases. The associated pain is typically substernal with radiation to the back and left shoulder, usually is exacerbated by deep breathing or turning, and may be diminished by the patient sitting up. A pericardial rub can be heard on auscultation, although it is often evanescent and may be misdiagnosed as a heart murmur. Pericarditis associated with AMI has been reported to be a marker of extensive myocardial damage and may be accompanied by atrial dysrhythmias, commonly atrial fibrillation or flutter (91). Symptomatic relief of pain with aspirin or other nonsteroidal anti-inflammatory agents is the usual treatment with close observation for findings of pericardial tamponade. Corticosteroids are usually not necessary and should be avoided if possible.

(h). Cardiogenic Shock. See Chapter 11.

II. ACUTE CARDIOGENIC PULMONARY EDEMA

Acute cardiogenic pulmonary edema is the sudden accumulation of fluid in the lungs caused by the rapid rise of pulmonary capillary hydrostatic pressure greater than 25 to 30 mm Hg. A sudden rise of pulmonary capillary pressure is not uncommon in elderly patients and may be related to various cardiac causes (Table 6). The most common cause in elderly patients is acute left ventricular dysfunction, either systolic or diastolic, resulting from AMI or myocardial ischemia. Not infrequently, the sudden onset of pulmonary edema will be the first manifestation of coronary artery disease in elderly patients. Many of these elderly patients will be without chest pain at time of the pulmonary edema, even though three-vessel coronary disease is present. Left ventricular systolic function will usually be only moderately depressed if there has not been an associated AMI; the sudden left ventricular impairment will be due to diastolic dysfunction as a result of acute myocardial ischemia (92,93). In most of these elderly patients, a history of hypertension and left ventricular hypertrophy is present (92).

Another cause of cardiogenic pulmonary edema in elderly patients is a sudden left ventricular volume overload resulting from acute mitral or aortic valvular regurgitation. The acute valvular regurgitation may be caused by coronary artery disease (AMI or ischemia), trauma, infective endocarditis, or spontaneous valvular disruption. The most common cause of acute mitral regurgitation with resultant heart failure is mitral valve prolapse (MVP). Although MVP is usually considered a benign disorder, in certain elderly patients with MVP, particularly older males, chordae tendinae will rupture, producing acute mitral regurgitation

Table 6 Etiology of Cardiogenic Pulmonary Edema

Coronary artery disease
Acute myocardial infarction
Acute myocardial ischemia
Acute ventricular volume overload
Acute valvular regurgitation (MR, AR)
Acute interventricular septal rupture
Accelerated hypertension*
Acute tachycardia*
Aortic valvular stenosis
Mechanical diastolic restrictive disorder
Mitral stenosis

AR, Aortic valvular regurgitation; LV, left ventricle; LVH, left ventricular hypertrophy; MR, mitral valvular regurgitation.

* In conjunction with underlying LVH or LV dysfunction.

with resultant pulmonary edema (94–96). Another cause of an acute left ventricular volume overload in elderly patients is an interventricular septal rupture as a result of an AMI.

Other cardiogenic causes of acute left ventricular dysfunction with resultant pulmonary edema in elderly patients are accelerated hypertension, tachycardia, or rarely aortic valvular stenosis. In most of these elderly patients, long-standing underlying left ventricular hypertrophy or dysfunction is present.

In some elderly patients with acute cardiogenic pulmonary edema, pulmonary capillary pressure may abruptly rise in the absence of myocardial impairment, as in the patient with mitral stenosis who develops a rapid heart rate, which impairs left ventricular filling.

A. Clinical Manifestations

Acute cardiogenic pulmonary edema is one of the most dramatic cardiac syndromes and is a terrifying experience for both the patient and the bystander. Usually extreme breathlessness develops suddenly, often preceded by coughing, productive of pink frothy fluid. The patient quickly feels suffocated with an oppression in the chest, which further intensifies the patient's fright and elevates the heart rate and blood pressure, usually associated with diffuse diaphoresis. Some patients will experience intense chest pain, particularly when the pulmonary edema is a result of an AMI or ischemia. Many elderly patients, however, will be without chest pain even in the setting of an acute infarction. The patient will sit upright, exhibit air hunger, and be severely dyspneic. Severe systolic hypertension with pressures greater than 200 mm Hg may be present. Such accelerated systemic hypertension may be the cause of the acute left ventricular failure, although more commonly, the hypertension reflects increased sympathetic nervous system activity with vasoconstriction as a result of the patient's acute distress.

Physical examination of the patient will demonstrate an elevated respiratory rate with inspiratory retraction of the intercostal spaces and supraclavicular fossae with the patient using accessory muscles of respiration. Respiration is noisy with gurgling sounds; auscultation demonstrates diffuse rhonchi, wheezing, and fine inspiratory rales. Cardiac auscultation will be difficult because of the harsh pulmonary sounds, although a gallop rhythm and loud pulmonic valve closure sound (P_2) are usually present. A heart murmur may be detected in those elderly patients whose acute left ventricular dysfunction is related to valvular dysfunction or interventricular septal defect. However, in many of these elderly patients the murmur may not be detected until the patients' pulmonary findings are resolved.

In certain elderly patients, it may be difficult to distinguish between acute cardiogenic pulmonary edema and an acute asthmatic attack. In both cases, the patients will be severely dyspneic associated with marked anxiety and demonstrate diffuse pulmonary wheezing. Fortunately, often a history of previous episodes in elderly patients with asthma is present and the patient may be aware of the diagnosis. Pulmonary auscultation may be helpful; the wheezes are usually more high pitched and musical in patients with asthma, and rhonchi and rales are less prominent.

B. Immediate Diagnostic Evaluation

Chest radiographic abnormalities are very helpful in diagnosing cardiogenic pulmonary edema. Cardiomegaly may be present, although in many elderly patients cardiac enlargement may be moderate only, and in some patients with acute MI or ischemia, the heart size will be within normal limits. Pulmonary radiographic findings include interstitial and perihilar engorgement, Kerly's B lines, and pleural effusion. The radiographic abnormalities may be several hours behind development of symptoms, and the elderly patient's physical findings may be much more impressive than the findings on the patient's chest x-ray film.

Arterial gases will usually demonstrate severe hypoxemia and often hypocapnia. In some elderly patients, however, hypercapnia with acute respiratory acidemia will be noted; these findings are usually present in the severe cases.

Electrocardiographic findings are often nonspecific and usually are not diagnostic of a specific cardiac disorder. The elderly patient may demonstrate nonspecific ST-T wave changes, an intraventricular conduction abnormality, or left ventricular hypertrophy. In other patients, low voltage will be noted, reflecting the patient's concomitant chronic pulmonary disease. ST-T wave changes of ischemia may be present, and in other patients an AMI will be diagnosed.

Echocardiography provides valuable bedside information when evaluating and managing the elderly patient with acute cardiogenic pulmonary edema. Besides assessing possible underlying cardiac causes for the acute ventricular dysfunction, such as valvular and interventricular shunting disorders, echocardiography can assess left ventricular wall motion and hypertrophy and differentiate between systolic and diastolic ventricular dysfunction. Because of these benefits, echocardiography is considered necessary in all patients who have heart failure (97).

Bedside right-heart catheterization with pulmonary pressure monitoring will usually not be necessary in most elderly patients with acute pulmonary edema but may be beneficial in patients whose condition is not quickly relieved with usual therapy or in patients who are hypotensive. Also, therapeutic doses of drugs can be better regulated with measurement of hemodynamics, including cardiac output and pulmonary pressures. Measurement of the pulmonary capillary wedge pressure will also differentiate between cardiogenic and noncardiogenic pulmonary edema and will be beneficial in diagnosing acute mitral regurgitation versus acute ventricular septal defect in patients with systolic heart murmurs.

C. Therapeutic Intervention

General principles should include placing the patient in a sitting position to promote venous pooling and to relieve the patient's anxiety. Administration of oxygen is necessary by nasal cannula or mask in a concentration to raise the arterial oxygen partial pressure (Po_2) to greater than 60 mm Hg. If adequate oxygenation is not possible by way of nasal cannula or mask, if significant hypercapnia coexists, or if the patient demonstrates signs of exhaustion, mechanical ventilation will be necessary.

Morphine sulfate reduces anxiety and pain and decreases pulmonary pressure by venodilation. Two to 5 mg of intravenous morphine can be given safely over several minutes and can be repeated every 10 to 15 minutes if the patient is not significantly improved. Intravenous furosemide is a potent diuretic and venodilator and should be administered quickly after diagnosing acute pulmonary edema. Because of its venodilator effects and the resultant decrease in pulmonary pressures, patients will often be relieved of the acute pulmonary distress before diuresis occurs. An initial dose of 20 to 40 mg should be given over several minutes and can be increased on the basis of the response.

Nitroglycerin will augment the venodilatory effects of morphine and furosemide. A sublingual dose can be followed by nitroglycerin topical ointment 2%, 1 to 2 inches, or the drug may be administered intravenously, particularly if myocardial ischemia is present.

Arterial vasodilatory therapy (afterload reduction) with nitroprusside may be beneficial in patients whose acute left ventricular dysfunction is a result of accelerated hypertension and in those patients whose condition has not improved with diuretics and venodilatory therapy, particularly in patients with acute valvular regurgitation. Nitroprusside is a potent arterial vasodilator, and close monitoring of blood pressure is necessary when the drug is used. Hemodynamic monitoring with pulmonary artery pressures and cardiac outputs is recommended by some when nitroprusside is used to treat patients with acute pulmonary edema. The initial dose of nitroprusside is 10 mg/min, slowly titrating to desired hemodynamic effect (maximum dose is 300 to 400 mg/min). Abrupt marked decrease in systolic blood pressure should be avoided, particularly in elderly patients with a hypertrophic left ventricle; catastrophic effects, including death, have been reported in such patients with the use of vasodilators (98).

In elderly patients with cardiogenic pulmonary edema and severe systolic ventricular dysfunction and whose condition fails to improve with usual therapy, the use of inotropic agents or intra-aortic balloon counterpulsation should be considered. Dobutamine is usually considered the inotropic agent of first choice. Dobutamine causes direct inotropic stimulation with reflex vasodilation, resulting in afterload reduction and augmentation of cardiac output. Blood pressure usually remains constant, but heart rate may increase minimally. If hypotension is present, dopamine infusion will need to be administered to correct hypotension, before dobutamine administration. Dobutamine should be administered as a constant infusion that is initiated at a rate of 1 to 2 mg/kg/min and is gradually increased to obtain the desired effect or until excessive tachycardia or ventricular irritability occur. Dobutamine should not be used in patients with predominantly diastolic ventricular dysfunction (hypertrophic cardiomyopathy). Dopamine is an endogenous catecholamine with positive inotropic properties at doses of 2 to 5 mg/kg/min. At lower doses (1–3 mg/kg/min) dopamine has a selective vasodilator effect on renal and mesenteric arterioles and may improve urine output. At doses greater than 5 to 10 mg/kg/min, peripheral vasoconstriction occurs with increases in systemic venous resistance, which may be deleterious in patients with low cardiac output and heart failure. The use of either dobutamine or dopamine in elderly patients with pulmonary edema should be guided by careful hemodynamic and electrocardiographic monitoring.

Another inotropic agent, milirone, may be beneficial in patients with cardiogenic pulmonary edema and low cardiac output. Milirone is a phosphodiesterase inhibitor that increases myocardial contractility by increasing intracellular cyclic adenosine monophosphate. Its net effect is similar to dobutamine. It is administered intravenously with an initial bolus of 0.75 mg/kg given over 2 to 3 minutes, followed by continuous infusion of 2.5 to 10 mg/kg/min. Sinus tachycardia, as well as atrial or ventricular tachyarrhythmias, may occur. Thrombocytopenia is another side effect, and serial determination of platelets will be necessary.

The benefits of ACE inhibitors in elderly patients with chronic heart failure and depressed left ventricular systolic function is well established. However, the use of ACE inhibitors in the setting of acute cardiogenic pulmonary edema is usually not recommended.

III. CONCLUSIONS

Acute AMI is a common disorder in elderly patients and is associated with high morbidity and mortality. The presentation of AMI may be atypical in elderly patients, and the diagnosis may be more difficult compared with younger patients. Early stratification of elderly AMI patients into high and low risk is necessary, as is early administration of proper therapies. Therapies and diagnostic interventions should not be deferred because of the patient's age alone.

Acute pulmonary edema is a life-threatening disorder and may be the first manifestation of heart disease in elderly patients. Prompt differentiation between cardiogenic and noncardiogenic pulmonary edema is mandatory in these patients, as is early determination of the specific cause of left ventricular impairment in those patients whose pulmonary edema is of cardiac orgin. Proper emergency therapy will be greatly beneficial and will quickly relieve symptoms in elderly patients with cardiogenic pulmonary edema.

REFERENCES

1. Gillum RF. Trends in acute myocardial infarction and coronary heart disease death in the United States. J Am Coll Cardiol 1993; 23:1273–1277.
2. Maggioni AP, Maseri A, Fresco C, Franzosi MG, Mauri F, Santiro E, Tognoni G. Age-related increase in mortality among patients with first myocardial infarctions treated with thrombolysis. N Engl J Med 1993; 329:1442–1448.
3. Backus RJ, Rangalos EG, Gersh BJ, Kottet E. Survival after acute myocardial infarction in patients 70 years and older J Am Coll Cardiol (abstr). 1991; 17:329A.
4. Rich MW, Bosner MS, Chung MT, Shen J, McKenzie JP. Is age an independent predictor of early and late mortality in patients with acute myocardial infarction? Am J Med 1992; 92:7–13.
5. Rosenthal GI, Fortinsky RH. Differences in the treatment of patients with acute myocardial infarction according to patient age. J Am Geriatr Soc 1994; 42:826–832.
6. Krumholz HM, Forman DE, Kuntz RE, Bain DS, Wei JY. Coronary revascularization after myocardial infarction in the very elderly: Outcomes and long-term follow-up. Ann Intern Med 1993; 119:1984–1090.
7. Kannel WB. Prevalence and clinical aspects of unrecognized myocardial infarction and sudden unexpected death. Circulation 1987; 75:114–115.

8. Sigurdsson E, Thorgeirsson G, Sigvaldason H, Sigfusson N. Unrecognized myocardial infarction: Epidemiology, clinical characteristics, and the prognostic role of angina pectoris. The Reykjavik Study. Ann Intern Med 1995; 122:96–102.
9. Tofler GH, Muller JE, Stone PH, Willich SN, Davis VG, Poole VK, Braunwald E. Factors leading to shorter survival after acute myocardial infarction in patients ages 65 to 75 years compared with younger patients. Am J Cardiol 1988; 62:860–867.
10. Smith SC Jr, Gilpin E, Ahnve S, Dittrich H, Nicod P, Henning H, Ross J. Outlook after acute myocardial infarction in the very elderly compared with that in patients aged 65 to 75 years. J Am Coll Cardiol 1990; 16:784–793.
11. Tresch DD. Management of the older patient with acute myocardial infarction: Difference in clinical presentations between older and younger patients. J Am Geriatr Soc 1998; 46:1157–1162.
12. Rodstein M. The characteristics of non-fatal myocardial infarction in the aged. Arch Intern Med 1956; 98:84–90.
13. Pathy MS. Clinical presentation of myocardial infarction in the elderly. Br Heart J 1967; 29:190–199.
14. Solomon CG, Lee TH, Cook EF, Weisberg MC, Branch DA, Rouan GW, Goldman L. Comparison of clinical presentation of acute myocardial infarction in patients older than 65 years of age to younger patients: The Multicenter Chest Pain Study experience. Am J Cardiol 1989; 63:772–776.
15. Limacher MC. Clinical features of coronary heart disease in the elderly. Cardiovasc Clin 1992; 22:63–73.
16. Paul SD, O'Gara PT, Mahjoub ZA, DiSalvo TG, O'Donnell CJ, Newell JB, Villareal-Levy G, Conrad-Smith AJ, Kondo NI, Cararach M, Ferrer L, Eagle KM. Geriatric patients with acute myocardial infarction: Cardiac risk factor profiles, presentation, thrombolysis, coronary interventions, and prognosis. Am Heart J 1991; 131: 710–715.
17. Bayer AJ, Chadha JS, Farag RR, Pathy J. Changing presentation of myocardial infarction with increasing old age. J Am Geriatr Soc 1986; 23:263–266.
18. Wroblewski M, Mikulowski P, Steen B. Symptoms of myocardial infarction in old age: Clinical case, retrospective and prospective studies. Age Ageing 1986; 15: 99–104.
19. Clemmensen P, Grande P, Saumamaki K, Pederson F, Svendsen JM, Wagner NB. Effect of IV streptokinase on relation between initial ST predicted size and final QRS estimated size of acute MI. J Am Coll Cardiol 1990; 16:1252–1257.
20. Lie KI, Wellens HJ, Schuilenburg RM, Becker AE, Durrer DV. Factors influencing prognosis of bundle branch block complicating acute antero-septal infarction. The value of His bundle recordings. Circulation 1974; 50:935–941.
21. Braat SH, Gorgels APM, Bar FW, Wellens HJ. Value of the ST-T segment in lead V_4R in inferior wall acute myocardial infarction to predict the site of coronary artery occlusion. Am J Cardiol 1988; 62:140–142.
22. Braat SH, deZwaan C, Brugada P, Coenegracht JM, Wellens HJ. Right ventricular involvement with acute inferior wall myocardial infarction identifies high risk of developing atrioventricular nodal conduction disturbances. Am Heart J 1984; 107: 1183–1187.
23. Yusuf S, Collins R, MacMahon S, Peto R. Effect of intravenous nitrates on mortality

in acute myocardial infarction: An overview of randomized trials. Lancet 1988; 1: 1088–1092.

24. ISIS-2 (Second International Study of Infarct Survival) Collaborative Group: Randomized trial of intravenous streptokinase, oral aspirin, both or neither among 17,187 cases of suspected myocardial infarction. Lancet 1988; 2:349–360.
25. Yusuf S, Wittes J, Friedman L. Overview of results of randomized clinical trial in heart disease. I. Treatments following myocardial infarction. JAMA 1988; 260: 2088–2093.
26. Fibrinolytic Therapy Trialists' (FTT) Collaborative Group. Indications for fibrinolytic therapy in suspected acute myocardial infarction: Collaborative overview of early mortality and major morbidity results from all randomized trials of more than 1000 patients. Lancet 1994; 343:311–322.
27. Gruppo Italiano per lo Studio della Streptochinasi nell' Infarto Miocardio (GISSI). Effectiveness of intravenous thrombolytic treatment in acute myocardial infarction. Lancet 1986; 1:397–401.
28. AIMS Trial Study Group. Effect of intravenous APSAC on mortality after acute myocardial infarction: Preliminary report of placebo-controlled clinical trial. Lancet 1988; 314:1465–1471.
29. Wilcox RG, Olsson CG, Skene AM, von der Leepe G, Jensen G, Hampton JR. Trial of tissue plasminogen activator for mortality reduction in acute myocardial infarction: Anglo-Scandinavian Study of Early Thrombolysis (ASSET). Lancet 1988; 2:525–530.
30. Forman DE, Gutierrez-Bernal JL, Wei JY. Management of acute myocardial infarction in the very elderly. Am J Med 1992; 93:315–326.
31. International Study Group. In-hospital mortality and clinical course of 20,891 patients with suspected acute myocardial infarction randomized between alteplase and streptokinase with or without heparin. Lancet 1990; 336:71–75.
32. Rich MW. Acute myocardial infarction in the elderly. Cardiology 1990; 7(10): 79–86, 90, 120.
33. Stone GW, Grines CL, Browne KF, Marco J, Rothbaum D, O'Keefe J, Hartzler GO, Overlie P, Donohue B, Chelliah N. Predictors of in-hospital and 6 month outcome after acute MI in the reperfusion era: The primary angioplasty in MI Trial (PAMI). J Am Coll Cardiol 1995; 25:370–377.
34. Grines CL, Browne KF, Marco J, Rothbaum D, Stone GW, O'Keefe J, Overlie P, Donohue B, Cheillah N, Timmis GC, Vlietstra RE, Strzalecki M, Puchrowicz-Ochoki S, O'Neil WW. A comparison of immediate angioplasty with thrombolytic therapy for acute myocardial infarction. N Engl J Med 1993; 328:673–679.
35. Stone GW, Grines CL, Browne KF, Marco J, Rothbaum D, O'Keefe J, Hartzler GO, Overlie P, Donohue B, Chelliah N, Vlietstra R, Puchrowicz-Ochoki S, O'Neil WW. Comparison of in-hospital outcomes in men versus women treated by either thrombolytic therapy or primary coronary angioplasty for acute myocardial infarction. Am J Cardiol 1995; 75:987–992.
36. Laster SB, Rutherford BD, Giorgi LV, Shimshar TM, McConahay DR, Johnson WL, Huber KC, Ligon RW, Hartzler GO. Results of direct percutaneous transluminal coronary angioplasty. Am J Cardiol 1996; 77:10–13.
37. Hochman JS, Boland J, Sleeper L. Current spectrum of cardiogenic shock and effect

of early revascularization on mortality. Results of an International Registry. SHOCK Registry Investigators. Circulation 1995; 91:873–881.
38. The Global Use of Strategies to Open Occluded Coronary Arteries in Acute Coronary Syndromes (GUSTO) IIB) Angioplasty Substudy Investigators. A clinical trial comparing primary coronary angioplasty with tissue plasminogen activator for acute myocardial infarction. N Engl J Med 1997; 336:1621–1628.
39. Hjalmarson A, Herlitz J, Holmberg S, Ryden L, Svedberg K, Vedin A, Waagstein F, Waldenstrom A, Waldenstrom J, Wedel H, Wilhelmsen L, Wilhelmsen C. The Goteborg Metoprolol Trial: Effects on mortality and morbidity in acute myocardial infarction. Circulation 1983; 67:126–131.
40. ISIS-1 Collaborative Group. Randomized trial of intravenous atenolol among 16,027 cases of suspected acute myocardial infarction: ISIS-1. Lancet 1986; 2:57–65.
41. MIAMI Trial Research Group. Metoprolol in acute myocardial infarction (MIAMI): A randomized placebo-controlled international trial: Eur Heart J 1985; 6:199–226.
42. Gruppo Italiano per lo Studio della Sopravvivenza nell'Infarto Miocardioco. Six-month effects of early treatment with lisinopril and transdermal glyceryl trinitrate singly and together withdrawn six weeks after myocardial infarction: The GISSI-3 Trial. J Am Coll Cardiol 1996; 27:337–344.
43. Ambrosioni E, Borghi C, Magnani B, and the Survival of Myocardial Infarction Long-term Evaluation (SMILE) Study Investigators. The effect of the angiotensin-converting-enzyme inhibitor zofenopril on mortality and morbidity after anterior myocardial infarction. N Engl J Med 1995; 332:80–85.
44. Swedburg K, Held P, Kjekshus J, Rasmussen K, Ryden L, Wedel H. Effects of early administration of enalapril on mortality in patients with acute myocardial infarction. Results of the Cooperative New Scandinavian Enalapril Survival Study II (CONSENSUS II). N Engl J Med 1992; 327:678–684.
45. Pfeffer MA, Braunwald E, Moye L, Baste L, Brown EJ, Cuddy TE, Davis BR, Geltman S, Flaker GC, Klein M, Lamas GA, Parker M, Rouleau JL, Rutherford JD, Wertheimer JH, Hawkins CM. Effect of captopril on mortality and morbidity in patients with left ventricular dysfunction after myocardial infarction. Results of the Survival and Ventricular Enlargement Trial. N Engl J Med 1992; 327:669–677.
46. The Acute Infarction Ramipril Efficacy (AIRE) Study Investigators. Effect of ramipril on mortality and morbidity of survivors of acute myocardial infarction with clinical evidence of heart failure. Lancet 1993; 342:821–828.
47. The Trace Study Group. The Trandolapril Cardiac Evaluation (TRACE) study: Rationale, design, and baseline characteristics of the screened population. Am J Cardiol 73: 44C–50C, 1994.
48. Ryan TJ, Anderson JL, Antman EM, Braniff BA, Brook NH, Califf RM, Hillis LD, Hiratzka LF, Rapaport E, Riegel BJ, Russell RO, Smith EE III, Weaver WD. ACC/AHA guidelines for the management of patients with acute myocardial infarction. J Am Coll Cardiol 1996; 28:1328–1428.
49. Furberg CD, Psaty BM, Meyer JV. Nifedipine: Dose-related increase in mortality in patients with coronary heart disease. Circulation 1995; 92:1326–1331.
50. Yusuf S, Held P, Furberg C. Update of effects of calcium antagonists in myocardial infarction or angina in light of the second Danish Verapamil Infarction Trial (DAVIT-II) and other recent studies. Am J Cardiol 1991; 67:1295–1297.

51. Gibson RS, Boden WE, Theroux P, Strauss HD, Pratt CM, Gheorghiade M, Capone RJ, Crawford MH, Schlant RC, Kleiger RE. Diltiazem and reinfarction in patients with non-Q-wave myocardial infarction. Results of a double-blind, randomized, multicenter trial. N Engl J Med 1986; 315:423–429.
52. The Multicenter Diltiazem Postinfarction Trial Research Group. The effect of diltiazem on mortality and reinfarction after myocardial infarction. N Engl J Med 1988; 319:385–392.
53. Woods KL, Fletcher S. Long-term outcome after intravenous magnesium sulphate in acute MI. The second Leicesheg Intravenous Magnesium Intervention Trial (LIMIT-2). Lancet 1994; 343:816–819.
54. ISIS-4 (Fourth International Study of Infarct Survival) Collaborative Group. ISIS-4: A randomized factorial trial assessing early oral captopril, oral mononitrate, and intravenous magnesium sulphate in 58,059 patients with suspected acute myocardial infarction. Lancet 1995; 345:669–685.
55. Nicod P, Gilpin E, Dittrich H, Polikar R, Hjalmarson A, Blacky R, Henning H, Ross J. Short- and long-term clinical outcome after Q wave and non-Q wave myocardial infarction in a large patient population. Circulation 1989; 79:528–536.
56. Tresch DD, Brady WJ, Aufderheide TP, Lawrence SW, Williams KJ. Comparison of elderly and younger patients with out-of-hospital chest pain. Arch Intern Med 1996; 156:1089–1093.
57. Chung MK, Bosner MS, McKenzie JP, Shen J, Rich MW. Prognosis of patients ≥ 70 years of age with non-Q-wave acute myocardial infarction compared with younger patients with similar infarcts and with patients ≥ 70 years of age with Q-wave acute myocardial infarction. Am J Cardiol 1995; 75:18–22.
58. Inhibition of the platelet glycoprotein IIb/IIIa receptor with tirofiban in unstable angina and non-Q wave MI. Platelet receptor inhibition in ischemic syndrome management in patients limited by unstable signs and symptoms (PRISM-PLUS) Study Investigators. N Engl J Med 1998; 338:1488–1497.
59. The Pursuit Trial Investigators. Platelet glycoprotein-IIb/IIIa in unstable angina: receptor suppression using integrilin therapy. N Engl J Med 1998; 339:436–443.
60. The TIMI IIIB Investigators. Effects of tissue plasminogen activator and a comparison of early invasive and conservative strategies in unstable angina and non-Q-wave myocardial infarction. Results of the TIMI IIIB Trial. Circulation 1994; 89:1545–1556.
61. Ambrose JA, Hjemdahl-Monsen C, Borrico S, Sherman K, Cohen M, Grelin R, Fuster V. Quantitative and qualitative effects of intracoronary streptokinase in unstable angina and non-Q wave infarction. J Am Coll Cardiol 1987; 9:1156–1165.
62. O'Doherty M, Tayler DI, Quinn E, Vincent R, Chamberlain DA. Five hundred patients with myocardial infarction monitored within one hour of symptoms. Br Med J 1983; 286:1405–1408.
63. Boden WE, O'Rourke RA, Crawford MH, Blaustein AS, Deedwania PC, Zable RG, Wexler LF, Kleiger RL, Pepine CJ, Ferry DR, Chow BK, Lavori PW. Outcomes in patients with acute non-Q wave myocardial infarction randomly assigned to an invasive as compared with a conservative management strategy. N Engl J Med 1998; 338:1785–1792.
64. Weinberg B, Zipes D. Strategies to manage the post-MI patient with ventricular arrhythmias. Clin Cardiol 1989; 12:1186–1190.

65. Warnica JW. Pharmacologic management of acute myocardial infarction. In: Rahimtoola SH, ed. Current Topics in Cardiology: Acute Myocardial Infarction. New York: Elsevier, 1991, pp 205–217.
66. Hine LK, Laird N, Hewitt P, Chalmer TC. Meta-analytic evidence against prophylactic use of lidocaine in acute myocardial infarction. Arch Intern Med 1989; 149: 2694–2698.
67. Eldar M, Sievner Z, Goldbourt U, Reicher-Reiss M, Kaplinsky E, Behar S. Primary ventricular tachycardia in acute myocardial infarction: Clinical characteristics and mortality: The SPRINT Study Group. Ann Intern Med 1992; 117:31–36.
68. Campbell RWF, Murray A, Julian DG. Ventricular arrhythmias in first 12 hours of acute myocardial infarction: Natural history study. Br Heart J 1981; 46:351–357.
69. Tofler GH, Stone PH, Muller JE, and the MILIS Study Group. Prognosis after cardiac arrest due to ventricular tachycardia or ventricular fibrillation associated with acute myocardial infarction (MILIS Study). Am J Cardiol 1987; 60:755–761.
70. Behar S, Reicher Ress H, Schedhter M, Rabinowitz B, Kaplinsky E, Abinader J, Friedman Y, Barzilai J, Kauli N. Frequency and prognostic significance of secondary ventricular fibrillation complicating acute myocardial infarction. Am J Cardiol 1993; 71(2):152–156.
71. Emergency Cardiac Care Committee and Subcommittees, American Heart Association. Guidelines for cardiopulmonary resuscitation and emergency cardiac care: III. Adult advanced cardiac life support. JAMA 1992; 268:2199–2241.
72. Six AJ, Louwenburg JH, Kingma, JH, Robles de Medina EO, Van Hemel NM. Predictive value of ventricular arrhythmias for patency of infarct-related coronary artery after thrombolytic therapy. Br Heart J 1991; 66:143–146.
73. Ganz LI, Freidman PL. Supraventricular tachycardia. N Engl J Med 1995; 332(3): 162–173.
74. Behar S, Zahari Z, Goldboust U, Reicher-Reiss H. Long-term prognosis of patients with paroxysmal atrial fibrillation complicating acute myocardial infarction. Eur Heart J 1992; 13(1):45–50.
75. Pantridge JF, Webb SW, Adgey AAJ. Arrhythmias in the first hours of acute myocardial infarction. Prog Cardiovasc Dis 1981; 23:265–278.
76. Graver LE, Gershen BJ, Orlando MM, Epstein SE. Bradycardia and its complications in the pre-hospital phase of acute MI. Am J Cardiol 1973; 32:607–610.
77. Brown RW, Hunt D, Sloman JG. The natural history of atrioventricular conduction defects in acute myocardial infarction. Am Heart J 1969; 78:460–466.
78. Behar S. Zissman E, Zion M, Golbourt V, Reicher-Reiss H, Shaler Y, Hod H, Kaplinsky E, Caspi A. Complete AV block complicating inferior wall acute myocardial infarction: Short and long-term prognosis. Am Heart J 1993; 125(6):1622–1627.
79. Goldberg RJ, Zevalloe JC, Yarzebski J, Alpert JS, Gore JM, Chen Z, Dalen JE. Prognosis of acute MI complicated by complete heart block (The Worcester Heart Attack Study) Am J Cardiol 1992; 69(14):1135–1141.
80. Tresch DD, Amirani H. Cardiopulmonary resuscitation: Beneficial or an exercise in futility? In: Wenger NK, ed. Cardiovascular Disease in the Octogenarian and Beyond. London: Martin Dunitz Ltd., 1999, pp 291–304.
81. Bedell SE, Delbanco TL, Cook EF, Epstein FH. Survival after cardiopulmonary resuscitation in the hospital. N Engl J Med 1983; 309:569–575.

82. Tresch DD, Thakur R, Hoffman R, Brooks HL. Should the elderly be resuscitated following out-of-hospital cardiac arrest? Am J Med 1989; 86:145–150.
83. Longstreth WT Jr, Cobb LA, Fahrenbruch CE, Copas MK. Does age affect outcomes of out of hospital cardiopulmonary resuscitation? JAMA 1990; 264:2109–2110.
84. Murphy DI, Murry AM, Robinson BE, Campion EU. Outcomes of cardiopulmonary resuscitation in the elderly. Ann Intern Med 1989; 111:199–205.
85. Tresch DD, Heudebert G, Kutty K, Ohlert S, Van Beck K, Masi A. Cardiopulmonary resuscitation in elderly patients hospitalized in the 1990s: a favorable outcome. J Am Geriatr Soc 1994; 42:137–41.
86. Shah PK, Maddahi J, Berman DS, Pichler M, Swan HJ. Scintigraphically detected predominant right ventricular dysfunction in acute myocardial infarction: Clinical and hemodynamic correlates and implications for therapy and prognosis. J Am Coll Cardiol 1985; 6:1264–1272.
87. Zehender M, Kasper W, Kauder E, Schonthaler M, Geibel A, Olschewski M, Just H. Right ventricular infarction as an independent predictor of prognosis after acute inferior myocardial infarction. N Engl J Med 1993; 328:981–988.
88. Bueno H, Lopez-Palop R, Bermejo Javier, Lopez-Sendon JL, Delcan JL. In-hospital outcome of elderly patients with acute inferior myocardial infarction and right ventricular involvement. Circulation 1997; 96:436–441.
89. Shapira I, Isabov A, Burke M, Almog C. Cardiac rupture in patients in acute MI. Chest 1987; 92(2):219–223.
90. Held AC, Cole PL, Lipton B, Gore JM, Antman EM, Hockman JS, Carraro J, Goldberg RJ, Alpert JS. Rupture of the interventricular septum complicating acute MI: A multicenter analysis of clinical findings and outcome. Am Heart J 1988; 116: 1330–1334.
91. Wall TC, Califf RM, Harrelson-Woodlief L, Mark DB, Honan M, Abbottsmith CW, Candela R, Berrio SE, Phillips HR, Topol EJ. Usefulness of a pericardial friction rub after thrombolytic therapy during acute myocardial infarction in predicting amount of myocardial damage. Am J Cardiol 1990; 66:1418–1420.
92. Siegel R, Clemens T, Wingo M, Tresch D. Acute heart failure in the elderly: Another manifestation of unstable ''angina.'' J Am Coll Cardiol (abstr) 1991; 17:149A.
93. Kunis R, Greenberg H, Yeoh CB, Garfein OB, Pepe AJ. Coronary revascularization for recurrent pulmonary edema in elderly patients with ischemic heart disease and preserved ventricular function. N Engl J Med 1985; 313:1207–1209.
94. Tresch DD, Doyle TP, Boncheck LI, Siegel R, Keelan MH, Olinger GN, Brooks HL. Mitral valve prolapse requiring surgery. Am J Med 1985; 78:245–250.
95. Kolibash AJ, Kilman JW, Bush CA, Ryan JM, Fontana ME, Wooley CF. Evidence of progression from mild to severe mitral regurgitation in mitral valve prolapse. Am J Cardiol 1986; 58:762–727.
96. Devereux RB, Hawkins I, Kramer-Fox R. Complications of mitral valve prolapse. Disproportionate occurrence in men and older patients. Am J Med 1986; 81:751–758.
97. Aronow WS. Echocardiography should be performed in all elderly patients with congestive heart failure. J Am Geriatr Soc 1994; 423:1300–1302.
98. Topol EJ, Traill TA, Fortuin NJ. Hypertension hypertrophic cardiomyopathy of the elderly. N Engl J Med 1985; 312:277–307.

13
Hypertensive Crises

Ronald L. Fong
Charles R. Drew University of Medicine and Science, and Martin Luther King, Jr.–Charles R. Drew Medical Center, Los Angeles, California

Keith C. Norris
Charles R. Drew University of Medicine and Science, Martin Luther King, Jr.–Charles R. Drew Medical Center, and UCLA School of Medicine, Los Angeles, California

I. CLINICAL RELEVANCE

A. Epidemiology

It is universally appreciated that elderly patients merit special consideration in the diagnosis, evaluation, and treatment of hypertension. However, this germane facet of patient care has not been extended to the specific issue of hypertensive crises in the elderly. It is common for review articles dealing with hypertensive crises to ignore the subtleties of treating the geriatric patient (1–3). Few studies have focused on the effective and safe treatment for dangerously high blood pressure levels in this extremely vulnerable population. This is alarming in view of the rapidly growing geriatric population in the United States. In 1990, this group made up 12.6% of the population (31.4 million), with a projected increase to 19.6% of the population (58.9 million) by the year 2025 (4,5). Over the past four decades the elderly subset of the oldest-old individuals, aged 85 years and older, has increased its numbers by 232% compared with a growth of 39% in the general population (5). Moreover, hypertension is disproportionately represented in the elderly, with a prevalence of more than 50% (6,7). The impact of hypertension on mortality and morbidity in the United States is dramatic and substantial. Hypertension is a major risk factor for both coronary artery disease and cerebrovascular accidents, the first and third leading causes of death annually respectively. Despite this dire state of affairs, many health care providers have not earmarked blood pressure control as a priority for their elderly patients. More than half of this population remains untreated, and in more than half of the treated patients blood pressure levels are not adequately controlled (8–11). Inadequate blood pressure control increases the risk of detrimental sequelae developing in these individuals. Cautious encouragement comes from one study of patients enrolled in a large health maintenance organization (HMO). From a period from 1967 to 1988, the organization identified between 44% and 53% of its hypertensive enrollees. Treatment for these patients during this period increased from 25% to 60%, and the proportion of patients on treatment and controlled increased from 8% to 34% (9). Despite this report, it is still unclear whether HMOs differ from their fee-for-service counterparts in the quality of care provided to older hypertensive patients (12–14).

B. Benefits of Blood Pressure Control

The benefits of proper blood pressure control have been clearly established in the elderly population. In fact, older patients treated for hypertension derive greater absolute and relative benefits with respect to risk reduction for coronary artery disease and cerebrovascular events than their younger counterparts (15). Blood pressure control for older adults is estimated to reduce all-cause mortality by 12%, coronary heart disease by 20%, and stroke by 36% (8). However, despite the documented benefits from treating elderly hypertensive patients and heightened treatment recommendations over the past decade (16–19), physicians still hesitate to treat elderly hypertensive patients with well-established guidelines. Kilander and coworkers reported that more than half of a group of Swedish geriatricians delineated a systolic blood pressure (SBP) of 180 mm Hg or a diastolic blood pressure (DBP) of 100 mm Hg as the cut-off points for initiation of pharmacological intervention (20). This is in stark contrast to the results of the Systolic Hypertension in the Elderly Program (SHEP); blood pressure reduction to a mean SBP of 143 mm Hg and a mean DBP of 68 mm Hg significantly reduced the risk of fatal and nonfatal myocardial infarction and stroke (21). The recent recommendations by The Sixth Report on the Joint National Committee on Prevention, Detection, Evaluation, and Treatment of High Blood Pressure (JNC VI) targeted blood pressure levels in the elderly to a SBP <140 mm Hg and DBP <90 mm Hg, if tolerated, although an interim SBP goal of <160 mm Hg may be appropriate (22).

II. IMMEDIATE DIAGNOSTIC APPROACH

A. Definition of Hypertensive Crisis

A hypertensive crisis is defined as a severe elevation in blood pressure requiring immediate attention and is now commonly classified as either a hypertensive urgency or emergency (23,24). The terms accelerated hypertension and malignant hypertension have largely been abandoned in favor of these more clinically descriptive terms, urgency or emergency, that convey a clinical assessment that accompanies a markedly high blood pressure. Often a hypertensive crisis is associated with a SBP of 210 to 220 mm Hg or greater and DBP of 120 to 130 mm Hg or greater. However, the level of blood pressure is not the sole determinant. Both the rate of blood pressure rise and the degree of elevation above a given baseline lead to wide variations in the level of blood pressure at which a designation of hypertensive crisis is given.

In a hypertensive urgency no evidence of acute end-organ injury and no evidence to support that rapid lowering of blood pressure is beneficial exists. In fact, rapid blood pressure reduction may be deleterious and lead to relative or absolute hypotension, stroke, or myocardial infarction. In hypertensive urgencies, blood pressure should be lowered gradually, over 24 to 48 hours, with oral antihypertensives in most instances. By contrast, in a hypertensive emergency acute end-organ involvement, such as ophthalmological, cerebral, cardiac, or renal injury is present, and in such a situation the immediate lowering of blood pressure is critical to help avoid permanent and debilitating end-organ damage.

B. Altered Cognition and Severe Hypertension

An alteration in mental status caused by severe hypertension qualifies as hypertensive encephalopathy and a medical emergency. However, the elderly patient is prone to disorders of cognition independent of hypertension. Changes in cognitive function in elderly patients are common, and decline is almost universal in at least one cognitive area among patients older than 85 years of age (25). Among patients aged 55 to 88 from the Framingham Heart study, increasing levels of blood pressure were associated with lower average levels of cognitive function (26,27). If unaccompanied to the emergency room, the elderly patient with a hypertensive urgency may be misclassified as having a hypertensive emergency because of the combination of an elevated blood pressure and neurological signs, if the latter is mistaken as acute in nature. A thorough history including assessment of the baseline neuropsychiatric status, careful examination of the fundus, and judicious use of computed tomography can alleviate the potential confusion regarding misdiagnosis of hypertensive encephalopathy and in many cases the premature initiation of a more risky treatment plan of immediate blood pressure reduction.

Impaired cognition can also affect adherence to a prescribed treatment program. Lack of adherence and subsequent hypertensive crisis is an important clinical issue among many geriatric patients and is due to multiple factors including cognitive dysfunction, economic depravity, and polypharmacy (22). Diuretic or calcium channel blockers have been suggested as placing the older hypertensive patient at greater risk for cognitive dysfunction (28), although this remains an area of great debate (21,29). Physician sensitivity toward and awareness of diverse ethnic and cultural factors plays an important role in recognizing cognitive changes in the older patient and greatly influences adherence to both nonpharmacological and pharmacological recommendations. Older minority patients may be at an even greater risk of poor blood pressure control (14,30), in large part because of adverse socioeconomic conditions or influences from an urban environment (13,31,32). For the hypertensive patient, poor blood pressure control itself may contribute to adherence difficulties by means of cognitive impairment. Thus, a vicious positive circles ensues: the patient forgets to take his/her medication, the blood pressure increases, and the rise in blood pressure leads to a further deterioration in cognitive function (33).

C. Clinical and Laboratory Assessment

Several key clinical characteristics must be critically assessed in a patient with markedly elevated blood pressure. Symptoms such as chest pain, dyspnea, blurred vision, headaches, or overt neurological symptoms herald the presence of a hypertensive emergency.

The treating physician should repeat the blood pressure preferably in both arms to confirm the findings. A careful cardiac examination should be undertaken for clinical evidence of cardiac involvement, such as the presence of a S_3 or S_4 gallop consistent with left ventricular dysfunction and/or murmur of mitral regurgitation consistent with papillary muscle dysfunction. The pulmonary examination should focus on evidence of pulmonary vascular congestion. A careful funduscopic examination should be performed, and if any concern exists about the inability to adequately examine the fundus, the pupils should be dilated to allow a more thorough assessment. Evidence of retinal hemorrhages or papilledema mandate immediate blood pressure reduction in a controlled setting.

Neurological symptoms including headaches and dizziness are often the initial complaint in malignant hypertension, whereas the classic symptoms of hypertensive encephalopathy characterized by headache, nausea, vomiting, and visual blurring, together with impaired cognitive function, generalized seizures, or cortical blindness are much less common (24). A thorough neurological examination should be performed including a neurocognitive assessment for evidence of a mild stroke, transient ischemia attack, or subtle mental status changes. Overt manifestations such as coma or seizures are readily recognized. In some instances computed tomography or magnetic resonance imaging of the head should be performed to exclude intracerebral bleeding or other focal lesions, or when uncertainty exists as to whether central nervous manifestations in an older person represent acute pathology.

An electrocardiogram and a radiograph of the chest should be obtained to assess for evidence of acute cardiac injury and/or pulmonary vascular congestion. Serum chemistries and urine should be tested to check electrolyte abnormalities for presence of elevated blood urea nitrogen and creatinine levels, heavy proteinuria, or hematuria, which if new, signal acute renal damage resulting from severe hypertension. Also, in the presence of renal dysfunction, intravenous contrast should not be given if possible to avoid precipitating acute renal failure. Renal doppler ultrasonography may be useful if a suspicion of renal artery stenosis exists and to determine renal size. A complete blood count and peripheral smear should also be evaluated for evidence of microangiopathic hemolytic anemia (red cell fragments, thrombocytopenia, increased fibrin degradation products, and increased fibrinogen). A strong clinical suspicion of acute cardiac, neurological, ophthalmological, or renal damage in the presence of severe hypertension should prompt a diagnosis of hypertensive emergency and the initiation of immediate treatment as described later. Careful monitoring of blood pressure, fluid balance, electrolytes, and renal function is necessary, but invasive monitoring is not required in all cases.

III. PATHOPHYSIOLOGY AND EVOLVING CONCEPTS

Another important aspect of treating the elderly patient with severe hypertension begins with the proper assessment of the mean arterial pressure (MAP). Franklin et al. have proposed a modification of the MAP calculation for hypertensive individuals older than 50 that has a greater correlation with cardiovascular and cerebrovascular outcomes than either SBP or DBP, termed the vascular overload index (VOI) (34). Studies have also indicated a better correlation between Franklin's VOI compared with the conventional MAP as a predictor of declining renal function in patients with hypertensive nephrosclerosis (35). This VOI is calculated as the sum of half pulse pressure (PP) and DBP (34,35). For example, a 66-year-old patient with a blood pressure of 220/130 mm Hg would have a MAP of 160 mm Hg with the conventional MAP calculation (one third SBP plus two third DBP). However, the VOI yields a value of 175 mm Hg, suggesting an even greater risk for cardiovascular-related complications and likely a greater shift to the right in the patient's blood pressure–blood flow curve (Figure 1), which increases susceptibility to target organ ischemia if the initial blood pressure reduction is too great. Thus, the initial blood pressure goal of a 25% reduction in MAP in 2 to 4 hours (22) would lead to an even greater absolute fall of the VOI. Because the VOI is often 10% to 20% greater than the standard MAP in older persons, a more appropriate goal of acute blood pressure reduction should be 15% to 20% of the initial MAP so as to attenuate the fall in the patient's VOI and improve each patient's safety profile. This attenuation of acute MAP reduction is especially critical in the elderly patient with hypertensive crisis because an excessive acute blood pressure reduction is more likely to impair end-organ hypoperfusion and cause irreversible complications in this high-risk population.

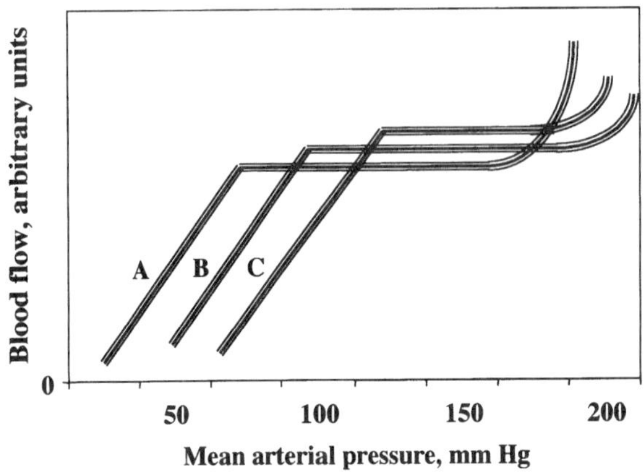

Figure 1 Blood pressure–blood flow curves for patients with (A) normal blood pressure, (B) chronic hypertension, and (C) hypertensive emergency.

IV. THERAPEUTIC INTERVENTION

A. General Guidelines

With regard to the rate and extent of blood pressure reduction, as well as specific medications for the treatment of hypertensive emergencies in the elderly, a few general guidelines should be followed until prospective studies provide clear evidenced-based recommendations. The most important aspect of treating a hypertensive emergency is to lower blood pressure slowly in a controlled manner with a continuous infusion in a monitored setting in contrast to intermittent boluses, which are more likely to produce inadvertent hypotension. The initial blood pressure goal and choice of therapy should achieve a reduction in blood pressure no more than 15% to 20% of the MAP over the first 2 to 4 h with minimal or no reduction in cardiac output to avoid ischemia-induced target organ damage. The medication selected should not induce significant reflex tachycardia, which may aggravate previously diagnosed or underlying coronary disease. Antihypertensive therapy should be initiated within the lower range of recommended doses and then titrated upward as necessary (Table 1). In addition, the choice of therapy should be modified to address specific comorbidities. Although acceleration of essential hypertension remains the leading cause of hypertensive emergencies, one should consider specific causes of accelerated hypertension, including acute antihypertensive drug withdrawal, autonomic hyperactivity, collagen vascular diseases and vasculitis, pheochromocytoma, renal vascular disease and renal failure and substance abuse (Table 2). Finally, specific cautions need to be observed because the elderly are more susceptible to a variety of medication-induced side

Table 1 Commonly Used Intravenous Medications for Hypertensive Crises, Dosing, and the Mechanism of Action (Doses Adjusted for Elderly Patients)

Medication	Common initial dosing	Mechanism of action
Nitroprusside[a]	0.5 μg/kg/min	Direct arterial > venous dilation
Labetolol[a]	5 mg IV then 1–2 mg/min	Beta and alpha-receptor blocker
Nitroglycerin[a]	5 μg/min; ↑ by 5 μg q 5 min	Direct venous > arterial dilation
Esmolol[a]	500 μg/kg loading, 25 μg/kg/min	Beta-receptor blocker
Trimethaphan	1–2 mg/min	Ganglionic blocker
Nicardipine	5–10 mg/h	Calcium channel blocker
Diazoxide[b]	30 mg IV boluses every 20–30 min	Direct arterial vasodilator
Hydralazine[b]	5 mg IV; then 5 mg q 20–30 min	Direct arterial vasodilator
Furosemide	40–80 mg IV	Diuresis and venodilatation
Enalaprilat	0.625 mg IV q6 h	ACE[c] inhibition
Methyldopa	250 mg IV q4–6 h	Central alpha-agonist
Phentolamine	5–15 mg IV bolus	Alpha-receptor blocker
Fenoldopam	0.1 μg/kg/min	Dopamine agonist

[a] Preferred medication for elderly considering overall effectiveness and safety profile.
[b] Use with extreme caution or not at all in elderly.
[c] Angiotensin converting enzyme.

Table 2 Special Considerations in Hypertensive Urgencies in the Elderly

Lower blood pressure slowly in a controlled manner using a continuous infusion in a monitored setting
No or minimal reduction in cardiac output
No or minimal reflex tachycardia
Modify for specific comorbidities
Consider specific causes of accelerated hypertension
Antihypertensive drug withdrawal
Collagen vascular disease, vasculitis
Renal vascular disease, renal failure
Autonomic hyperactivity
Neoplasias (i.e., pheochromocytoma)
Drug use (cocaine, alcohol, amphetamines)

Table 3 Cautions with Commonly used Intravenous Medications for Hypertensive Crises

Medication	Caution
Nitroprusside	Liver and renal failure; cyanide and thiocyanate toxicity may develop
Labetolol/esmolol	Bronchospasms, heart failure, heart block
Enalaprilat	Bilateral renovascular disease; may precipitate acute renal failure
Methyldopa	Hypertensive encephalopathy; may reduce mental acuity

effects (Table 3). Baseline and serial blood chemistries, including renal function, must be closely monitored because the kidney excretes many medications used to treat hypertensive crises. The presence of renal impairment could lead to drug accumulation and subsequent hypotension or other side effects such as thiocyanate toxicity in patients receiving nitroprusside infusion. Also, a list of commonly used parenteral medications with their preferred medical conditions(s) for use and mechanism of action are listed in Table 4. In general, most clinicians use nitroprusside, labetolol, nitroglycerin as the initial therapy for acute blood pressure reduction.

B. Hypertension Control in Selected Medical Conditions

Although arterial vasodilation is the preferred treatment strategy in most states of hypertensive crises, because of the significant increase in total peripheral resistance, extra caution must be applied in considering potential confounding overt and subclinical conditions that may exist in the older patient, such as a dissecting aneurysm or secondary hypertension. In general, vasodilators tend to have a lesser effect on the cerebral circulation in contrast to other vascular beds, making them primary choices for patients with hypertensive encephalopathy. Sodium nitro-

Table 4 Medications for Selected Conditions of Hypertensive Emergencies in the Elderly

Condition	Medication of choice	Contraindicated
Encephalopathy	Nitroprusside	Central agonists
Subarachnoid hemorrhage	Nimodipine	
Aortic dissection	Labetolol, nitroprusside	Hydralazine, diazoxide
Heart failure	Nitroprusside, nitroglycerin	Beta-blocker
Cardiac ischemia	Nitroglycerin, labetolol	Hydralazine, diazoxide
Acute renal failure	Labetolol, nitroprusside	Nitroprusside $>$ 24–48 h

prusside is the ''gold standard'' and probably the most commonly used medication for treating hypertensive emergencies (36,37) because of its rapid onset of action, being the most potent of all vasodilators, and a proven track record of efficacy. However, even sodium nitroprusside must be used with special care in the elderly because it crosses the blood-brain barrier and may lead to uneven cerebral perfusion, especially in border zones of the cerebral arterial supply, which increases the risk of complications (38).

Selecting a specific treatment to counteract the suspected pathophysiological abnormality in a given clinical situation can yield a safe and effective outcome (Table 4). Patients with hyperadrenergic states will respond well to alpha-adrenergic blockade. Elderly patients with hypertensive crisis and chest pain, where in which a greater likelihood of overt or subclinical coronary atherosclerosis exists, should be treated with nitroglycerin or beta-blockade, whereas aortic dissection responds well to a combination of alpha- and beta-adrenergic blockade (labetolol), nitroprusside, or ganglionic blockade (trimethaphan). A combination of nitroglycerin and alpha-adrenergic and beta-adrenergic blockade is particularly effective in the elderly patient with ischemic-type chest pain and hypertensive crisis when the diagnosis of aortic dissection has yet to be excluded. Patients with renovascular hypertension respond well to inhibition of the renin-angiotensin system. Indeed, hypertensive crisis in many patients with idiopathic hypertension is characterized by elevated renin and angiotensin levels, and therefore often responds well to angiotensin converting enzyme inhibitor (ACEI) therapy (39). With the case of enalaprilat (intravenous form of enalapril), the responses among a group of treated patients with hypertensive crises to only 0.625 mg intravenously was no different than the 1.25-mg, 2.5-mg, and 5-mg groups, demonstrating that blood pressure response in many of these patients is sensitive to even small doses of an ACEI (40). Unfortunately, it is difficult to achieve well-controlled minute-to-minute regulation of blood pressure reduction with intravenous ACEI therapy and, in general, it is better reserved for use after the initial 24 to 48 h of strictly monitored blood pressure reduction. A recently developed dopamine agonist, fenoldopam, has also been reported to be both effective and safe for treating hypertensive emergencies in patients up to 80 years of age; however, it has not been widely used in clinical practice (41). Although hypertensive crises often respond well to vasodilator therapy, in instances of overt volume overload the co-administration of a loop diuretic, which has both natriuretic and venodilatory properties, may be helpful. However, a careful clinical assessment is necessary because diuretic-induced volume depletion may elevate renin or angiotensin levels and paradoxically exacerbate the hypertensive crisis.

V. FOLLOW-UP MANAGEMENT

Once the immediate control of blood pressure has been achieved, the use of intermittent intravenous therapy or oral medications can be initiated judiciously

Table 5 Commonly Used Medications After Initial Blood Pressure Control (Doses Adjusted for Elderly Patients)

Medication	Common dosing
Clonidine	0.1 mg po q30–60 min
Enaliprat	0.625 mg IV q6 h
Aldomet	250 mg IV q4–6 h
Nifedipine	10 mg po q30–60 min
Labetalol	200 mg po q2–4 h
Minoxidil	2.5 mg po q4 h
Captopril	12.5 mg po q4 h

to maintain adequate blood pressure control while the continuous infusion therapy is slowly discontinued. These same agents are commonly used in the management of hypertensive urgencies when prompt but not immediate blood pressure reduction is warranted. The choice of therapy for this period may or may not be the ultimate medication that the clinician intends for the patient to resume on discharge. A variety of options are available and again the choice should depend on the patient's overall clinical picture. For example, clonidine or other central-acting agents are extremely effective in controlling dangerously high blood pressure but may be problematic if mental acuity or preservation of cognitive function is a concern (42). Intermittent intravenous or oral ACEI can be particularly effective but must be used with care or withheld if the patient has co-existing renal impairment. A list of common options for treating hypertensive urgencies is presented in Table 5, with doses adjusted for elderly patients. Careful monitoring of the patient is still warranted during this phase for the signs or symptoms of retinal, cerebral, coronary, or renal ischemia that may alert the physician to institute any appropriate management changes to optimize the patient's immediate and long-term prognosis. With careful clinical assessment, thoughtful selection of therapy, and close monitoring (Table 2), many older patients with a hypertensive emergency will recover with minimal or no adverse sequelae.

ACKNOWLEDGMENT

This chapter was supported in part by P20-RR11145-03 NIH/RCMI Clinical Research Center Grant and G12-RR03026-11 Biomedical Infrastructure Development Grant.

REFERENCES

1. Calhoun DA, Oparil S. Treatment of hypertensive crisis. N Engl J Med 1990; 323: 1177–1183.
2. Sanders AB. Hypertensive emergencies. Am Fam Physician 1991; 44:1767–1774.
3. Amsterdam EA, Mathews JJ, Messerili FH, Pitts S, Ram VS. Urgent, emergent- and safe-BP reduction. Patient Care 1994; Sept. 15:80–111.
4. Chelluri L, Pinsky MR, Donahoe M, Grenvik A. Long-term outcome of critically ill elderly patients requiring intensive care. JAMA 1993; 269:3119–3123.
5. Randall T. Demographers ponder the aging of the aged and await unprecedented looming elder boom. JAMA 1993; 269:2331–2332.
6. Ooi HH, Coleman PL, Duggan J, O'Meara YM. Treatment of hypertension in the elderly. Curr Opin Nephrol Hypertens 1997; 6(5):504–509.
7. Vetter W. Treatment of senile hypertension. The Fosinopril in Old Patients Study (FOPS). Am J Hypertens 1997; 10:255S–261S.
8. Prince MJ. The treatment of hypertension in older people and its effect on cognitive function. Biomed Pharmacol 1997; 51:208–212.
9. Barker WH, Mullooly JP, Linton KL. Trends in hypertension prevalence, treatment and control in a well-defined older population. Hypertension 1998; 31[part 2]:552–559.
10. Burt VL, Whelton P, Roccella EJ, Brown C, Cutler JA, Higgins M, Horan MJ, Labarthe D. Prevalence of hypertension in the US adult population: results from the third National Health and Nutrition Examination Survey, 1988–1991. Hypertension 1995; 25:305–313.
11. Berlowitz DR, Ash AS, Hickey EC, Friedman RH, Glickman M, Kader B, Moskowitz MA. Inadequate management of blood pressure in a hypertensive population. N Engl J Med 1998; 339(27):1957–1963.
12. Preston JA. Management of geriatric hypertension in health maintenance organizations. J Am Geriatr Soc 1991; 39:683–690.
13. Saag KG, Doebbeling BN, Rohrer JE, Kolluri S, Peterson R, Hermann ME, Wallace RB. Variation in tertiary prevention and health service utilization among the elderly: the role of urban-rural residence and supplemental insurance. Med Care 1998; 36(7): 965–976.
14. Ware JE Jr, Bayliss MS, Rogers WH, Kosinski M, Tarlov AR. Differences in 4-year health outcomes for elderly and poor, chronically ill patients treated in HMO and fee-for-service systems. Results from the Medical Outcomes Study. JAMA 1996; 276(13):1039–1047.
15. Mulrow CD, Cornell JA, Herrera CR. Hypertension in the elderly. Implications and generalization of randomized trials. JAMA 1994; 272:1932–1938.
16. Applegate WB. Hypertension in the elderly. Geriatrics 1987; 12:16–19.
17. Working Group on Hypertension in the Elderly. Statement on hypertension in the elderly. JAMA 1986; 256:70–74.
18. Borhani NO. Prevalence and prognostic significance of hypertension in the elderly. J Am Geriatr Soc 1986; 34:112–114.
19. Norris KC, Fong RL. Hypertension in the African-American elderly. Clin Geriatr 1997; 5(9):56–71.

20. Kilander L, Boberg M, Lithell H. How do we treat, or not treat, high blood pressure in the oldest old? A practice study in Swedish geriatricians. Blood Pressures 1997; 6:372–376.
21. SHEP Cooperative Research Group. Prevention of stroke by antihypertensive drug treatment in older persons with isolated systolic hypertension. Final results of the Systolic Hypertension in the Elderly Program (SHEP). JAMA 1991; 265:3255–3264.
22. The sixth report of the Joint National Committee on prevention, detection, evaluation, and treatment of high blood pressure. Arch Intern Med 1997; 157(21):2413–2446.
23. The fifth report of the Joint National Committee on prevention, detection, evaluation, and treatment of high blood pressure. Arch Intern Med 1993; 153:154–183.
24. Kitiyakara C, Guzman NJ. Malignant hypertension and hypertensive emergencies. J Am Soc Nephrol 1998; 9(1):133–142.
25. Korten AE, Henderson AS, Christensen H, Jorm AF, Rodgers B, Jacomb P, Mackinnon AJ. A prospective study of cognitive function in the elderly. Psychol Med 1997; 27:919–930.
26. Elias MF, D'Agostino RB, Elias PK, Wolf PA. Neuropsychological test performance, cognitive functioning, blood pressure, and age: the Framingham Heart Study. Exp Aging Res 1995; 21:369–391.
27. Muldoon MF, Waldstein SR, Jennings JR. Neuropsychological consequences of antihypertensive medication use. Exp Aging Res 1995; 21:353–368.
28. Heckbert SR, Longstreth WT Jr, Psaty BM, Murros KE, Smith NL, Newman AB, Williamson JD, Bernick C, Furberg CD. The association of antihypertensive agents with MRI white matter findings and the Modified Mini-Mental State Examination in older adults. J Am Geriatr Soc 1997; 45(12):1423–1433.
29. Staessen JA, Birkenhäger WH, Fagard R, Forette F. Antihypertensive drugs and cognitive function in older people (letter). J Am Geriatr Soc 1998; 46(6):791.
30. Svetkey LP, George LK, Tyroler HA, Timmons PZ, Burchett BM, Blazer DG. Effects of gender and ethnic group on blood pressure control in the elderly. Am J Hypertens 1996; (6):529–535.
31. Satish S, Markides KS, Zhang D, Goodwin JS. Factors influencing unawareness of hypertension among older Mexican Americans. Prev Med 1997; (5 Pt 1):645–650.
32. Shakoor-Abdullah B, Kotchen JM, Walker WE, Chelius TH, Hoffmann RG. Incorporating socio-economic and risk factor diversity into the development of an African-American community blood pressure control program. Ethn Dis 1997; 7(3): 175–183.
33. Kunze M. Psychological background of noncompliance in old age. Gerontology 1982; 28(suppl 1):116–122.
34. Franklin SS, Weber MA. Measuring hypertensive cardiovascular risk: the vascular overload concept. Am Heart J 1994; 128(4):793–803.
35. Fong RL, Norris KC, Pan D, Ward HJ. The correlation between renal function and age-related changes in blood pressure in an inner city minority population. Ethn Dis 1998; 8:2;265A.
36. Rubenstein EB, Escalante C. Hypertensive crisis. Crit Care Clin 1989; 5(3):477–495.

37. Reuler JB, Magarian GJ. Hypertensive emergencies and urgencies: definition, recognition, and management. J Gen Intern Med 1988; 3(1):64–74.
38. Reed G, Devous M. Cerebral blood flow autoregulation and hypertension. Am J Med Sci 1985; 289:37–44.
39. Case DB, Atlas SA, Sullivan PA, Laragh JH. Acute and chronic treatment of severe and malignant hypertension with the oral angiotensin-converting enzyme inhibitor captopril. Circulation 1981; 64(4):765–771.
40. Hirschl MM, Binder M, Bur A, Herkner H, Brunner M, Mullner M, Sterz F, Laggner AN. Clinical evaluation of different doses of intravenous enalaprilat in patients with hypertensive crises. Arch Intern Med 1995; 155:2217–2223.
41. Panacek EA, Bednarczyk EM, Dunbar LM, Foulke GE Holcslaw TL. Randomized, prospective trial of fenoldopam vs sodium nitroprusside in the treatment of acute severe hypertension. Acad Emerg Med 1995; 2(11):959–965.
42. Grossman E, Ironi AN, Messeril FH. Comparative tolerability profile of hypertensive crisis treatments. Drug Safety 1998;19:99–122.

14
Acute Respiratory Failure

Darryl Y. Sue
Harbor–UCLA Medical Center, and UCLA School of Medicine, Torrance, California

Acute respiratory failure is a broad and complex topic that describes suboptimal function of any of the components of the respiratory system from a large potential mix of clinical disorders. Patients with respiratory failure may have clinical disorders ranging from underlying chronic lung diseases, such as emphysema and chronic bronchitis, to acute lung disorders, such as pneumonia in patients with no underlying lung disease, to other acute and chronic problems with the respiratory system including central nervous system dysfunction, upper airway obstruction, and abnormal control of ventilation, or to catastrophic disruption of normal gas exchange as a result of an enormous list of predisposing conditions that lead to a single common pathway of acute lung injury (i.e., noncardiogenic pulmonary edema or acute respiratory distress syndrome [ARDS]). A comprehensive discussion of respiratory failure is well beyond the scope of this chapter. Instead, this chapter will focus on the potential increased likelihood of respiratory failure developing in the elderly patient, mechanisms disrupting the balance between the capacity of the respiratory system and the demands placed on it in the older patient, and clinical features of several specific types of respiratory failure.

I. CLINICAL RELEVANCE

A. Defining Respiratory Failure

Respiratory failure occurs when the normal physiological homeostasis maintained by the respiratory system is disrupted. The markers of lack of success include hypoxemia, hypercapnia, or both; in addition, inability to compensate appropriately for metabolic acidosis (i.e., to hyperventilate in response to metabolic acidosis) would also be considered respiratory failure. Most definitions of respiratory failure use arterial blood gases, and respiratory failure is present when the arterial partial pressure of oxygen (Pa_{O_2}) is <60 mm Hg or when the arterial partial pressure of carbon dioxide (Pa_{CO_2}) is >45 to 46 mm Hg, except when compensating for metabolic alkalosis. Confounding this relatively simple definition is the role of oxygen therapy—what if the patient has a Pa_{O_2} >60 mm Hg but needs supplemental oxygen (O_2) to achieve this? Similarly, when a patient is receiving mechanical ventilatory support and has a normal Pa_{CO_2}, does he have respiratory failure? In fact, most clinicians would accept a patient as having respiratory failure if either of the arterial blood gas definitions is met, but also if the patient requires significant supportive care to maintain blood gases at normal levels.

It is important to keep in mind that the respiratory system includes much more than the lungs. Respiratory homeostasis requires an apparatus that controls the rate and depth of breathing, and that in turn needs sensors (chemoreceptors and lung and chest wall mechanoreceptors) for proper feedback. The controller must be able to send signals to the periphery, that is, to the respiratory muscles. Therefore, an intact central and peripheral nervous system and musculoskeletal system are needed. The proper amount of ventilation must be made available and matched to the proper amount of pulmonary blood flow (i.e., the pulmonary circulation and right ventricular function). Finally, the large amount of gas exchanging surface of the alveoli and alveolar capillaries needs to be intact and functioning. Respiratory failure can occur from any defect of any part of the system. In other words, respiratory failure may result from lung failure, but normal ''lung function'' does not guarantee the absence of respiratory system failure.

Respiratory failure results when the physiological capacity of the respiratory system is less than the physiological requirements. Physiological capacity is compromised by disease of any part of the respiratory system, including disorders of control of ventilation, the connections to the respiratory muscles (neurological disease), muscular disease or dysfunction, lung mechanical derangements, or abnormalities of lung gas exchange. In other situations, capacity is more or less normal, but the physiological requirement is increased. An example of the latter occurs with the stress of increased metabolic demands, as seen during exercise or with infection or metabolic acidosis. In anyone, excessive demand not capable of being met by the respiratory system results in ''respiratory failure.''

B. Impact of Aging on Respiratory Physiology and Function

Aging alone does not alter the normal physiological requirements at rest or the normal requirements during exercise by appreciable amounts, although the proportion of body weight made up of metabolically active tissues does change. However, the normal physiological changes with aging can contribute to decreased capacity of the respiratory system to meet increases in requirement, making the elderly more likely to face a situation in which demand exceeds capacity. This must be true regardless of whether the person has no prior history of lung disease or if the patient has had chronic lung disease for many years.

Physiological changes caused by aging affect the respiratory system in several ways (1–3), including alterations in lung mechanics, lung gas exchange, respiratory muscle strength and endurance, control of ventilation, and the pulmonary circulation. In addition, the heart and systemic circulation play key roles in facilitating ''cellular respiration,'' and, thereby, are major contributors to the patient's physiological capacity. Decreased lung defense mechanisms and impaired host immunity also increase the chance of respiratory failure developing.

Cross-sectional and longitudinal studies done as long as 150 years ago have consistently demonstrated reduction in vital capacity with age after normal subjects reach their early 20s. Similarly, the maximum voluntary ventilation decreases with age. These variables reflect a combination of decreased lung elastic recoil and increased outward recoil of the chest wall, decreased respiratory muscle strength, and a slight increase in lung tissue resistance. Total lung capacity, on the other hand, decreases somewhat less with aging. Because vital capacity decreases more, this must mean that the residual volume is maintained or even increases with advancing age. This may be explained by decreased elastic recoil of the lungs, resulting in ''air trapping,'' and increased outward recoil of the chest wall. Flow rates of gas, both inspiratory and expiratory, are critically dependent on lung and chest wall compliance, airway resistance, and inspiratory and expiratory muscle strength. Airway resistance changes very little with age when related to lung volume. Therefore, the reduction in forced expiratory flow in 1 second (FEV_1) seen with aging is likely due to a combination of other mechanical alterations along with a decrease in respiratory muscle strength.

The simplest estimates of respiratory muscle strength are the maximal inspiratory and expiratory pressures measured at the mouth (4). Although affected by subject effort and the lung volume at which they are measured, and allowing for the confounding effects of lung and chest wall compliance, these indirect measures of muscle strength nonetheless show a decline of about 15% (5) during adulthood with the greatest decline after age 55. Attempts to partition the pressure generation decline between diaphragmatic and nondiaphragmatic respiratory muscles have suggested that both muscle groups are affected. Studies of respiratory muscle endurance have been more difficult to interpret. In normal elderly, endurance is not greatly different. But, the true measure of endurance is reflected by the ability to sustain contraction in the face of increased load (increased pressure generation or change in length) and increased rate of contraction, that is, an increase in tension-time index. Extrapolation from data in normal subjects would suggest that a decrease in maximum strength generation would be translated into decreased endurance time with muscle loading, exactly the situation that might be faced with increased metabolic requirement. This predisposition to respiratory muscle fatigue would thereby contribute to respiratory failure.

Interestingly, the ventilatory response to carbon dioxide (CO_2) in older normal persons is difficult to distinguish from younger persons. Thus, in general $Paco_2$ is well maintained and pH homeostasis is achieved; this suggests that control of ventilation is normal in these persons. However, the normal $Paco_2$ is attained at the expense of slightly higher minute ventilation ($\dot{V}E$) both at rest and during exercise when CO_2 production increases, indicating higher physiological dead space in older individuals. Any increase in $\dot{V}E$ at a given $Paco_2$ translates into decreased ventilatory reserve, higher work of breathing, and an increase in the difference between end-tidal and arterial Pco_2.

Increased physiological dead space is a marker of increased inhomogeneity of ventilation and perfusion in the lungs that is seen with aging. The other important marker of greater ventilation-perfusion inequality in older individuals is the decrease in Pao_2 and increase in the difference between estimated mean alveolar Po_2 and arterial Po_2 (alveolar-arterial Po_2 difference). A normal age-related decline in Pao_2 of about 0.4 mm Hg per year occurs in healthy adults. The normal alveolar-arterial Po_2 difference is <12 mm Hg in young adults but may still be normal when as great as 25 to 30 mm Hg in the elderly. The fall in Pao_2 is thought to be due to closure of lung air spaces at higher lung volume such as may be seen with a larger closing volume. Mechanisms explaining increased physiological dead space include decreased cardiac output relative to ventilation, more heterogeneity of local pulmonary vascular resistance, and smaller tidal volume as a result of mechanical constraints of the lung or chest wall.

Because it is essential that gas exchange with the atmosphere takes place, the respiratory system is highly vulnerable to infection. The defense mechanisms of the lung play a major role in keeping infections under control. As expected, the aging lung becomes less able to defend against infection. Part of this effect is due to decreased mechanical function, such as impaired cough, poorer ciliary function, and altered mucous gland activity, but the immune system may also be compromised with aging. Of particular interest are the effects of aging on antioxidant levels needed for optimal immune function because of decreased dietary intake of antioxidants, such as vitamin C and vitamin E, in many elderly subjects and decreased synthesis of glutathione.

Malnutrition from protein-calorie insufficiency, vitamin deficiency, or trace element deficiency is not uncommonly seen in the elderly population for a variety of reasons, including disinterest in eating, social problems, financial limitations, chronic illness, and gastrointestinal problems. Malnutrition contributes to the likelihood of respiratory failure in several ways. First, decreased respiratory muscle strength is a consequence of protein-calorie insufficiency. Second, infections, including pneumonia, are seen as a result of impaired cellular and humoral immunity seen in malnourished patients. Third, lack of antioxidant vitamins and trace elements has been associated with lung injury and altered immune status. In animal studies, starvation leads to decreased respiratory muscle strength and increased rate of respiratory infections. Among patients with chronic lung diseases, those who have respiratory failure are more likely to be malnourished, and malnourished patients are more likely to have respiratory failure. For example, some 25% to 65% of patients with emphysema weigh <90% of ideal body weight, and the severity of airway obstruction is generally proportional to the degree of weight loss. These and other patients with chronic lung disease have decreased lean body weight, fat stores, biochemical markers of nutritional status such as serum albumin, and immune response as seen in malnourished patients. The mechanism of malnutrition in these patients is not clear but may be due to increased work of breathing, impaired gastrointestinal function, depression, or the presence of circulating factors reflecting chronic inflammation such as tumor necrosis factor.

Table 1 summarizes some of the features of aging on the respiratory system and how these contribute to decreased reserve to meet the needs of increased

Table 1 Changes in Respiratory System with Aging

Physiological alteration with aging	Clinical consequence
Decreased vital capacity	Decreased tidal volume, decreased maximum sustained minute ventilation (VE)
Decreased maximal voluntary ventilation	Decreased maximum sustained VE
Decreased lung elastic recoil	Impaired cough, increased airway resistance, increased likelihood of hyperinflation
Decreased inspiratory muscle strength	Impaired cough, decreased VE, decreased compensation for obstructive and restrictive lung diseases
Decreased expiratory muscle strength	Impaired cough, decreased VE, decreased compensation potential for obstructive lung disease
Decreased respiratory muscle endurance with resistive loading	Decreased maximum sustained VE in face of obstructive or restrictive disease
Normal ventilatory response to CO_2	Increased ventilatory requirement for given CO_2 production rate
Higher dead space/tidal volume ratio	Increased ventilatory requirement for given CO_2 production rate
Increased alveolar-arterial PO_2 difference	Decreased physiological reserve, less tolerance for hypoxemic respiratory diseases

demands on the respiratory system. Briefly, decreased vital capacity and maximum voluntary ventilation mark the limits of the ability of the patient to increase tidal volume and minute ventilation. When faced with higher CO_2 production or worsening of ventilation-perfusion matching, the elderly patient is more likely to be unable to increase ventilation than a younger subject, and hypercapnia ensues. Second, the combination of decreased inspiratory and expiratory muscle strength and decreased lung elastic recoil attenuates the effectiveness of cough in clearing respiratory secretions. This is because the most effective cough occurs at high lung volumes, when airway resistance is minimal and lung recoil forces are maximal and when there are strong expiratory muscles capable of generating high positive intrathoracic pressures. These in turn increase alveolar pressure and cause dynamic compression of the airways. Third, decreased muscle function with loading is a marker of decreased muscle function in the face of high airway resistance seen in obstructive lung disease or pulmonary edema and ARDS, stiff lungs (ARDS, interstitial lung disease, obstructive lung disease), or a stiff chest wall. Finally, abnormal gas exchange contributes to the inefficiency of the lungs, thereby leading to the need to increase minute ventilation out of proportion to the metabolic rate.

II. IMMEDIATE DIAGNOSTIC APPROACH

A. Clinical Features of Respiratory Failure

Respiratory failure often is initially seen with relatively nonspecific symptoms and signs, and this feature may be even more common in the elderly patient. Hypoxemia is the major immediate problem faced by all patients with respiratory failure regardless of cause, type, severity, and extent of disease. Patients with hypoxemia may rapidly have acute severe organ system dysfunction develop, sometimes irreversibly. The elderly patient who may have concomitant heart, central nervous system, renal, or peripheral vascular disease is likely to be more susceptible to this problem, particularly when hypoxemia is compounded by anemia and poor systemic perfusion. Symptoms of hypoxemia include altered mental status, including agitation, confusion, disorientation, lethargy, and coma; dyspnea; and chest pain from myocardial ischemia. Patients with hypoxemia may have tachycardia, tachypnea, dilated pupils, cyanosis, seizures, and diaphoresis. Prolonged severe hypoxemia may lead to permanent central nervous system (CNS) deficits, myocardial infarction, ischemic bowel, and other organ system failures. Hypercapnia in contrast is a CNS depressant, and patients in whom elevated P_{CO_2} develops rapidly (acute respiratory acidosis with low pH) become lethargic, stuporous, and comatose. Carbon dioxide retention may be confused with other syndromes with CNS depression, such as hypothyroidism, sedative-hypnotic drugs, other toxic-metabolic encephalopathies, and focal or diffuse structural CNS disorders. Of course, hypercapnia may be seen as part of these conditions as well.

Respiratory failure is seen in three distinct populations of patients. First, patients with chronic lung diseases such as chronic obstructive pulmonary disease (COPD), idiopathic pulmonary fibrosis, asthma, and sarcoidosis may initially be seen with respiratory failure. The underlying disease diminishes the reserve capacity of the respiratory system. These patients may experience episodic exacerbations of the underlying lung disease, or they may experience complicating conditions, such as superimposed infection, heart failure, renal failure, or metabolic acidosis. A second population consists of patients who have an underlying disease of a nonrespiratory component of the respiratory system. These patients may have chronic neurological disease (stroke, Parkinson's disease, decreased level of consciousness), abnormal chest wall mechanics (severe kyphoscoliosis, obesity), or impaired control of ventilation (obesity-hypoventilation syndrome, central nervous system disorder). The largest group of patients, however, has no underlying disease but has respiratory failure develop because of an acute disorder of one or more components of the respiratory system. This group includes patients with acute neurological problems such as stroke, Guillain-Barré syndrome, spinal cord compression from tumor, or myasthenia gravis. Others have acute lung disease, such as pneumonia, aspiration of gastric contents, pulmonary edema, pulmonary embolism, or ARDS.

The elderly are more likely to encounter one of the major precipitating causes of respiratory failure and are less likely to have sufficient reserve function to avoid respiratory failure. Precipitating factors directly involving the lungs and associated more often with aging include increased risk of aspiration, impaired gag and cough reflexes, and impaired immunity. Furthermore, because of the decreased likelihood that the elderly patient will enjoy an independent life style, more older patients will have gram-negative bacillary colonization of the oropharynx, predisposing them to more serious pneumonia. Among nonrespiratory causes, elderly patients are more likely to have sepsis syndrome; stroke; heart failure; immobilizing disorders of the lower extremities, such as hip fractures, cellulitis, or arthritis; higher frequency of adverse medication reactions; high incidence of protein-calorie malnutrition; and higher prevalence of gastroesophageal reflux disease. The presence of respiratory symptoms and the decline in pulmonary function have been associated with increased risk of death in older populations, as shown in an analysis of the Framingham Study data (6).

Although any cause of respiratory failure may be seen in the older population, several acute precipitating disorders deserve attention. The combination of decreased pulmonary system reserve with normal aging, effects of chronic underlying disease, and the impact of acute disorders on respiratory failure is schematically shown in Figure 1. First, pneumonia is probably the most common precipitating cause of respiratory failure in this population, occurring in patients with

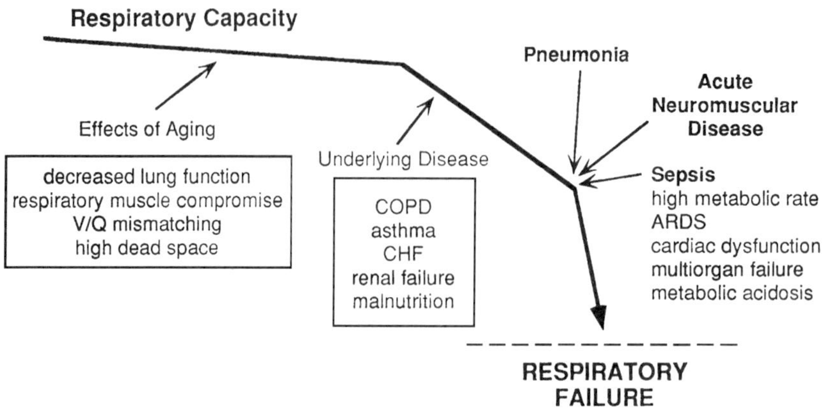

Figure 1 Decline in respiratory system capacity is shown schematically. The detrimental effects of underlying diseases, if any, on respiratory capacity are accelerated by aging, thereby diminishing the system's reserve. One or more major precipitating events (pneumonia, acute neuromuscular disease, and sepsis) further compromise respiratory function and may add considerably to the demand on the system. The combination of underlying disease, aging, and acute events may lead to respiratory failure. V/Q = ventilation/perfusion; COPD = chronic obstructive pulmonary disease; CHF = congestive heart failure; ARDS = acute respiratory distress syndrome.

and without chronic lung or other diseases. Medical problems associated with advanced age are risk factors for development of pneumonia (7,8), and advanced age is one of several factors associated with poor outcome in patients with community-acquired pneumonia (9–12). Second, ARDS is an example of hypoxemic respiratory failure that is associated with a wide variety of causes and clinical conditions, many of which are seen in the elderly population. In particular, sepsis, aspiration pneumonia, severe pneumonia, and fat embolism syndrome account for a significant number of cases of ARDS. The syndrome is also important because of the disproportional amount of time and effort devoted to the care of these patients in the intensive care unit. Third, exacerbation of chronic lung disease is a frequent cause of respiratory failure, especially in patients with chronic obstructive pulmonary disease. Finally, neurological disease leading to respiratory failure is a major cause in the elderly population, and pneumonia and respiratory failure are the most commonly encountered complications of stroke.

B. Acute Respiratory Distress Syndrome

Acute respiratory distress syndrome, sometimes previously called adult respiratory distress syndrome, is a severe form of primarily hypoxemic respiratory failure with a variety of causes and associated conditions. The histological picture is of acute lung injury with a combination of alveolar epithelial damage, destruction of type I alveolar epithelium, a variable inflammatory response, pulmonary interstitial and alveolar edema, and a spectrum of development of pulmonary fibrosis. Grossly, nonhomogeneous edema, atelectasis, and consolidation are seen. The physiological findings correlate with the pathological changes, the key features being severe hypoxemia that responds poorly to increased inspired O_2 concentrations (''refractory hypoxemia'') and decreased global lung and respiratory system compliance. Evidence indicates that acute lung injury and ARDS are a common final pathway when the lungs are damaged by a vast number of insults seen in association with many different kinds of local and systemic disorders.

Recent consensus conferences have simplified the criteria for ARDS needed for inclusion in multicenter trials, and these criteria are useful for clinical purposes as well (13). Patients are considered to have ARDS if they have hypoxemia, require high concentrations of supplemental oxygen, have diffuse infiltrates on chest roentgenogram, and have no evidence of cardiac disease.

Despite suggestions that a host of clinical conditions are associated with ARDS, approximately 70% of all cases are caused by or associated with extrapulmonary sepsis, aspiration pneumonia, severe pneumonia, or trauma with or without blunt or penetrating lung damage (14,15). The ARDS attack rate for patients who have one of these common conditions is highly variable, ranging from 5% to 70%. In some situations, such as pneumonia, toxic gas exposure, or aspiration of gastric contents, the mechanism of lung damage is obvious. In others, however, it appears that the lung injury must be due to products that reach the lung through the circulation, and almost every potential product has been accused of participation in lung injury. Some of these include activated polymorphonuclear leukocytes, complement components, interleukins, other cytokines, tumor necrosis factor, leukotrienes, immune complexes, endotoxin, and other bacterial products or components. A single common mechanism of lung injury has not been identified, and it is highly likely that multiple mechanisms play a role in some if not all ARDS cases.

The major concern about ARDS, of course, is the high mortality associated with this syndrome, ranging from 30% to 80% in studies beginning in the late 1960s. For some time, there has been debate about the cause of death in ARDS. One study suggested that respiratory failure was seldom the proximate cause of death, despite the severe hypoxemia, in patients who received aggressive respiratory supportive care (16–18). Instead, most deaths were associated with sepsis and nonrespiratory organ system dysfunction such as renal failure. These data are supported by other investigations that have found poor correlation between the severity of respiratory failure and mortality. On the other hand, other studies do find that inability to reverse the respiratory compromise is the cause of death in substantial numbers of ARDS patients. This debate is not insignificant because it asks fundamental questions about ARDS management. Is ARDS a systemic disorder that somehow affects the lungs disproportionately? Or is ARDS primarily a lung injury for which our vigorous mechanical ventilatory support contributes to multiorgan system failure? The former viewpoint would argue that treatment should not only address the lungs but that we should be trying to understand and treat nonrespiratory failure simultaneously. If the answer to the latter question is affirmative, we might wish to adapt a strategy that minimizes support of the respiratory system to minimize damage to other organs.

Potential mechanisms for increased mortality in the elderly patient with ARDS can be proposed. First, because nonrespiratory organ system failure is the causative event in many patients with ARDS, underlying renal, CNS, or cardiac disease would almost certainly increase mortality. Similarly, decreased physiological reserve of these organ systems as seen in normal aging would be expected to play a role. Second, aggressive treatment with antibiotics, diuretics, vasopressors, and other drugs in an attempt to reverse the gas exchange abnormalities, pulmonary edema, underlying infection, and other clinical features of ARDS may be more detrimental in the elderly. Next, because sepsis is the most common proximate cause of death in ARDS, studies showing higher mortality in older patients are relevant to the mechanism of the ARDS outcome. Finally, older patients may have lower tolerance for currently used ventilatory support modalities. That is, they may be more at risk for barotrauma (pneumothorax, subcutaneous emphysema), pulmonary O_2 toxicity, and hemodynamic compromise from positive-pressure ventilation and positive end-expiratory pressure (PEEP) than a younger group of patients with similar severity of ARDS.

Several studies have found a higher mortality in older patients with ARDS, with death rates ranging from 66% to 82% in this population. Recently, Suchyta et al (19) reviewed their data for 256 ARDS patients identified over a 3-year period, including 112 patients >55 years. They found that mortality was 64% in the older group compared with 45% in the 144 patients <55 years. When analyzed in terms of potential factors contributing to higher mortality, the authors found that neither gender, smoking history, ARDS risk factors, Acute Physiology and Chronic Health Evaluation (APACHE II) score, organ failure, or the incidence of sepsis were different between the two groups. Interestingly, the level of ventilatory support required in the older patients was somewhat less, with lower inspired fraction of oxygen (FIO_2) and PEEP levels during the 48 hours preceding death. They concluded that a potential was present for the increased mortality to be associated with age bias, basing this conclusion on the greater likelihood of a decision to withdraw care in the older population. Notably, 50% of nonsurvivors <55 years had support withdrawn compared with 73% of older nonsurvivors ($P < .05$), and this proportion seemed to be independent of the presence of a chronic disease state. In contrast, Gee and colleagues (20) prospectively studied 39 patients with ARDS, including 17 patients <60 years old and

16 patients ≥60 years old (mean age, 73 years). Mortality rates were 12% and 69%, respectively. Because of indirect evidence that the older patients had less severe lung disease as judged by FIO_2 and PEEP requirements, they suggested that the higher mortality in older patients might have been contributed to by impaired cardiovascular function and smaller renal reserve as a result of aging. These data are compatible with other studies of ARDS outcome that suggest that multiorgan system failure is the major association with death in ARDS patients.

Some additional issues regarding treatment of ARDS are discussed below. Treatment of ARDS focuses on (1) support of gas exchange, (2) minimizing complications of support, (3) prevention of multiorgan system failure, and (4) treatment of the underlying disease. Gas exchange support is provided by supplemental oxygen, often initially requiring concentrations of 60% to 100%, and PEEP. Almost always, patients require intubation and mechanical ventilation because of the high work of breathing and easier application of high O_2 concentrations and PEEP. Oxygen toxicity and pulmonary barotrauma are complications of therapy. Newer modalities of mechanical ventilation have shown variable degrees of success in improving gas exchange and minimizing complications. These include such techniques as pressure-controlled ventilation, inverse-ratio ventilation, tracheal gas insufflation, and high-frequency oscillation. Recently, interest has increased in inhaled nitric oxide as a means of improving PaO_2 and minimizing lung injury, but data are inconclusive.

As discussed in the following, complications of positive-pressure ventilation and oxygen should be minimized by the use of the least O_2 concentration possible and, although controversial, low tidal volume and PEEP. In addition to minimizing further lung damage, low tidal volume and low PEEP strategies may also reduce damage to nonpulmonary organ systems (multiorgan system failure). Finally, treatment of the underlying disease(s) may reduce ongoing lung injury and diminish the degree of lung permeability.

C. Respiratory Failure from Chronic Obstructive Pulmonary Disease

Chronic obstructive pulmonary disease includes chronic bronchitis, emphysema, and asthma. Chronic bronchitis is characterized primarily by airway obstruction caused by increased output of mucus-secreting glands in the airway epithelium and is highly associated with cigarette smoking, generally progressive, and associated in some studies with hypoxemia, hypercarbia, and right ventricular failure (cor pulmonale). Emphysema is a destructive process of the lungs, the precise cause of which is unclear except in a small number of patients who have insufficient or absent quantities of anti-proteases ($alpha_1$-antitrypsin deficiency) or those with exposure to certain metal fumes. The obstruction is caused by the markedly decreased lung elastic recoil, resulting in decreased transpulmonary pressure at any lung volume and thereby decreased caliber of the airways, especially during exhalation. In practice, features of chronic bronchitis and emphysema are commonly seen together. Finally, asthma is a disease characterized by airway obstruction caused by a combination of increased bronchial smooth muscle tone or reactivity, increased mucous gland secretion sometimes with thick or viscous qualities, and airway inflammation often with an eosinophilic or mixed inflammatory reaction.

As described previously, vital capacity (VC) and forced expiratory volume in 1 second (FEV_1) decline with aging. In smokers, the decline in lung volume and flow rates is accelerated. Patients with chronic bronchitis have a more rapid decline in VC and FEV_1 than those without this disease; apportioning the amount caused by smoking and that caused by chronic airway inflammation and excessive respiratory secretions is difficult. Asthma, often thought to be a reversible disease of younger patients, may have a more progressive, chronic, and less reversible course in the elderly (21,22), and features of asthma may overlap considerably with those of chronic bronchitis and emphysema. In addition, asthma symptoms and signs in the elderly patient may be mistaken for congestive heart failure or upper airway obstruction.

The elderly population may be prone to the development of asthma and chronic bronchitis for a variety of reasons. First, the cumulative effects of long-term continued smoking are obviously going to be manifest more with advanced age and longer history of smoking. Second, considerable evidence exists that asthma is far from a reversible disease; repeated attacks of asthma or chronic inflammation from asthma leads to progressive decline in lung function. Braman et al found that asthma of new onset in the elderly was similar in clinical features to asthma of long duration, but those with asthma with a mean duration of 31 years had significantly worse pulmonary function (21). These and other data suggest that the clinical manifestations of asthma are not confined to ''attacks'' or ''episodes'' only. Finally, the role of chronic gastroesophageal reflux disease as a contributor to chronic lung disease has been investigated, and this disorder is not infrequently seen in the older population. Estimates of asthma in the population 65 years or older are in the 7% to 10% range, whereas COPD among elderly populations may be as much as 35%. Although most of these patients manage to maintain function and are compromised on a chronic basis, one estimate is that 2% to 3% require hospitalization for exacerbations leading to respiratory failure (23).

Patients with COPD and asthma have respiratory failure develop because of the inability to maintain adequate ventilation in the face of increased work of breathing and worsening efficiency of ventilation (high dead space/tidal volume ratio). In other words, maintenance of arterial blood gas homeostasis is made more difficult because for a given quantity of CO_2 produced, the higher dead space/tidal volume ratio demands a higher minute ventilation. When the higher minute ventilation must be achieved despite increased airway resistance, the patient compensates by breathing at a higher relative lung volume, resulting in "air-trapping" with a higher than normal functional residual capacity. At the higher lung volume, airway resistance is minimized but at the expense of less compliant lungs and chest wall. Finally, because expiratory airway resistance is higher than inspiratory resistance, the patient further compensates by increasing inspiratory airflow to maximize the amount of expiratory time. The net effect is a progressive increase in the work of breathing that may or may not be met by the respiratory muscles; respiratory failure ensues when inspiratory muscle fatigue results in failure to compensate.

Therefore, an elderly patient with obstructive lung disease would be predicted to be more likely to have respiratory failure develop for several reasons. First, the older patient will have higher airway resistance because of the progressive nature of these disorders. Second, the older patient will generally have more inefficiency of ventilation (higher VD/VT). Third, the ability to compensate for acute exacerbation of obstruction should be more limited because of decreased strength and endurance of the inspiratory muscles.

A Finnish study found that in men and women with COPD, the need for hospitalization increased with advanced age (24). By reviewing a discharge database, they found that the need for hospital treatment began to increase at age 50, increasing to a peak at age 73 for men and age 68 for women. Their analysis led to the conclusion that heavy use of hospital resources should be anticipated in the elderly with COPD, especially for repeated admissions necessary for treatment of recurrent exacerbations. A large epidemiological study (23) reviewed the impact of asthma and COPD in the elderly patient by identifying patients with exacerbations from either of these diseases that led to hospitalization for patients >65 years. By analysis of cohorts of such patients, these investigators determined that the rehospitalization rate, duration of hospitalization, and discharge rate to a nonindependent living facility increased as patients aged. Overall, for all patients regardless of age, prognosis for acute exacerbation of severe COPD is poor. A recent report of the SUPPORT trial examined a cohort of 1016 adult patients of all ages admitted with COPD and a Pa_{CO_2} ≥50 mm Hg (25). Only 11% of patients died during the hospitalization but 33% had died by 6 months, 43% at 1 year, and 49% at 2 years. Furthermore, after discharge, 446 patients required readmission 754 times in the first 6 months after discharge. Survival time was independently associated with severity of respiratory disease, body mass index, age, prior functional status, severity of hypoxemia, and the presence of congestive heart failure, low serum albumin, or cor pulmonale.

Acute exacerbations of COPD leading to respiratory failure have been associated with variable prognosis in elderly patients. Moran et al found that among 75 patients with a mean age of 68.5 ± 7 years with 100 intensive care unit (ICU) admissions for exacerbations, most had an acceptable outcome (26). Many of the patients were severely limited before ICU admission, and, at the time of admission, mean $Paco_2$ was 86 ± 28 mm Hg, pH 7.24 ± 0.11. However, only 43 of the patients were treated by mechanical ventilation for a median of 4 days. Only 1 patient died in the ICU, although 11% died in the hospital. Seneff and colleagues (27) described a prospective multicenter cohort trial that looked at 362 admissions for COPD exacerbation from a database of 17,440 admissions to 42 ICUs in 40 hospitals. Hospital mortality overall was 24%, but for those age 65 years or older, hospital mortality was 30%, and 90-day cumulative death rate was 41%. Mortality was 47% at 180 days and 59% at 1 year. Variables associated with increased risk of hospital death included age, severity of respiratory failure or nonrespiratory organ system failure, and hospitalization time before ICU admission. Interestingly, their analysis found that mechanical ventilation at ICU admission was not associated with hospital or subsequent mortality. These authors remarked on what they considered poor prognosis, noting that 30% mortality was found during hospitalization but a further 30% of the cohort died during the next year's follow-up.

Management of exacerbations of COPD and asthma leading to respiratory failure is directed at (1) decreasing the airway obstruction, (2) restoring the strength and endurance of fatigued respiratory muscles, and (3) minimizing complications. Some issues regarding treatment are discussed in the following. Patients are most often given combinations of bronchodilators including beta-agonists, theophylline, and anticholinergics (ipratropium), often in high doses. In general, response should be guided by clinical improvement along with peak flow or FEV_1 measurements. As described later, elderly patients may be particularly sensitive to the side effects of these agents. Because airway obstruction is also caused by inflammation and mucus secretions, corticosteroids are given to asthmatics and often used with variable effects in chronic bronchitis. Attention should be paid to suctioning, effective coughing, and, in selected patients, mucolytic therapy to address the issue of airway obstruction from secretions. Appropriate antibiotics effective against *Streptococcus pneumoniae* and *Hemophilius influenzae* are usually given to patients with acute exacerbation of COPD, although the benefit of this common practice has been questioned.

Respiratory muscle fatigue is the common pathway leading to respiratory failure in obstructive lung disease. These muscles will benefit from "unloading" by decreasing airway resistance with bronchodilators and decreasing excessive air trapping. Many patients with respiratory muscle fatigue require noninvasive positive-pressure ventilation or, more often, intubation and mechanical ventilation to maintain adequate gas exchange. Particular complications of mechanical ventilation in COPD and asthma include pneumothorax and hypotension. These problems can be avoided if excessive airway pressures are minimized by using low tidal volumes (5–8 mL/kg) and high inspiratory flow rates (>60–70 L/min) to keep air trapping at a minimum. Regaining sufficient respiratory muscle function to discontinue mechanical ventilation continues to be a major problem in a number of patients with COPD and asthma. To optimize respiratory muscle function, patients should be given adequate nutritional support, maintain normal serum potassium and phosphorus, and minimize the doses of corticosteroids. Studies of weaning patients from mechanical ventilation have not shown conclusively the superiority of any technique.

D. Respiratory Failure from Neuromuscular Disorders

Neuromuscular disease, especially stroke, is commonly seen in elderly populations, and a common complication is acute respiratory failure. In addition, neurological complications of acute illness contribute to respiratory problems and may delay or preclude weaning from mechanical ventilation.

The most frequently encountered respiratory problem that results from neuromuscular weakness from any cause that affects the respiratory muscles is pneumonia and atelectasis. Impaired cough results from decreased ability to reach high lung volumes and develop high positive intrathoracic pressure because of weakness. This is why pneumonia is so often a complication of patients with strokes, Parkinson's disease and other extrapyramidal disorders, and spinal cord injury. Pneumonia is also a problem in those with a decreased level of consciousness, cranial nerve dysfunction, or sedating drugs. Respiratory failure can be seen in stroke patients. In a recent study, 24 mechanically ventilated patients with ischemic hemispheric strokes were reported (28). Mechanical ventilation was initiated as needed for generalized seizures, progression to stupor, need for hyperventilation to decrease cerebral edema, airway protection, or, most commonly, for cardiac and noncardiac pulmonary edema. Mortality was high in this group, with 17 nonsurvivors of a total of 24.

A common complication of acute severe illness, especially sepsis with hypotension and multiorgan system failure, is a disorder known as critical illness polyneuropathy (29,30). This is a peripheral nerve dysfunction with axonal degeneration seen in a high percentage of ICU patients hospitalized for more than 2 weeks. It is associated with sepsis, when there are at least two organ systems failing, low serum albumin, failure to wean from mechanical ventilation, muscle atrophy, and diminished reflexes. It is not associated with nutritional deficiency, corticosteroids, or an inflammatory condition of the nerves; the most likely explanation is that critical illness polyneuropathy is the peripheral nerves' response to generalized hypoperfusion and tissue hypoxia. Critical illness polyneuropathy should be considered when patients have weakness of the extremities or have difficult weaning because of profound respiratory muscle weakness. This disorder should not be confused with patients who have been treated with corticosteroids and nondepolarizing muscle relaxants, such as atracurium or vecuronium, who have muscle weakness develop from a severe myopathy. These patients lack sensory nerve dysfunction.

Treatment of patients with neuromuscular disease is entirely supportive and directed at prevention of further complications, and resolution of the underlying disease is the key to restoration of pulmonary function. Efforts to minimize development of pneumonia should be attempted.

III. THERAPEUTIC INTERVENTION

Acute respiratory failure is treated with a multipronged attack that can be divided into (1) supportive care until the underlying disease and exacerbating factors are resolved, (2) treatment aimed at reversing the acute disorder, and (3) maintenance of other organ systems during the acute phase of illness. In the elderly patient, treatment must be adjusted to account for differences in physiology and function, including greater sensitivity to the effects of mechanical ventilation, oxygen, respiratory medications, antibiotics, diuretics, and other drugs.

A. Supportive Care

1. Oxygen

The mechanism of hypoxemia determines the response to oxygen therapy. Patients most commonly have ventilation-perfusion inequality that allows adequate arterial Po_2 to be achieved with increased inspired O_2 between 30% and 50% (COPD, asthma, pneumonia, pulmonary edema), but patients with severe right-to-left shunting as a cause of hypoxemia (ARDS, severe pneumonia, aspiration of gastric contents, fat embolism syndrome) have refractory hypoxemia. In the latter situations, 80% to 100% inspired O_2 may be required. Supplemental O_2 may be given by nasal cannula, simple O_2 masks, or by Venturi-type masks. Higher concentrations are administered by nonrebreathing reservoir-type masks or by other special high-flow systems. In patients receiving mechanical ventilation, supplemental O_2 is usually administered at between 30% and 100% concentrations. Higher concentrations of O_2 are considered toxic to the lungs because of increased likelihood of oxidant damage to tissues. This seems to be especially true in the face of inflammation with increased production of superoxide anion, hydoxyl radicals, and hypochlorous acid enhanced by the high O_2 environment. Experimental studies have suggested that intrinsic antioxidant defenses play a major role in ameliorating O_2 toxicity. Because elderly patients have diminished antioxidant defenses, either because of antioxidant deficiency or other reasons, such as decreased reduced glutathione production, they may be more susceptible to lung O_2 toxicity, but data are not available. In any case, recommendations for O_2 therapy are to give the minimal amount of O_2 necessary to achieve a Pao_2

>60 mm Hg (O_2 saturation >90%), and to attempt to use, if possible, less than 50% inspired O_2.

2. Mechanical Ventilation

Mechanical ventilation with positive-pressure ventilation is a mainstay of supportive care for respiratory failure. In simplest terms, mechanical ventilation provides sufficient minute ventilation to patients whose ventilatory requirements exceed their sustained ventilatory capacity because of increased work of breathing, fatigue of the respiratory muscles, and inefficient lung gas exchange. In addition, mechanical ventilation may allow improvement in oxygenation by the use of adjunctive techniques such as PEEP in suitable patients. Many new and different methods of ventilation, increasingly specific techniques for particular kinds of respiratory failure, and increased understanding of the physiology and complications of mechanical ventilation characterize the current state of the art. A comprehensive review of mechanical ventilation is beyond the scope of this chapter, but several new concepts can be explored as they relate to treatment of older patients.

Nearly all positive-pressure ventilation has been provided to patients by means of cuffed endotracheal tubes. However, recent studies have indicated that noninvasive positive pressure ventilation given by a moderately tight-fitting mask may be successful in some patients who would otherwise require intubation. Patients with COPD, obesity-hypoventilation syndrome, reversible neurological diseases, asthma, ARDS, and cardiogenic pulmonary edema may benefit from several hours to days of noninvasive ventilation with this technique. Caution should be used in terms of universal application, particularly in the elderly patient. First, patients should generally be awake, alert, able to protect their airway from aspiration of secretions or gastric contents, and able to generate an appropriate rate and depth of ventilation. Second, many patients are unable to tolerate the noninvasive mask because of facial discomfort, feelings of suffocation, and other symptoms. Third, the amount of positive pressure that can be generated may be inadequate in some patients, especially those with the highest airway resistance or lowest lung and chest wall compliance. Finally, some studies have pointed out that the increased monitoring and supportive care for these patients precludes use of noninvasive positive pressure in their facility. This technique should only be used by those highly experienced in setting up, adjusting, and monitoring noninvasive ventilation.

Positive-pressure ventilation and PEEP have been in widespread use for more than 40 years, and from the earliest application, these techniques have been associated with complications such as barotrauma. In recent years, increasing evidence exists that positive-pressure ventilation and PEEP may cause other forms of lung damage and adversely affect outcome even while providing life-sustaining supportive care, especially in patients with ARDS and asthma. Although currently a somewhat controversial subject, many investigators and clinicians have adopted various strategies to minimize the potential for lung injury. A variety of methods have been advocated, but most are based on the idea that excessive stretching of the lung during ventilation is the cause of injury. Therefore, some have recommended that tidal volume be constrained to 5 to 7 mL/kg ideal body weight instead of 8 to 10 mL/kg as previously suggested, with a goal of limiting peak airway pressure to 30 cm H_2O or less. In some cases, lowering tidal volume has resulted in hypercapnia, and because a mild to moderate degree of hypercapnia is often well tolerated, ''permissive hypercapnia'' as a means of minimizing lung injury has been proposed. Recently, this view has been challenged by data suggesting that hypercapnia may be associated with organ system dysfunction (31). In addition, the amount of PEEP recommended has undergone changes. Some continue to advocate the least amount of PEEP needed to achieve the goal of adequate arterial oxygenation with minimal effects on cardiac output. But a new strategy is based on the possibility that too low a PEEP setting also contributes to lung injury and suggests that sufficient PEEP be given to avoid repeated lung closure and reopening during each respiratory cycle (32,33). Despite the attractiveness of this method to reduce lung injury, recent trials have not been conclusive (31,33–35). These new concepts may have important implications for management of respiratory failure in the elderly because this population has disproportionate alterations in lung mechanics, potential for greater risk of barotrauma, possibly greater sensitivity of cardiac function to PEEP, and perhaps higher risk of organ system dysfunction from hypercapnia. Clinical trials conducted thus far have not sought to determine whether differences exist in the older population's response to these strategies of mechanical ventilation.

It might be assumed that mechanical ventilation is an aggressive support modality that would be poorly tolerated by elderly patients with limited organ system reserve (because positive-pressure ventilation is associated with lowering cardiac output) or because of preexisting changes in lung anatomy or lung function brought about by aging. In fact, data support this concept, but subsets of elderly patients who undergo mechanical ventilation may have a good outcome. Studies that have found a poor overall prognosis include two retrospective reports. In a study of 612 mechanically ventilated Department of Veterans Affairs patients (97% men), hospital mortality was 64%, whereas 1-year mortality was 77% (36). When separated by age, those >70 years had 76% in-hospital and 94% 1-year mortality. Those with low serum albumin (<2 g/100 mL), high APACHE II scores, and postcardiopulmonary resuscitation had the poorest prognosis. Of note is that these patients had a wide range of acute and chronic illnesses and required mechanical ventilation for different reasons. Overall mortality was also high regardless of age. Those <60 years were 180 patients who had a 60%

in-hospital death rate, and only 29% survived 1 year. In another retrospective review, 59 patients >80 years were followed up after mechanical ventilation was initiated (37). In-hospital mortality was 78%. Those who required more than 100 days of mechanical ventilation, a subgroup of 22 patients, had only 2 patients survive to discharge.

It is clear that age has an important effect on outcome of mechanical ventilation, but other factors influence results as well, and age should not be used as the only factor in making a decision to use mechanical ventilation (38). Subgroup analyses in more recent studies suggest that prognosis may not be poor for all patients. For example, a study by Dardaine and coworkers (39) found that among 110 patients aged 70 or older who required ventilatory support in the ICU, the mortality in the ICU was 38%. Subsequent mortality was 60% at 6 months, 63% at 12 months, and 67% at 18 months. The presence of shock and previous health status predicted mortality at 6 months. The leveling off of mortality suggests that a subset of patients with good prognoses exists; this is supported by examination of surviving patients at 18 months. Among these, 92% had the same residence, 75% had the same health status as before the ICU admission, and 78% had the same degree of independent living as before. The authors concluded that age itself was a poor predictor of outcome, whereas physiological status (presence of chronic disease) and shock (acute deterioration) were more important determinants. Similarly, Swinburne et al (40) retrospectively reviewed 1860 patients treated with mechanical ventilation for more than 3 hours. Separating out patients 80 years and older, they determined that 31% of these 282 survived to discharge compared with 44% of 1578 younger patients. A combination of advanced age and pre-existing renal disease, liver disease, cancer, other systemic illness, or malnutrition has a much poorer survival, as low as 7% compared with 29% for younger patients with these conditions, whereas the absence of these conditions led to survival of 38% in the older patients versus 49% in the younger patients. These authors concluded that for adults aged 80 and older who are mechanically ventilated, prognosis for the short term is very good to excellent unless patients have severe underlying illness or malnutrition. Importantly, the duration of mechanical ventilation did not affect the likelihood of a good outcome, and age did not appear to be a factor in survival up to the point of ventilator weaning. In a 5-year retrospective review of 383 men with acute respiratory failure requiring mechanical ventilation, however, survival to hospital discharge was only 50% and only 30.1% at 1 year (41). These authors also reviewed data from 10 previously reported studies and found a pooled survival rate of 46% to ICU discharge, 43% to hospital discharge, and 30% at 1 year. They also found that age did have a significant effect on survival; younger patients had better survival along with patients who required mechanical ventilation for COPD or postoperatively compared with those after cardiac or respiratory arrest.

B. Specific Therapy

Relatively few treatments are aimed at reversing the underlying cause of respiratory failure. Of course, antibiotics are given for pneumonia and sepsis, and antibiotics have variable success in affecting the outcome of acute bronchitis. For treatment of primary lung diseases, bronchodilators and corticosteroids are commonly given to patients with respiratory failure from obstructive pulmonary diseases such as chronic bronchitis and asthma.

1. Bronchodilators

The three major classes of bronchodilators are beta-adrenergic agonists, anticholinergics, and theophylline or methylxanthine. Beta-agonists, such as albuterol, are sympathomimetic agents that have potent relatively short-acting bronchodilator effects in most patients when given by inhalation of an aerosol. Recent recommendations have suggested a more favorable therapeutic ratio when given by inhalation compared with orally. Long-acting beta-agonists such as salmeterol are useful in many patients. The most commonly used beta-agonists have some degree of selectivity for beta-$_2$-receptors, thereby minimizing tachycardia and increased myocardial oxygen demand, important considerations in the elderly. These drugs may cause tremors at moderate to high doses, and at higher doses do not exhibit perfect beta-$_2$-selectivity. Several studies in recent years have suggested potential adverse effects on airway function when short-acting beta-agonists are given routinely to patients with asthma. This has led to the recommendation that these drugs should be used primarily for occasional short-term relief, whereas anti-inflammatory therapy becomes the mainstay of asthma therapy. New long-acting beta-agonists such as salmeterol are intended for maintenance therapy and should not be used in acute exacerbations.

Anticholinergic drugs have been shown to be of greatest benefit in chronic bronchitis and have variable efficacy in asthma. Ipratropium bromide is available for inhalation. Side effects are relatively few, but, importantly for the elderly, may rarely include urinary retention and dry mouth.

Inhaled bronchodilators have been shown to be highly effective, largely because the dose delivered to the airways can be enhanced while minimizing systemic side effects. However, many patients prescribed inhaled bronchodilators by metered-dose inhalers are unable to use these devices effectively because they are poorly instructed, lack coordination, or are unable to remember the steps necessary. Such shortcomings are especially relevant to older patients. Moreover, many caregivers may be unable to operate metered-dose inhalers properly. Such older patients and their caregivers should be carefully taught and asked to demonstrate proper use. They should understand the purpose of the drugs, including whether the drugs should be used on a regular or intermittent basis.

Particular care must be observed when giving elderly patients theophylline, a mild bronchodilator useful in some patients as adjunctive therapy. Recent data have suggested that theophylline may have anti-inflammatory properties or act as an immunomodulatory agent. Theophylline can be given orally in time-released form and intravenously. This drug must be given with careful consideration of dose and elimination rates because of the high potential for adverse effects such as tachycardia, dysrhythmia, nausea, vomiting, and seizures. Decreased clearance of theophylline is seen with advanced age, congestive heart failure, liver disease, and in the presence of such drugs as erythromycin, fluoroquinolones, cimetidine, and others. Increased clearance may be seen in smokers and patients taking phenobarbital or other drugs that stimulate the cytochrome P450 system.

2. Corticosteroids

These potent anti-inflammatory agents are most often given to respiratory failure patients with asthma for which there is strong evidence of benefit. Evidence for benefit in exacerbations of chronic bronchitis is considerably weaker. About 15% to 25% of patients with chronic bronchitis have some clinical response to corticosteroids; therefore, these drugs should probably be tried when patients have acute exacerbations. But they should be withdrawn quickly in the absence of response before complications occur. In most reported studies, ARDS patients do not benefit from corticosteroids. Corticosteroids may be tried in selected patients with sarcoidosis or interstitial pulmonary fibrosis. Although potent corticosteroids may be given by inhalation, respiratory failure patients should be given corticosteroids orally or intravenously in moderately high doses to ensure adequate delivery in respiratory failure. Although all patients are prone to side effects of corticosteroids, the elderly patient is particularly susceptible acutely to hypokalemia with cardiac dysrhythmia, metabolic alkalosis, salt and water retention, hyperglycemia, and acute steroid myopathy with weakness. Over a longer time, corticosteroids contribute to calcium mobilization from bone, osteoporosis and fractures, infections with opportunistic organisms, and cataracts. In patients given these chronically, adrenal cortical hormone production is suppressed, and adrenal insufficiency may result if the drugs are withdrawn rapidly.

3. Other Drugs

Patients with asthma and chronic bronchitis may be given drugs that modify the effects of certain leukotrienes, either as a receptor antagonist or by interfering with synthesis of these products of arachidonic acid (5-lipo-oxygenase inhibitor). Leukotrienes have multiple effects, including participating in inflammation, airway smooth muscle contraction, and response to inhalation challenges. These drugs are most often given orally as maintenance therapy and to spare the use of corticosteroids. Their use in patients during acute respiratory failure is unclear.

C. Support of Nonrespiratory Systems

Patients with respiratory failure in the ICU should have attention paid to prevention of aspiration pneumonia (elevation of head of bed), pressure ulcers because of immobilization, anemia, other nosocomial infections (urinary bladder catheters, intravenous lines), prevention of deep venous thrombosis (anticoagulation, intermittent pneumatic compression of the legs), and prevention of fluid overloading. Psychosocial needs should be addressed, in particular the difficulty with communication in patients with endotracheal tubes and the extreme dependence of patients needing mechanical ventilation. In addition, three areas are specific to patients with acute respiratory failure: nutritional support, prevention of upper gastrointestinal bleeding, and prevention and treatment of ventilator-associated pneumonia (VAP).

1. Nutritional Support

Patients should be assessed for the degree and nature of nutritional depletion by standard methods, and nutritional support should be started as soon as possible to minimize further loss of respiratory muscle function. This is especially important in elderly patients because of the higher prevalence of undernutrition or malnutrition associated with increasing age. In most patients who require mechanical ventilation, enteral feeding is preferred and feasible with a variety of commercially available preparations. These are generally high in quality protein, include easily absorbed carbohydrate and fat, and contain vitamins and trace elements. Some patients will require parenteral nutrition with central venous catheters. The choice of feeding formula is usually not critical, but some investigators have called attention to increased CO_2 production seen with high-carbohydrate feedings, although most of these patients were studied after rapid infusion of highly concentrated glucose solutions. The increased CO_2 necessitates either an increase in minute ventilation, sometimes precipitating respiratory failure, or an increase in Pa_{CO_2}. It is unclear, however, whether high-fat, low-carbohydrate formulas have an advantage in respiratory failure patients. Complications of enteral feeding include aspiration of gastric contents and diarrhea, both of which tend to be more problematic in the elderly. Parenteral nutrition is associated with certain complications that are particularly devastating to elderly patients (i.e., higher infection rates, fluid overload, electrolyte disturbances, and acid-base imbalance). Careful calculation of nutritional requirements and how they can be met are essential, usually with the help of nutritional support staff.

2. Gastrointestinal Bleeding Prophylaxis

The incidence of upper gastrointestinal bleeding from gastritis has declined considerably in recent years in association with routine administration of antacids, acid-secretion inhibitors (H_2-blockers or proton pump inhibitors), or sucralfate, an agent that works without changing gastric pH. Recent studies support the use of these agents in patients with a coagulopathy or thrombocytopenia or those who are receiving mechanical ventilation (42). One controversy centers around whether an increase in pneumonia is associated with gastric acid inhibition, in which case sucralfate may be preferred, but this issue remains unresolved. A recent multicenter randomized trial of sucralfate compared with ranitidine found that the H_2-blocker was superior in preventing clinically important gastrointestinal bleeding, whereas no significant differences occurred in the incidence of ventilator-associated pneumonia, duration of ICU stay, or mortality (43). However, the data were not evaluated on the basis of increasing age.

3. Ventilator-Associated Pneumonia

Pneumonia developing during mechanical ventilation is a common complication of endotracheal intubation and, especially, prolonged mechanical ventilation (44,45). The upper airways become colonized with bacteria soon after intubation. Often, these are gram-negative bacilli and *Staphylococcus aureus*. In many ICUs, these bacteria have acquired resistance to multiple antibiotics, and when pneumonia develops, treatment is difficult, prolonged, and poorly tolerated (46). Patients with ventilator-associated pneumonia (VAP) have increased mortality, longer ICU and hospital stays, higher costs, and longer duration of mechanical ventilation. Prevention of VAP by use of a variety of techniques, including oral administration of poorly absorbable antibiotics, avoidance of gastric acid inhibition, and frequent changing of ventilator-patient tubing circuits, has not been shown to have clear benefits. Decreasing the duration of mechanical ventilation is likely to be the best prevention of VAP, but, if not possible, careful attention must be paid to endotracheal tube suctioning technique, proper drainage of water condensing in the circuit, prevention of aspiration of gastric contents, consideration of type and duration of antibiotic treatment, and patient positioning. Some hospitals have found that special beds that provide rotational therapy and automated chest percussion can decrease the incidence of hospital-acquired pneumonia and VAP; these beds might be considered in selected patients.

REFERENCES

1. Campbell EJ, Lefrak SS. How aging affects the structure and function of the respiratory system. Geriatrics 1978;33:68–74.

2. Griffith D, Idell S. Approach to adult respiratory distress syndrome and respiratory failure in elderly patients. Clin Chest Med 1993;14:571–582.
3. Mahler DA, Rosello RA, Loke J. The aging lung. Clin Geriatr Med 1986;2:215–225.
4. Enright PL, Kronmal RA, Manolio TA, Schenker MB, Hyatt RE. Respiratory muscle strength in the elderly. Correlates and reference values. Am J Respir Crit Care Med 1994;149(2 Pt1):430–438.
5. Tolep K, Kelsen SG. Effect of aging on respiratory skeletal muscles. Clin Chest Med 1993;14:363–378.
6. Sorlie PD, Kannel WB, O'Connor G. Mortality associated with respiratory function and symptoms in advanced age. The Framingham Study. Am Rev Respir Dis 1989; 140:379–384.
7. Koivula I, Sten M, Makela PH. Risk factors for pneumonia in the elderly. Am J Med 1994;96:313–320.
8. Riquelme R, Torres A, El-Ebiary M, de la Bellacasa JP, Estruch R, Mensa J, Fernandez-Sola J, Hernandez C, Rodriguez-Roisin R. Community-acquired pneumonia in the elderly: a multivariate analysis of risk and prognostic factors. Am J Respir Crit Care Med 1996;154:1450–1455.
9. Niederman MS, Bass JB, Campbell GD, Fein AM, Grossman RF, Mandell LA, Marrie TJ, Sarosi GA, Torres A, Yu VL. Guidelines for the initial empiric therapy of community-acquired pneumonia: proceedings of an American Thoracic Society Consensus Conference. Am Rev Respir Dis 1993;148:1418–1426.
10. Fine MJ, Auble TE, Yealy DM, Hanusa BH, Weissfeld LA, Singer DE, Coley CM, Marrie TJ, Kapoor WN. A prediction rule to identify low-risk patients with community-acquired pneumonia. N Engl J Med 1997;336:243–250.
11. Fine MJ, Smith MA, Carson CA, Mutha SS, Sankey SS, Weissfeld LA, Kapoor WN. Prognosis and outcomes of patients with community-acquired pneumonia. A meta-analysis. JAMA 1996;275:134–141.
12. Bartlett JG, Breiman RF, Mandell LA, File TM. Community-acquired pneumonia in adults: Guidelines for management. Clin Infect Dis 1998;26:811–838.
13. Milberg JA, Davis DR, Steinberg KP, Hudson LD. Improved survival of patients with Acute Respiratory Distress Syndrome (ARDS): 1983–1993. JAMA 1995;273: 310–312.
14. Fowler AA, Hamman RF, Good JT, Benson KN, Baird M, Eberle DJ, Petty TL, Hyers TM. Adult respiratory distress syndrome: risk with common predispositions. Ann Intern Med 1983;98:593–597.
15. Hudson LD, Milberg JA, Anardi D, Maunder RJ. Clinical risks for development of the acute respiratory distress syndrome. Am J Respir Crit Care Med 1995;121(2 Pt 1):293–301.
16. Bell RC, Coalson JJ, Smith JD, Johanson WG Jr. Multiple organ system failure and infection in the adult respiratory distress syndrome. Ann Intern Med 1983;99:293–298.
17. Montgomery AB, Stager MA, Carrico CJ, Hudson LD. Causes of mortality in patients with adult respiratory distress syndrome. Am Rev Respir Dis 1985;132:485–489.
18. Seidenfeld JJ, Pohl DF, Bell RC, Harris GD, Johanson WG Jr. Incidence, site and

outcome of infections in patients with the adult respiratory distress syndrome. Am Rev Respir Dis 1986;134:12–16.
19. Suchyta MR, Clemmer TP, Elliott CG, Orme JF, Morris AH, Jacobson J, Menlove R. Increased mortality of older patients with acute respiratory distress syndrome. Chest 1997;111:1334–1339.
20. Gee MH, Gottlieb GE, Albertine KH, Kubis JM, Peters SP, Fish JE. Physiology of aging related outcome in the adult respiratory distress syndrome. J Appl Physiol 1990;69:822–829.
21. Braman SS, Kaemmerlen JT, Davis SM. Asthma in the elderly. A comparison between patients with recently acquired and long-standing disease. Am Rev Respir Dis 1991;143:336–340.
22. Braman SS. Asthma in the elderly patient. Clin Chest Med 1993;14:413–422.
23. Cydulka RK, McFadden ER, Emerman CL, Sivinski LD, Pisanelli W, Rimm AA. Patterns of hospitalization in elderly patients with asthma and chronic obstructive pulmonary disease. Am J Respir Crit Care Med 1997;156:1807–1812.
24. Vilkman S, Keistinen T, Tuuponen T, Kivela SL. Survival and cause of death among elderly chronic obstructive pulmonary disease patients after first admission to hospital. Respiration 1997;64:281–284.
25. Connors AF Jr, Dawson NV, Thomas C, Harrell FE Jr, Desbiens N, Fulkerson WJ, Kussin P, Bellamy P, Goldman L, Knaus WA. Outcomes following acute exacerbation of severe chronic obstructive lung disease. The SUPPORT investigators. Am J Respir Crit Care Med 1996;154 (4 Pt 1):959–967.
26. Moran JL, Green JV, Homan SD, Leeson RJ, Leppard PI. Acute exacerbations of chronic obstructive pulmonary disease and mechanical ventilation. A reevaluation. Crit Care Med 1998;26:71–78.
27. Seneff MG, Wagner DP, Wagner RP, Zimmerman JE, Knaus WA. Hospital and 1-year survival of patients admitted to intensive care units with acute exacerbation of chronic obstructive pulmonary disease. JAMA 1995;274:1852–1857.
28. Wijdicks EF, Scott JP. Causes and outcome of mechanical ventilation in patients with hemispheric stroke. Mayo Clin Proc 1997;72:210–213.
29. Zochodne DW, Bolton CF, Wells GA, Gilbert JJ, Hahn AF, Brown JD, Sibbald WA. Critical illness polyneuropathy: a complication of sepsis and multiple organ failure. Brain 1987;110:819–841.
30. Witt NJ, Zochodne DW, Bolton CF, Grand'Maison F, Wells G, Young GB, Sibbald WJ. Peripheral nerve function in sepsis and multiple organ failure. Chest 1991;99: 176–184.
31. Stewart TE, Meade MO, Cook DJ, Granton JT, Hodder RV, Lapinsky SE, Mazer CD, McLean RF, Rogovein TS, Schouten BD, Todd TRJ, Slutsky AS and the Pressure- and Volume-Limited Ventilation Strategy Group. Evaluation of a ventilation strategy to prevent barotrauma in patients at high risk for acute respiratory distress syndrome. N Engl J Med 1998;338:355–361.
32. Amato MBP, Barbas CSV, Medeiros DM, Schettino GdePP, Filho GL, Kairalla RA, Deheinzelin D, Morais C, Fernandes EdeO, Takagaki TY, De Carvalho CRR. Beneficial effects of the "open lung approach" with low distending pressures in acute respiratory distress syndrome: a prospective randomized study on mechanical ventilation. Am J Respir Crit Care Med 1995;152:1835–1846.

33. Amato MBP, Barbas CSV, Medieros DM, Magaldi RB, Schettino GdePP, Lorenzi-Filho G, Kairalla RA, Deheinzelin D, Munoz C, Oliveira R, Takagaki TY, Carvalho CRR. Effect of a protective ventilation strategy on mortality in the acute respiratory distress syndrome. N Engl J Med 1998;338:347–354.
34. Weg JG, Anzueto A, Balk RA, Wiedemann HP, Pattishall EN, Schork MA, Wagner LA. The relation of pneumothorax and other air leaks to mortality in the acute respiratory distress syndrome. N Engl J Med 1998;338:341–346.
35. Hudson LD. Protective ventilation for patients with acute respiratory distress syndrome (editorial). N Engl J Med 1998;338:385–387.
36. Papadakis MA, Lee KK, Browner WS, Kent DL, Matchar DB, Kagawa MK, Hallenbeck J, Lee D, Onishi R, Charles G. Prognosis of mechanically ventilated patients. West J Med 1993;159:659–664.
37. Cohen IL, Lambrions J, Fein IA. Mechanical ventilation for the elderly patient in intensive care. Incremental changes and benefits. JAMA 1993;269:1025–1029.
38. Cohen IL, Lambrinos J. Investigating the impact of age on outcome of mechanical ventilation using a population of 41,848 patients from a statewide database. Chest 1995;107:1673–1680.
39. Dardaine V, Constans T, Lasfargues G, Perrotin D, Ginies G. Outcome of elderly patients requiring ventilatory support in intensive care. Aging (Milano) 1995;7:221–227.
40. Swinburne AJ, Fedullo AJ, Bixby K, Lee DK, Wahl GW. Respiratory failure in the elderly. Analysis of outcome after treatment with mechanical ventilation. Arch Intern Med 1993;153:1657–1662.
41. Stauffer JL, Fayter NA, Graves B, Cromb M, Lynch JC, Goebgel P. Survival following mechanical ventilation for acute respiratory failure in adult men. Chest 1993;104:1222–1229.
42. Cook DJ, Fuller HD, Guyatt GH, Marshall JC, Leasa D, Hall R, Winton TL, Rutledge F, Todd TJ, Roy P. Risk factors for gastrointestinal bleeding in critically ill patients. N Engl J Med 1994;330:377–381.
43. Cook D, Guyatt G, Marshall J, Leasa D, Fuller H, Hall R, Peters S, Rutledge F, Griffith L, McLellan A, Wood G, Kirby A, Tweeddale M, Pagliarello J, Johnston R, for the Canadian Critical Care Trials Group. A comparison of sucralfate and ranitidine for the prevention of upper gastrointestinal bleeding in patients requiring mechanical ventilation. N Engl J Med 1998;338:791–797.
44. American Thoracic Society. Hospital-acquired pneumonia in adults: Diagnosis, assessment of severity, initial antimicrobial therapy, and preventative strategies. Am J Respir Crit Care Med 1995;153:1711–1725.
45. Meduri GU. Diagnosis and differential diagnosis of ventilator-associated pneumonia. Clin Chest Med 1995;16:61–93.
46. Wunderink RG. Ventilator-associated pneumonia. Failure to respond to antibiotic therapy. Clin Chest Med 1995;16:173–193.

15
Acute Renal Failure

Dean T. Yamaguchi
VA Greater Los Angeles Healthcare System, and UCLA School of Medicine, Los Angeles, California

I. INTRODUCTION

In this review the more commonly observed causes of acute renal failure in the elderly will be discussed. The great spectrum of causes of acute renal failure that can occur in both young and in older patients will not be elaborated on. The physiological alterations in the kidney that occur with aging will be highlighted to explain the potential susceptibility of the older kidney to insults resulting in acute renal failure. A practical diagnostic approach based on the history, physical examination, and simple biochemical tests will be outlined, followed by discussions regarding specific, common causes of acute renal failure in the elderly (Table 1) and a brief description of therapeutic options.

II. PHYSIOLOGICAL ALTERATIONS IN RENAL FUNCTION WITH AGE

To understand why the aging kidney may be more prone to a variety of causes of acute renal failure, renal and cardiovascular changes that occur with age should be delineated. An excellent review of aging renal physiology is given by Epstein (1).

In general renal mass decreases with age. From young adulthood to the ninth decade, an approximate 25% decrement in renal mass occurs, mainly as a result of renal cortical loss with sparing of the medulla. Sclerosis and subsequent loss of glomeruli (up to 10%–30% of total glomeruli by the eighth decade) occur with the subsequent hypertrophy of remaining glomeruli. Renal perfusion has

Table 1 Common Causes of Acute Renal Failure in the Elderly

Prerenal	Renal	Postrenal
Dehydration	Vascular	Bladder outlet obstruction
Congestive heart failure	Acute tubular necrosis	Prostatic hypertrophy or neoplasm
	Atheroemboli	Anticholinergic medication
	Radiocontrast	Upper tract obstruction
	Angiotensin-converting enzyme inhibition	Retroperitoneal tumors, lymph node hypertrophy, hematoma, nephrolithiasis
	NSAIDs	
	Glomerular	
	Rapidly progressive glomerulonephritis	
	Tubulointerstitial	
	Acute allergic interstitial nephritis	
	Aminoglycoside nephrotoxicity	
	Multiple myeloma	

NSAIDS = nonsteroidal antiinflammatory drugs.

also been shown to decrease by approximately 10% per decade after the fourth decade of life, with increases in renal vascular resistance and an increase in filtration fraction (glomerular filtration rate/renal blood flow). The decrease in renal blood flow occurs predominantly in the cortex. Structural vascular changes in interlobar, arcuate, and interlobular arteries with advancing age (increased tortuosity of vessels) and increased effects of renal vasoconstrictors such as angiotensin II, endothelin, and thromboxane A_2; decreases in vasodilatory substances, such as prostacyclin (PGI_2) and nitric oxide; and impaired vascular response to nitric oxide account for the increase in renal vascular resistance (2).

Glomerular filtration rate also decreases approximately after the fourth decade of life. On the average, Lindeman, et al (3) reported an approximate decrease in glomerular filtration rate of 1 mL/min per 1.73 m^2 per year beginning from about age 50. However, it should be noted that approximately a third of the elderly subjects in this study had a stable creatinine clearance for more than 20 years of this longtitudinal study, suggesting that a decrease in renal function may not be totally a consequence of age but perhaps linked to the dietary intake of protein (4). A decrement in total urinary creatinine excretion occurs with age, reflecting decreased muscle mass in the elderly in general. However, serum creatinine may remain in the normal range even with the fall in creatinine clearance. Thus serum creatinine levels may not accurately reflect true glomerular filtration rate in older individuals.

In addition to decrements in glomerular filtration rate, tubular function in the elderly is compromised. Marcias-Nunez et al (5) reported that elderly patients infused with sodium chloride showed a decrease in distal sodium reabsorption. In response to dietary sodium intake, healthy elderly subjects older than 60 years of age are significantly slower in reducing urinary sodium excretion than subjects younger than 25 years of age (1). Similarly Fish et al (6) concluded that older individuals given saline infusions had a delay in sodium excretion. This suggests that response time for sodium conservation is longer in elderly subjects, and thus elderly patients may be prone to states that result in volume depletion. The defect seen in renal sodium conservation may be due to diminished response to angiotensin II and aldosterone. It has been shown that with aging, renin synthesis and release decrease, which may result in decreased angiotensin II levels and subsequent aldosterone secretion under basal, posture-stimulated, and volume-depleted conditions. Basal atrial natriuretic peptide in general has been found to be increased in older individuals compared with younger individuals and may be a compensatory mechanism in response to the renal tubular impairment in excretion of a sodium load.

Renal concentration ability also declines in older individuals as demonstrated by lower urinary osmolality after dehydration. Differences in basal and stimulated plasma arginine vasopression (AVP) in old versus young individuals are controversial. In earlier studies, AVP was found to be increased by approximately twofold in the elderly compared with younger subjects in response to increases in serum osmolality. The sensitivity of osmoreceptors appears to be greater with age, leading to increases in AVP release; thus, higher AVP levels in the elderly per unit change in serum osmolality may be a compensatory mechanism for the reduction in the ability of the aging kidney to concentrate urine. Interestingly, the AVP response to orthostasis and presumably volume depeletion differs from the response to increased osmolality in that elderly subjects show diminished plasma AVP levels compared with younger subjects. However, other studies have failed to demonstrate a significant change in basal or osmolality-stimulated AVP levels in older versus younger individuals (7). Still others have reported that older subjects deprived of fluids had lower plasma AVP levels than younger subjects (8).

All the above changes in glomerular and tubular function and in the renal vasculature are important determinants for the susceptibility of elderly individuals to have acute renal failure develop. In addition, male gender is an important determinant of age-related changes in glomeruli, where the presence of androgens appears to promote age-dependent glomerular damage in rats (9). In rats chronic structural and functional renal changes increase suseptibility of the aged kidney to nephrotoxic insults (10). For instance, acute tubular necrosis was observed more frequently in kidneys of middle-aged (12–14 months) and aged (22–25 months) rats given acetaminophen (11,12). Recent studies in aging rats have demonstrated that the decrement in glomerular filtration rate caused by renal arterial clamping was greater in old than in young rats, whereas the time for recovery of acute renal failure was more protracted (13). Similarly, in humans, it has been reported that older patients with prerenal acute renal failure take longer to recover renal function than younger patients, and the number of older patients with acute tubular necrosis whose renal function does not return to normal is greater than in younger patients (14).

III. IMMEDIATE DIAGNOSTIC APPROACH

A. Initial Assessment

In various studies examining acute renal failure in the elderly, the criteria to define acute renal failure have been varied. Some have defined acute renal failure as an increase in serum creatinine levels to >2.0 mg/dL from previously normal renal function or unstated baseline renal function (14,15), an increase in serum creatinine levels >3.0 mg/dL from previously normal renal function (16,17), a serum creatinine level ≥1.85 mg/dL (18), an increase in serum creatinine level by 0.5 mg/dL (19), or a doubling of the patient's serum creatinine level in those with pre-existing chronic renal insufficiency defined as serum creatinine levels >1.7 mg/dL (16). In the elderly, normal renal function as defined by baseline serum creatinine levels can be in the range of 0.5 mg/dL up to 1.0 mg/dL, depending on muscle mass; thus creatinine level rises that still fall within the normal range need to be closely scrutinized for the possibility of beginning acute renal failure. It is recommended that a rise in the serum creatinine level usually ≥0.3 to 0.5 mg/dL from the patient's baseline serum creatinine level be carefully examined as potentially being indicative of early acute renal failure. Confirmation of the serum creatinine rise should be done by repeating the test or by serial determinations. Certain medications such as trimethoprim and cimetidine may cause a rise in serum creatinine as a result of inhibition of tubular secretion of creatinine (20,21). However, as in the case of a true decrement in renal function, no change is seen in blood urea nitrogen (BUN) levels from baseline.

Once it has been established that a bona fide change from the patient's baseline creatinine level has occured, it is prudent to first search for potentially reversible forms of renal disease. The three most common categories accounting for acute renal failure include (1) alterations in intravascular volume, (2) nephrotoxins, and (3) urinary obstruction.

A directed history should include a search for potential conditions that can either decrease intravascular volume (e.g., gastrointestinal loss as in diarrhea, vomiting; renal loss as in diuretic use) or increase intravascular volume (e.g., congestive heart failure). The sensation of thirst is always important historically because it may be one of the earliest symptoms found in intravascular volume depeletion. However, elderly patients may have a decreased sensation of thirst

(22). A review of the medications that the patient has been taking, especially newer medications begun 1 to 2 weeks before the observation of the serum creatinine level rise, should be done to screen for potential nephrotoxic drugs. In the case of the elderly who usually are taking multiple medications, potential drug interactions could occur to enhance renal toxicity. Over-the-counter medications should also be reviewed and ''health food/supplements'' examined for potential nephrotoxicity because the elderly may use food supplements and not always acknowledge such supplements as medications.

Change in urinary habits should be queried to include symptoms of prostatism in men, which include urgency, poor urinary stream, hesitancy, and incomplete voiding, and pelvic symptoms including vaginal bleeding in women. Urinary incontinence or increased frequency of urination, including nocturia resulting from the loss of renal concentration ability, may be an early finding in obstructive uropathy. Clues as to the cause and temporal occurrence of acute renal failure can be ascertained by a careful review of nursing notes, operative reports, and anesthesia records of hospitalized patients. Again, symptoms or signs of drug nephrotoxicity, alterations in vital signs such as acute decrements in blood pressure, or decreased oral intake may be gleaned from such records.

The physical examination is focused on vital signs including orthostatic changes in blood pressure, cardiovascular signs of congestive heart failure, and skin findings to help determine volume status and rashes that may indicate a drug reaction, as well as a prostate or pelvic examination to ascertain potential causes of obstruction. Because of the scarcity of subcutaneous tissue in many elderly patients, it is difficult to clearly assess skin turgor because skin ''tenting'' can be commonly found in the extremities of even euvolemic elderly patients. However, skin over the inner thighs may be useful in the assessment of turgor. In addition, lack of axillary moistness may be indicative of a volume-depleted patient. Caution should be exercised in the use of mucous membrane assessment for volume depletion in elderly patients who mouth breathe because mucous membranes in these types of patients may appear dry even in the absence of volume depletion. Finally, weighing the patient and finding a significant difference from the patient's usual weight may suggest volume depletion.

Important simple laboratory tests can be done in the initial workup of the patient with acute renal failure. Foremost is the urinalysis, which includes both qualitative (dipstick) and microscopic examination for cells, casts, and crystals. In volume depletion from nonrenal causes, the specific gravity is usually >1.025 g/ml with a benign urinary sediment except for hyaline casts. In urinary obstruction or intrinsic renal causes of acute renal failure, the specific gravity can be either isosthenuric or less than isosthenuric (≤ 1.010). With obstruction, little or no cells are in the urinary sediment unless a superimposed urinary tract infection occurs or the obstruction has resulted in loss of functioning nephrons, in which case coarse granular casts may be present. In nephrotoxic disease, white cells may be in the urine with an increase in urine eosinophils shown by Hansell stain in the case of acute allergic interstitial nephritis in its early course or round cell infiltrate later in the course of the interstitial nephritis. The finding of many renal tubular epithelial cells or renal tubular epithelial cell casts is significant for intrinsic renal disease such as acute tubular necrosis. The presence of crystalluria may suggest urinary tract obstruction from stones. Dysmorphic red blood cells, red blood cell casts, white blood cell casts, or mixed cellular casts may suggest the presence of glomerulonephritis. Assessment of proteinuria can be done qualitatively by dipstick, which detects albumin. It should be cautioned that dipstick determination of protein yields a protein concentration. Thus, dilute urine in large volumes having protein in the nephrotic range (greater than 3.0 to 3.5 g or more of protein per 24 hours per 1.73 m^2) may be represented by lower urine protein concentrations assessed by dipstick. All proteins including albumin can be precipitated with a strong acid such as 20% sulfosalicylic acid. A strongly positive sulfosalicylic acid protein precipitation reaction in the absence or presence of only a small amount of albumin by dipstick could be suggestive of paraproteinemia by such a bedside technique.

Assessment of residual urine after voiding is an important diagnostic procedure, especially in the elderly with acute renal failure. Residual urine after voiding can be determined immediately after voluntary voiding by either bedside ultrasonography or by straight catheterization. Volumes greater than 200 mL can be considered to be significant and should alert the practitioner to the possibility of bladder outlet obstruction. However, even lesser amounts of residual urine after voiding could suggest obstruction and warrant further workup if the history and physical examination are still suggestive of obstructive disease. Straight catheterization, while being more invasive, has the advantage of uncovering potential urethral stricture as a cause of urinary obstruction.

B. Further Diagnostic Evaluation

1. Chemistry Evaluation

Urine chemistry evaluation may be helpful in the case of oliguric renal failure (urine volume <400 mL/24 h). Urinary chemistry assessment should include creatinine, sodium, potassium, and chloride, as well as osmolality. Several urinary indices can be calculated from these chemistries as shown in Table 2 and their suggested prerenal, renal, or postrenal diagnoses (23,24). Caution should be exercised in trying to interpret urinary electrolytes when the patient has taken a diuretic within 48 hours of urinary electrolyte examination. Concomitant serum electrolytes should be obtained with urine electrolytes.

Examining serum electrolyte patterns can also give diagnostic clues as to the cause of the acute renal failure. In prerenal conditions, the serum BUN/creati-

Table 2 Urinary Indices Useful in Oliguric Acute Renal Failure

Index	Prerenal	Renal	Postrenal
U_{Na} (mEq/L)	<20	>40	>40
$U_{Chloride}$ (mEq/L)	<20	>40	>40
$U_{Creatinine}$ (mg/dL)	>100	<40	<40
FENa (%)	<1	>3	>3
$U_{Creatinine}/P_{Creatinine}$	>40/1	<20/1	<20/1
$U_{Osmolality}/P_{Osmolality}$	≥1.5	<1.35	<1.35
BUN/creatinine	>20/1	<20/1	<20/1

Source: Adapted in part from Ref. 23 and Ref. 24.

U_{Na} and U_{Cl}, may be higher and U_{Osm} may be lower in older patients with volume depletion who may not be able to conserve sodium and chloride or have loss of renal concentrating ability, respectively. Thus the values entered in Table 1 and the calculated indices such as the FENa and $U_{Osmolality}/P_{Osmolality}$ may differ in older subjects. A systematic study of urinary indices in elderly oliguric patients with various causes of acute renal failure has yet to be done.

U = urine; FENa = fractional excretion of sodium; P = plasma; BUN = blood urea nitrogen.

nine ratio may be greater than 20:1, although catabolic states including multiorgan system dysfunction or the administration of tetracyclines or corticosteroids can also raise the BUN out of proportion to the serum creatinine. Gastrointestinal bleeding, urinary tract obstruction, and acute glomerulonephritis are other entities that can cause disproportionate increases in the BUN over serum creatinine. It should be cautioned that the volume-depleted elderly patient with poor oral intake or whose intake includes foods with a decreased solute load (tea and toast diet) may have a lower BUN/creatinine ratio than expected for volume depletion. Although the presence of hypernatremia in the elderly is commonly associated with hyperosmolar states and volume depletion, hyponatremia could be associated with prerenal states such as congestive heart failure or volume depeletion where there is stimulated release of antidiuretic hormone caused by a decrease in effective circulating volume or untoward effects from medications.

The presence of metabolic alkalosis may be suspect for the presence of volume alterations in the elderly, whereas the presence of a hyperchloremic non-anion gap metabolic acidosis may be a clue to the presence of tubulointerstitial disease that can be seen with medication-induced acute allergic interstitial nephritis or urinary tract obstruction. Details of such electrolyte and acid-base disturbances are described elsewhere. (See Chapter 16.) The presence of hypercalcemia in the face of polyuria may suggest volume depletion or lead to other clues suggesting the presence of a paraproteinemia, which should be entertained in elderly patients with hypercalcemia and acute renal failure.

2. Imaging Studies

After the history, physical examination, urinalysis, and evaluation of serum and urine electrolytes suggest a differential diagnosis, imaging studies may be valuable in confirming various causes of acute renal failure. Ultrasonography should be the first imaging technique chosen in the evaluation. Renal size, cortical thickness, echogenicity, and evidence of urinary obstruction can be ascertained from ultrasonography. Depending on the size of the patient, normal renal size may be in the range of 9 to 12 cm in length, and cortical thickness is approximately 1 cm. Asymmetry of kidney size is suggestive of renal ischemic disease (renal artery stenosis), whereas small kidneys in general suggest underlying chronic renal disease, although in infiltrative diseases such as diabetes mellitus, multiple myeloma, or amyloidosis, the kidneys may appear larger than normal even in the face of significant renal failure. Normal kidney size with rising creatinine is suggestive of acute renal failure. In general, the kidney is less echogenic than liver parenchyma, and renal echogenicity similar to that of the liver is suggestive of intrinsic renal disease. Dilated calyces, renal pelvis, or ureters are found in urinary tract obstruction. It should be cautioned that ultrasonography may appear normal when acute obstruction is less than 24 hours in duration. In cases of suspected urinary tract obstruction but with a normal ultrasonogram, the study should be repeated within the next 48 hours. Renal stones as a cause for urinary obstruction may be suggested by ultrasonic ''shadowing,'' when a collimated loss of echoes is posterior to a suspected stone. Correlation can be made with a plain x-ray films of the kidneys, ureters, and bladder in the case of calcium-containing stones (approximately 80% of renal stones are visualized by plain x-ray film), whereas the x-ray findings may be negative with uric acid stones, although the ultrasonogram would still demonstrate ''shadowing.''

Renal blood flow alone can be evaluated with a radionuclide such as techetium diethylenetriamine pentaacetic acid (^{99}Tc-DTPA) or other substances that give an assessment of both renal blood flow and tubular function such as ^{99}Tc-glucoheptonate. Such studies may give clues as to the presence of renal arterial disease when combined with angiotensin-converting enzyme (ACE) inhibitors (25–27). Because the glomerular filtration rate may be sustained by glomerular efferent arteriolar vasoconstriction in the kidney affected by renal arterial stenosis and subsequent decreased renal perfusion, ACE inhibition will dilate the efferent arteriole and further decrease glomerular filtration rate. Thus, radionuclide renal scanning will show a poorer functioning kidney affected by significant renal arterial disease after administration of ACE inhibitors.

3. Other Diagnostic Procedures

Cystoscopy with retrograde pyelography is useful in the assessment of urinary tract obstruction. Trabeculations visualized in the bladder are suggestive of bladder outlet obstruction. Collection of urine from individual kidneys by retrograde catheters enables the determination of the contribution to total renal function from each kidney, urine culture, and cytological findings from individual kidneys in assessment for unilateral infections or tumors, respectively. Retrograde pyelography may be able to identify the level or source of upper tract obstruction.

In situations in which the cause of the acute renal failure is unclear, renal biopsy may be indicated to look for potentially treatable causes of the renal failure, such as vasculitis, acute interstitial nephritis, or rapidly progressive glomerulonephritis, or to determine the likelihood of the reversibility of the renal failure where oliguria is of longer than 3 to 4 weeks' duration or when anuria is not due to obstruction (28). Conditions that would preclude percutaneous renal biopsy are (1) solitary functioning kidney, (2) uncontrolled hypertension, (3) bleeding diathesis uncorrected by fresh frozen plasma or 1-desamino-8-D arginine vasopressin (dDAVP), or (4) a cognitively impaired patient who is unable to cooperate during the procedure. Open renal biopsy could be considered in those situations precluding percutaneous biopsy to aid in the diagnosis. Renal biopsy interpretation in elderly patients may have to be done with a background histological study of age-related changes or intercurrent disease such as arteriolar sclerosis and global sclerosis (29).

IV. SPECIFIC RENAL DISORDERS

A. Prerenal Acute Renal Failure

In the elderly, prerenal conditions such as congestive heart failure and fluid loss volume depletion are the most common causes of acute renal failure. Indeed, depending on the reported series of patients, prerenal causes of acute renal failure could be identified in 35% to more than 50% of elderly patients with acute renal failure (14,15,17,18,28,30). Volume depletion may occur in patients with acute infections such as pneumonia, in which insensible losses can be high because of increased ventilatory rate and fever in combination with inadequate oral intake. Insufficient oral intake may be observed in nursing home patients who are either restrained because of agitation or who have deficits in cognitive function where physical or mental barriers may exist in obtaining adequate fluids. It is not uncommon to find elderly patients with hyperosmolar and hypovolemic hypernatremic states who have an abnormal thirst mechanism, are unable to express the sensation of thirst, or who have physical barriers to obtain adequate fluids. The elderly may have physiological tubular changes that do not allow for as avid sodium retention in volume-depleted states as do younger individuals, and they may have deficits in urinary concentration, thus not allowing for maximal water reabsorption. Volume depletion either resulting from nonrenal causes (e.g., gastrointestinal loss) or renal causes (e.g., overzealous use of diuretics or chronic tubulointerstitial diseases causing "salt wasting") may be more rapid and of a greater degree in the elderly. Urinary sodium concentration in volume-depleted elderly patients may be greater than in younger patients because of the inability of the elderly to maximally retain sodium (28,30).

On the basis of the history and physical examination, estimates of intravascular volume depletion can be made. With orthostatic changes in blood pressure or pulse along with the patient's history helping to identify the cause of the volume depletion and in the absence of autonomic dysfunction, a conservative estimate of percent volume depletion can be placed at approximately 10% to 15%. This percent volume depletion can be multiplied by the patient's usual body weight to estimate the liters of 0.9% saline needed to correct volume depletion. Replacement of moderate to severe volume deficits is initially best done intravenously. In addition to replacing volume deficits, consideration should also be given to maintenance fluids, which in general are approximately 2500 mL of water, 50 to 70 mEq of sodium, 90 to 110 mEq of chloride, and 40 mEq of potassium (in the absence of hyperkalemia) per day. The initial treatment for volume depletion should be vigorous in severe deficits. Monitoring of vital signs, urinary output, and urinary and serum chemistries should be done during therapy. Fluid orders should be written on a 24-hour basis once hemodynamic stability has been achieved with initial fluid therapy because continuous fluid orders may predispose the elderly patient to volume overload, hyperkalemia, or water balance disorders such as hyponatremia.

B. Acute Tubular Necrosis

In the elderly, severe uncorrected intravascular volume depletion may lead to acute tubular necrosis. In fact, Macias-Nunez et al (28) have concluded that volume depletion leading to acute tubular necrosis occurred in 23% of elderly patients that they studied compared with 15% of younger patients. Alternately, hemodynamic instability with hypotension caused by medications, intraoperative complications, sepsis, or trauma may cause acute tubular necrosis. The diagnosis of acute tubular necrosis may be made on the basis of initial urinary and serum biochemical indices (Table 2), lack of response to a fluid challenge evidenced by lack of improvement in the serum creatinine and BUN, and absence of urinary tract obstruction in an appropriate clinical setting as described previously. In critically ill elderly patients in whom pre-existing cardiac compromise may exist because of myocardial dysfunction, rhythm disturbance, or pericardial disease, hemodynamic monitoring with pulmonary arterial catheterization may be necessary to optimize pulmonary capillary wedge pressure and subsequent cardiac index (31).

The use of renal-dose dopamine (<3 μg/kg/min) is controversial, and a recent review suggests that no evidence supports its routine use in acute renal failure (31). The use of loop diuretics with or without the potent thiazide diuretic, metolazone, has been advocated in trying to convert oliguric acute renal failure to nonoliguric renal failure in the hope of facilitating volume management and hyperkalemia in acute oliguric renal failure. However, care should be taken in the use of diuretics because their use in radiocontrast nephropathy or prerenal states could worsen the renal failure or precipitate acute tubular necrosis, respectively. Various strategies for diuretic use have been advocated in acute tubular necrosis. Bolus doses of furosemide may be given (up to 400 mg intravenously with or without 5 to 10 mg metolazone), or continuous furosemide infusion at 20 mg/h with or without concomitant infusion of dopamine may be administered (24,28). Extracorporeal therapy will be discussed later.

C. Acute Allergic Interstitial Nephritis

Acute allergic interstitial nephritis (AIN) is not an uncommon cause of acute renal failure seen in elderly patients. Antibiotics and nonsteroidal anti-inflammatory drugs (NSAIDs) lead the potential offending medications causing AIN, although other medications such as allopurinol and histamine receptor type 2 blockers (e.g., cimetidine) can also be implicated as causes of AIN in the elderly. The classical clinical presentation is that of fever, rash, and acute renal failure. The presence of eosinophiluria and peripheral eosinophilia is suggestive of AIN. Gallium scanning of the kidneys may show bilateral uptake. Again, cessation of the offending medication should reverse the process, and a short course of prednisone, 60 mg daily for 5 days, has been advocated to shorten the course of the renal failure. NSAIDs can also cause nephrotic syndrome (32–35) in which the glomerular pathosis is that of minimal change disease. The classes of NSAIDs usually associated with acute renal failure with nephrotic syndrome are the phenylpropionic and indoleacetic acid derivatives such as ibuprofen, naproxen, and indomethacin.

D. Aminoglycoside Nephrotoxicity

Aminoglycosides are a common cause of acute renal failure in the hospitalized elderly (30,35,36). Comorbid factors include volume depletion, hypokalemia, and hypomagnesemia. Although peak and trough levels of aminoglycosides can be drawn to guide dosing, maintaining such drug levels within the recommended limits is no guarantee of avoidance of nephrotoxicity. The clinical presentation is typically a finding of rising serum creatinine approximately 5 to 10 days after starting therapy. The renal failure is usually nonoliguric. Urinalysis may show mild proteinura, tubular epithelial cells, and some granular casts. Essentially, aminoglycosides are internalized into renal tubular epithelial cells and are localized to lysosomal compartments and bind to phospholipid bilayers. The intracellular phospholipid accumulation appears as myeloid bodies in electron micrographs. On cessation of aminoglycosides, recovery of renal function occurs within a few days. Renal ischemia may predispose to aminoglycoside toxicity only after short-term therapy or may be associated with oliguria when combined with other renal insults. Occasionally, renal potassium and magnesium wasting may be present with aminoglycoside nephrotoxicity.

E. Vascular Involvement in Acute Renal Failure

Structural changes in the renal vasculature that occur with age and alterations in vasoconstrictive and vasodilative factors as outlined previously leading to both glomerular and tubulointerstitial functional compromise predispose the aging kidney to acute renal failure. Although more implicated as a cause of chronic renal failure, ischemic nephrophathy caused by renal arterial stenosis from atherosclerosis is an important factor in the susceptibility of elderly patients to acute renal failure under a variety of insults. It has been estimated that the prevalence of renal artery stenosis in patients 65 years and older may be approximately 20%, with increasing prevalence up to 60% with further increase in age (37,38). Approximately 50% of patients with renal artery stenosis have bilateral disease. The following causes of acute renal failure can be categorized as being mainly vascular in origin, either caused by hemodynamic alterations in renal blood flow or by embolization from atherosclerotic plaques within blood vessels.

1. Medications Affecting Renal Circulation

Angiotensin-converting enzyme inhibitors are a class of medications that can cause acute renal failure in the elderly (24,28,30,36). In elderly patients with diffuse atherosclerotic cardiovascular disease or coronary artery disease and hypertension, ACE inhibition may lead to renal failure in patients with bilateral renal artery stenosis or renal artery stenosis in a solitary functioning kidney or in the case where most of a patient's glomerular filtration rate is being supplied predominantly by one kidney having significant renal arterial stenosis. In these situations, glomerular filtration rate is maintained by vasoconstriction of the glomerular efferent arteriole. Angiotensin-converting enzyme inhibition causes a vasodilation of the efferent arteriole with subsequent decrease in glomerular filtration rate. Thus, acute renal failure can occur with ACE inhibition even in the absence of a significant reduction in systemic blood pressure because of its effects on intrarenal hemodynamics. This acute renal failure is reversible on cessation of the ACE inhibitor.

In addition, in patients who are salt depleted from diuretics or a sodium-restricted diet or patients with chronic renal insufficiency with serum creatinine levels usually greater than 3.0 mg/dL, glomerular filtration rate again is maintained predominantly by glomerular efferent arteriolar vasoconstriction. Angiotensin-converting enzyme inhibition with the attendant efferent arteriolar vasodilation leads to acute decreases in glomerular filtration rate. Other risk factors identified that are associated with acute renal failure in patients who take ACE inhibitors are congestive heart failure, hypotension, and hyponatremia, which may reflect excessive diuretic use. Cessation of the ACE inhibitor usually reverses the acute renal failure.

NSAIDs are a common cause of acute renal failure in the elderly (24,28,30,36,39). The use of NSAIDs in the elderly population is widespread, especially as therapy for the various arthridities such as osteoarthritis and gout and general musculoskeletal complaints. The easy access to NSAIDs because of over-the-counter preparations has allowed this class of medications to become an important factor in acute renal failure. However, the incidence of impaired renal function caused by NSAIDs alone is $<1\%$ (24). What is important in the development of NSAID-induced acute renal failure is the identification of comorbid conditions. Such conditions include congestive heart failure, salt-depleted states resulting from diuretic therapy, diabetes mellitus, chronic renal insufficiency, and chronic hepatic disease. Inhibition of renal vasodilatory prostaglandins such as prostacyclin and prostaglandin E_2 result in a decrease in cortical renal blood flow and a decrease in glomerular filtration rate. Urinalysis is benign and urinary electrolytes generally reflect prerenal indices. Cessation of NSAIDs reverses the acute renal deterioration.

2. Radiocontrast-Induced Nephropathy

Radiocontrast-induced acute renal failure is seen more frequently in elderly patients perhaps because of age-related medical conditions requiring the use of contrast material in imaging procedures and, in general, renal functional decline observed with age. The pathophysiology of radiocontrast-induced acute renal failure is included in this section of vascular causes of acute renal failure because dye-induced vasoconstriction of renal blood vessels is a major contributor to the disease. However, direct tubular toxicity of radiocontrast agents also may contribute to the acute renal failure. The risk factors for radiocontrast-induced nephropathy include age, volume depletion or other low cardiac output states, diabetes mellitus, paraproteinemia, chronic renal insufficiency, and use of higher contrast doses. Rich and Crecelius (19) reported that 11% of patients older than 70 years had an increase in serum creatinine of approximately 0.5 mg/dL above baseline after receiving radiocontrast. However, in another study there was an incidence of approximately 0.15% of acute renal failure induced in a large series of patients receiving radiocontrast (24). Radiocontrast-initiated acute renal failure is typically characterized by an increase in serum creatinine levels within 24 hours after contrast is given. Creatinine levels peak within 3 to 5 days and resolve by 2 to 3 weeks. Urinary indicies can be compatible with a prerenal condition with low urinary sodium and fractional excretion of sodium <1%. The use of mannitol, low-dose dopamine or furosemide, or calcium channel antagonists have met with variable results in preventing radiocontrast-induced acute renal failure. In addition, a prospective trial of atrial natriuretic peptide to prevent radiocontrast nephropathy has not been shown to be efficacious (40). The use of low-osmolality contrast agents has also been associated with acute renal failure (41) and offers no improved prevention of acute renal failure (42). Hydration with 0.45% saline before and after radiocontrast administration to maintain volume expansion has been shown to be the most effective means of preventing radiocontrast-induced acute renal failure (43).

3. Atheroembolic Disease

Atheroembolic disease is generally a disease of older individuals. The mean age for the occurrence of atheroembolic renal disease has been reported to be between 66 and 70 years (44). The disease is more common in men and the incidence appears to be disproportionate in white compared with African-American patients (30:1). Cholesterol crystal emboli originate from atheromatous plaques in major arteries and can lodge in the arcuate, interlobular, and terminal arterioles of the kidney. Classically, the cholesterol crystals can be seen on light microscopic sections as biconcave needle-shaped clefts within the lumen of involved vessels. The cholesterol crystals provoke an inflammatory reaction within affected vasculature, leading to tissue ischemia and infarction and subsequent tubular atrophy, interstitial fibrosis, and hyalinization of glomeruli.

Atheroembolic renal disease is usually found in a patient with diffuse atherosclerotic cardiovascular disease with a recent history of arterial instrumentation for purposes of angiography, angioplasty, or thombolytic therapy. Other predisposing factors include vascular surgery, especially for abdominal aortic aneurysectomy, and anticoagulation (45). Manifestations of atheroembolic disease include fever and myalgia, cutaneous manifestations such as livedo reticularis, digital mottling, and cyanosis (purple or blue toes), and digital gangrene. Unlike major vessel arterial embolization, the distal pulses in cholesterol atheroembolization are usually intact. Nervous system involvement can take the form of stroke, altered mental status, or peripheral neuropathy. Examination of the retina may show cholesterol emboli at the bifurcations of retinal arterioles, which are called Hollenhorst's plaques. Gastrointestinal symptoms can include abdominal pain, pancreatitis, hepatitis, or gastrointestinal bleeding and bowel infarction. With renal involvement, accelerated or labile hypertension may be present. The course of the renal failure can be acute or subacute, occurring over a period of a few weeks. Daily urine output may be variable. The urinalysis is remarkable for coarse and fine granular casts and some white and red blood cells. Eosinophiluria may be present in up to a third of the patients with proven atheroemboli (46). Peripheral eosinophilia may be noted in up to 80% of cases (47). An increase in sedimentation rate and hypocomplementemia may also be observed. Thus, the varied constellation of clinical and laboratory findings suggests a wide differential diagnosis, including infective endocarditis, systemic vasculitis, acute allergic interstitial nephritis, and polymyositis.

The renal prognosis in general is poor. Mortality is high and reported to be between 64% and 81% (45,48). Morbidity is also high, with approximately 40% of patients requiring dialysis (45). At present, no effective therapy exists for renal atheroembolic disease. It is stressed that anticoagulation be avoided, and in fact, use of either heparin or coumadin anticoagulants could precipitate further atheroembolism.

F. Acute Glomerulonephritis

Glomerulonephritis can be found in up to 50% of the patients who have undergone renal biopsy to discern the cause of their acute renal failure (30). A variety of glomerular lesions demonstrating glomerular inflammatory changes resulting in acute renal failure can occur and include idiopathic rapidly progressive glomerulonephritis, mesangiocapillary glomerulonephritis, postinfectious glomerulonephritis, or other vasculitides. Of these, idiopathic rapidly progressive (crescentic) glomerulonephritis appears to be the most common type of glomerulonephritis seen in the elderly seen with acute renal failure with an incidence between 16% and 38% (49–51), whereas the overall incidence of rapidly progressive glomerulonephritis is approximately 2% to 4% of all cases of glomerulonephritis (52). Although the accuracy of these statistics may be somewhat in question because patients older than the age of 50 were considered ''elderly'' (49), Keller et al (53) showed that in their series of 64 patients with biopsy-proven rapidly progressive glomerulonephritis, a linear increase was found in the incidence of rapidly progressive glomerulonephritis with age, in which 26 of 64 patients (41%) with rapidly progressive glomerulonephritis were in the 60 to 80 age group.

The clinical presentation in idiopathic rapidly progressive glomerulonephritis may be nonspecific with symptoms similar to an upper respiratory tract infection with malaise and myalgias. Patients may have oligoanuria and new-onset renal failure. The urinalysis is characteristic of active glomerular inflammation with red blood cell casts or dysmorphic red blood cells, white blood cells, and white blood cell and granular casts. Proteinuria is present but usually not of nephrotic quantity. Histologically, crescent formation resulting from proliferation of glomerular parietal epithelial cells and mononuclear cells is the hallmark of the disease. In 20% of patients with rapidly progressive glomerulonephritis, a linear deposition of immunoglobulin is seen along the glomerular basement membrane, whereas in 30% of the cases a granular (''lumpy-bumpy'') pattern of immune deposits is seen in the glomeruli. In half of the patients, no immune deposits can be detected in the glomeruli (''pauci-immune disease''). Therapy with pulsed intravenous corticosteroids (methylprednisolone, 30 mg/kg IV for three consecutive doses) followed by prednisone, 2 mg/kg every other day for 2 months followed by a taper over 4 months (54), with or without the addition of cyclophosphamide, 2 mg/kg daily, has been advocated. The efficacy of plasmapheresis is unknown, although such therapy may be of more benefit in patients with antibodies to glomerular basement membrane. Features of rapidly progressive glomerulonephritis indicating poor renal prognosis (leading to renal replacement therapy) include oliguria of <500 mL/day and initial serum creatinine >5 to 6 mg/dL. Poor survival in patients with rapidly progressive glomerulonephritis has been shown to be correlated with age greater than 60 years and possibly as a result of infections and malignancies related to complications of immunosuppression (53).

A common clinical feature of acute glomerulonephritis in the elderly seen with acute renal failure is congestive heart failure (49). Perhaps the lesser capacity and protracted nature of the aging kidney to excrete a sodium load contribute to the occurrence of congestive heart failure in acute glomerulonephritis. Postinfectious glomerulonephritis and membranoproliferative glomerulonephritis can also be seen in elderly patients, although the former, at least with nephritogenic strains of streptococci, may be more commonly seen in children. In one study, older patients (>55 years) with poststreptococcal glomerulonephritis had higher levels of serum creatinine on admission compared with middle-aged (40–54 years) or younger patients (20–39 years) and had lower serum albumin concentrations and higher systolic blood pressures compared with that of younger patients (55). Visceral abscess, endocarditis, and catheter line infections are settings in which older patients may experience other causes of postinfectious glomerulonephritis. Complement levels, especially C3 and C4, are generally low in both postinfectious glomerulonephritis and membranoproliferative glomerulonephritis, unlike that of idiopathic rapidly progressive glomerulonephritis in which complement levels are normal. However, in postinfections glomerulonephritis resulting from methicillin-resistant *Staphylococcus aureus*, complement levels may also be normal (56). Complement levels remain low indefinitely in membranoproliferative glomerulonephritis, whereas in postinfectious glomerulonephritis, complement levels return to normal by 8 to 12 weeks. Therapy for postinfectious glomerulonephritis is aimed at treating the underlying infectious source and supportive therapy. In membranoproliferative glomerulonephritis, therapy with corticosteroids, cytotoxic agents, and antiplatelet medication have been advocated, although such therapy has not been universally shown to be efficacious in preserving renal function. Renal prognosis is excellent overall in postinfectious glomerulonephritis, whereas end-stage renal disease is a common sequela in membranoproliferative glomerulonephritis.

G. Obstructive Uropathy

Urinary tract obstruction is a significant cause of acute renal failure in the elderly. Various series describing elderly patients with acute renal failure have reported the incidence of obstructive uropathy as a cause of acute renal failure between 2% and 59%, with most of the studies reviewed reporting incidences between 8% and 20% (14–18,57). Men with benign prostatic hypertrophy and prostatic carcinoma should be considered as leading candidates in the cause of urinary obstruction. Prostate specific antigen determination may be helpful in following the course of prostatic carcinoma during and after treatment. Retroperitoneal involvement of lymph nodes in prostatic carcinoma or lymphoma or carcinomas of the bladder, cervix, uterus, ovaries, or rectum either by retroperitoneal lymph node involvement or by direct extension can be additional causes of urinary obstruction in women and men. Aside from mechanical obstruction, functional obstruction can also occur in elderly patients who may be taking multiple medications with anticholinergic effects, such as psychotropic agents, tricyclic antidepressants, or antihistamines.

Aside from bladder catheterization and ultrasonography to assess lower and upper urinary tract obstruction, some blood chemistries may serve as clues to the presence of urinary obstruction. A high BUN/creatinine ratio and an electrolyte pattern showing a hyperchloremic metabolic acidosis with a normal anion gap with either normal or elevated serum potassium levels is suggestive of obstructive uropathy (58). Urinary electrolytes and urinalysis are generally unremarkable in obstruction, although macroscopic and/or microscopic hematuria with or without pyuria may suggest tumor or nephrolithiasis as potential causes of the obstruction. In the absence of ultrasonographic findings of obstruction, duplex Doppler sonography showing a renal arterial resistive index greater than 0.7 may be suggestive of obstructive uropathy (59). Relief of obstruction either by bladder catheterization or, if upper tract obstruction exists, by retrograde placement of ureteral stents or by percutaneous nephrostomy generally leads to a prompt diuresis and rapid fall in serum creatinine levels. However, with long-standing urinary tract obstruction, tubulointerstitial damage may result in chronic renal insufficiency.

H. Multiple Myeloma

Multiple myeloma is included in this discussion because of its age prevalence in older adults and its many renal manifestations (60). Approximately 7% to 10%

of patients with multiple myeloma will be initially seen with acute renal failure. In elderly patients with acute renal failure, anemia, and back pain, multiple myeloma should be considered as a potential diagnosis. Volume depletion and NSAIDs used to relieve skeletal pains in such patients play a key role in the development of acute renal failure. In addition to prerenal acute renal failure, volume depletion and acidosis can lead to precipitation of myeloma proteins in renal tubules causing intratubular obstruction (myeloma kidney). Light chain glomerulopathy, which typically appears as a nodular glomerulosclerosis, can be found mainly with kappa light chains and is a cause of nephrotic syndrome in multiple myeloma. Amyloidosis, demonstrated by Congo red staining and apple-green birefringence of amyloid deposits under polarized light, is also a cause of nephrotic syndrome in multiple myeloma. Hypercalcemia and tubulointerstitial disease from hypercalcemia and proximal tubular disorders, including glycosuria, aminoaciduria, and phosphaturia, can occur as a result of direct tubular toxicity by myeloma proteins. Finally, multiple myeloma is a risk factor in the development of radiocontrast nephropathy. The use of plasmapheresis in addition to chemotherapy may be helpful in reducing quantities of nephrotoxic light chains specifically for light chain disease.

V. THERAPEUTIC INTERVENTION

Traditional indications for extracorporeal renal replacement therapy include (1) hypervolemia with symptoms and signs of congestive heart failure that is not amenable to medical management; (2) hyperkalemia that cannot be controlled by medical management; (3) acidosis unresponsive to medical therapy; (4) bleeding diathesis uncorrected with fresh frozen plasma or dDAVP; and (5) uremic signs and symptoms such as lethargy, seizures, myoclonus, asterixis, gastrointestinal symptoms, and findings of pericarditis. Overall, early renal replacement therapy should be considered in the elderly patient because serum creatinine may not correlate as well with the development of uremic symptoms. Early therapy may help to avert complications of a bleeding diathesis and volume overload in elderly patients with underlying heart disease.

Choice of extracorporeal therapy includes acute hemodialysis and continuous hemofiltration or hemofiltration in combination with dialysis (hemodiafiltration). Acute peritoneal dialysis, although useful in fluid removal, is more rarely used in adult patients because its efficiency for solute removal is much less than that of the other modalities, and albumin loss resulting in hypoalbuminemia can occur. Circulatory access for dialysis or hemofiltration is generally by venous access by way of femoral, subclavian, or internal jugular routes. The choice of dialyzer in the acutely ill patient should be aimed at using biocompatible membranes. Cellulose membranes can induce a proinflammatory response with the activation of complement, granulocyte, and monocyte with release of reactive oxygen species and other cytokines leading to hemodynamic instability (61). In addition, a bicarbonate-based dialysate is preferred over an acetate-based one to maintain hemodynamic stability and minimize hypotension associated with acetate dialysis. Because acute dialyses are generally done using a veno-venous route, it is important to maximize blood flow to improve solute clearance and to consider adequate time for dialysis. Generally, predialysis BUN should be kept to less than 80 mg/dL (31). If only volume control and not solute removal is the major concern, ''dry'' ultrafiltration (without dialysate application) may be done.

Continuous renal replacement therapy includes hemofiltration, which removes both solute and volume and is done on a slow, continuous basis, usually in an intensive care setting. The advantages of hemofiltration are that continuous removal of solutes and water does not allow for dramatic alterations of osmolality or electrolyte shifts as would be expected with intermittant dialysis, allows for more hemodynamic stability, and can be done without specialized personnel. Hemofiltration is thus an ideal therapy for hypercatabolic patients requiring parenteral or enteral nutritional support and is a favored means of renal replacement therapy in the elderly patient with acute renal failure (24,31,62,63). However, because adequate anticoagulation is necessary to prevent clotting of the hemofilter, active bleeding is a relative contraindication for this mode of therapy.

VI. PROGNOSIS AND OUTCOMES OF ACUTE RENAL FAILURE IN THE ELDERLY

Age as a risk factor in the prognosis of patients with acute renal failure has been controversial (30). Risk factors associated with poor outcome include hypotension requiring vasopressor, artificial ventilation, hypoalbuminemia, consciousness disturbance (coma), oliguria, level of BUN (usually >100 mg/dL), jaundice, sepsis, and multiple organ failure (24,28,30,64–67). In general, elderly patients may have a slightly worse prognosis than younger patients, and recovery of renal function after acute renal failure is generally slower and may not be complete (14). However, renal replacement therapy should not be withheld from elderly patients with acute renal failure who demonstrate these factors. Solid criteria have yet to be determined when renal replacement therapy may be terminated in those elderly patients who have not responded to a trial of intermittent or continuous extracorporeal therapy or for that matter what constitutes a sufficient trial of renal replacement therapy. Along these lines, various scoring systems such as the APACHE II scale have been used to try to predict survival and recovery of renal function (28,31,68,69). Nevertheless, mortality in the elderly patient with acute renal failure may be from 10% up to approximately 70% depending on the series reported, with higher mortality usually found in elderly patients hospitalized in an ICU setting (66–68,70,71).

REFERENCES

1. Epstein M. Aging and the kidney. J Am Soc Nephrol 1996;8:1106–1122.
2. Baylis C, Schmidt R. The aging glomerulus. Semin Nephrol 1996;16:265–276.
3. Lindeman RD, Tobin JD, Shock NW. Longitudinal studies on the rate of decline in renal function with age. J Am Geriatr Soc 1985;33:278–285.
4. Lew SQ, Bosch JP. Effect on diet on creatinine clearance and excretion in young and elderly healthy subjects and in patients with renal disease. J Am Soc Nephrol 1991;2:856–865.
5. Macias-Nunez JF, Iglesias CG, Bondia Roman A, Rodriguez Commes JL, Corbacho Becerra L, Tabernero Romo JM, De Castro Del Pozo S. Renal handling of sodium in old people: A functional study. Age Ageing 1978;7:178–181.
6. Fish LC, Murphy DJ, Elahi D, Minaker KL. Renal sodium excretion in normal aging: decreased excretion rates lead to delayed handling of sodium loads. Geriatr Nephrol Urol 1995;4:145–151.
7. Duggan J, Kilfeather S, Lightman SL. The association of age with plasma arginine vasopressin and plasma osmolality. Age Ageing 1993;22:332–336.
8. Faull CM, Holmes C, Baylis PH. Water balance in elderly people: Is there a deficiency of vasopressin? Age Ageing 1993;22:114–120.
9. Baylis C. Age-dependent glomerular damage in the rat: Dissociation between glomerular injury and both glomerular hypertension and hypertrophy. Male gender as a primary risk factor. J Clin Invest 1994;94:1823–1829.
10. Goldstein RS, Tarloff JB, Hook JB. Age-related nephropathy in laboratory rats. FASEB J 1988;2:2241–2251.
11. Beierschmitt WP, Keenan KP, Weiner M. Age-related increased susceptibility of male Fischer 344 rats to acetaminophen nephrotoxicity. Life Sci 1986;39:2335–2342.
12. Tarloff JB, Goldstein RS, Morgan DG, Hook JB. Acetaminophen and p-aminophenol nephrotoxicity in aging male Sprague-Dawlety and Fischer 344 rats. Fun Appl Toxicol 1989;12:78–91.
13. Sabbatini M, Sansone G, Uccello F, De Nicola L, Giliberti A, Sepe V, Margri P, Conte G, Andreucci VE. Functional versus structural changes in the pathophysiology of acute ischemic renal failure in aging rats. Kidney Int 1994;45:1355–1361.
14. Pascual J, Orofino L, Liano F, Marcen R, Naya MT, Orte L, Ortuno J. Incidence and prognosis of acute renal failure in older patients. J Am Geriatr Soc 1990;38: 25–30.
15. Prakash J, Gupta A, Malhotra V, Kumar O, Srivastava PK. Acute renal failure in the elderly: A demographic and clinical study of patients in Eastern India. Geriatr Nephrol Urol 1997;7:67–72.
16. Druml W, Lax F, Grimm G, Schneeweiss B, Lenz K, Laggner AN. Acute renal failure in the elderly 1975–1990. Clin Nephrol 1994;41:342–349.

17. Klouche K, Cristol JP, Kaaki M, Turc-Baron C, Canaud B, Beraud JJ. Prognosis of acute renal failure in the elderly. Nephrol Dial Transplant 1995;10:2240–2243.
18. McInnes EG, Levy DW, Chaudhuri MD, Bhan GL. Renal failure in the elderly. Q J Med 1987;64:583–588.
19. Rich MW, Crecelius CA. Incidence, risk factors and clinical course of acute renal insufficiency after cardiac catheterization in patients 70 years of age or older. Arch Intern Med 1990;150:1237–1242.
20. Naderer O, Nafziger AN, Bertino JS Jr. Effects of moderate-dose versus high-dose trimethoprim on serum creatinine and creatinine clearance and adverse reactions. Antimicrob Agents Chemother 1997;41:2466–2470.
21. Ixkes MC, Koopman MG, van Acker BA, Weber JA, Arisz L. Cimetidine improves GFR-estimation by the Cockcroft and Gault formula. Clin Nephrol 1997;47:229–236.
22. Phillips PA, Rolls BY, Ledingham JG, Forsling ML, Morton JJ, Crowe MJ. Reduced thirst after water deprivation in healthy elderly men. N Engl J Med 1984;311:753–759.
23. Miller TR, Anderson RJ, Linas SL, Henrich WL, Berns AS, Gabow PA, Schrier RW. Urinary diagnostic indices in acute renal failure: a prospective study. Ann Intern Med 1978;88:47–50.
24. Mandal AK, Baig M, Koutoubi Z. Management of acute renal failure in the elderly. Treatment options. Drugs Aging 1996;9:226–250.
25. Chen CC, Hoffer PB, Vahjen G, Gottschalk A, Koster K, Zubal IG, Setaro JF, Roer DA, Black HR. Patients at high risk for renal artery stenosis: a simple method of renal scintigraphic analysis with Tc-99m DTPA and captopril. Radiology 1990;176: 365–370.
26. Mann SJ, Pickering TG, Sos TA, Uzzo RG, Sarkar S, Friend K, Captopril renography in the diagnosis of renal artery stenosis: accuracy and limitations. Am J Med 1991; 90:30–40.
27. Abuelo JG. Diagnosing vascular causes of renal failure. Ann Intern Med 1995;123: 601–614.
28. Macias-Nunez JF, Lopez-Novoa JM, Martinez-Maldonado M. Acute renal failure in the aged. Semin Nephrol 1996;16:330–338.
29. Levison SP. Renal disease in the elderly: the role of the renal biopsy. Am J Kidney Dis 1990;16:300–306.
30. Pascual J, Liano F, Ortuno J. The elderly patient with acute renal failure. J Am Soc Nephrol 1995;6:144–153.
31. DuBose TD Jr, Warnock DG, Mehta RL, Bonventre JV, Hammerman MR, Molitoris BA, Paller MS, Siegel NJ, Scherbenske J, Striker GE. Acute renal failure in the 21st century: Recommendations for management and outcomes assessment. Am J Kidney Dis 1997;29:793–799.
32. Clive DM, Stoff JS. Renal syndromes associated with non-steroidal anti-inflammatory drugs. N Engl J Med 1984;310:563–572.
33. Lamy PP. Renal effects of non-steroidal anti-inflammatory drugs. Heightened risk in the elderly? J Am Geriatr Soc 1986;34:361–367.
34. Warren GV, Korbet SM, Schwartz MM, Lewis EJ. Minimal change glomerulopathy associated with non-steroidal anti-inflammatory drugs. Am J Kidney Dis 1989;13: 127–130.

35. Hock R, Anderson, RJ. Prevention of drug-induced nephrotoxicity in the intensive care unit. J Critical Care 1995;10:33–43.
36. Thomson NM. Drugs and the kidney in the elderly. Med J Aust 1995;162:543–547.
37. Greco BA, Breyer JA. The natural history of renal artery stenosis: Who should be evaluated for suspected ischemic nephropathy? Semin Nephrol 1996;16:2–11.
38. Preston RA, Epstein M. Ischemic renal disease: an emerging cause of chronic renal failure and end-stage renal disease. J Hypertens 1997;15:1365–1377.
39. Ailabouni W, Eknoyan G. Nonsteroidal anti-inflammatory drugs and acute renal failure in the elderly. Drugs Aging 1996;9:341–351.
40. Kurnik BR, Allgren RL, Genter FC, Solomon RJ, Bates ER, Weisberg LS. Prospective study of atrial natriuretic peptide for the prevention of radiocontrast-induced nephropathy. Am J Kidney Dis 1998;31:674–680.
41. Aron NB, Feinfeld DA, Peters AT, Lynn RI. Acute renal failure associated with ioxaglate, a low-osmolality radiocontrast agent. Am J Kidney Dis 1989;13:189–193.
42. Rudnick MR, Goldfarb S, Wexler L, Ludbrook PA, Murphy MJ, Halpern EF, Hill JA, Winniford M, Cohen MB, Van Fossen DB. Nephrotoxicity of ionic and nonionic contrast media in 1196 patients: A randomized trial: The Iohexal Cooperative Study. Kidney Int 1995;47:254–261.
43. Solomon R, Werner C, Mann D, D'Elia J, Silva P. Effects of saline, mannitol, and furosemide on acute decreases in renal function induced by radiocontrast agents. N Engl J Med 1994;331:1416–1420.
44. Saleem S, Lakkis FG, Martinez-Maldonado M. Atheroembolic renal disease. Semin Nephrol 1996;16:309–318.
45. Lye WC, Cheah JS, Sinniah R. Renal cholesterol embolic disease. Am J Nephrol 1993;13:489–493.
46. Wilson DM, Salazer TL, Farkouh ME. Eosinophiluria in atheroembolic renal disease. Am J Med 1991;91:186–189.
47. Kasinath BS, Corwin HL, Bidani AK, Korbet SM, Schwartz MM, Lewis EJ. Eosinophilia in the diagnosis of atheroembolic renal disease. Am J Nephrol 1987;7:173–177.
48. Fine M, Kapoor W, Falanga V. Cholesterol crystal embolization: A review of 221 cases in the English literature. Angiology 1987;38:769–784.
49. Arieff AI, Anderson RJ, Massry SG. Acute glomerulonephritis in the elderly. Geriatrics 1971;26:74–84.
50. Moorthy AV, Zimmerman SW. Renal disease in the elderly: clinicopathologic analysis of renal disease in 115 elderly patients. Clin Nephrol 1980;14:223–229.
51. Davison AM, Johnston PA. Glomerulonephritis in the elderly. Nephrol Dial Transplant 1996;11(suppl 9):34–37.
52. Hricik DE, Chung-Park M, Sedor JR. Glomerulonephritis. N Engl J Med 1998;339: 888–899.
53. Keller F, Michaelis C, Buttner P, Bennhold I, Schwarz A, Distler A. Risk factors for long-term survival and renal function in 64 patients with rapidly progressive glomerulonephritis (RPGN). Geriatr Nephrol Urol 1994;4:5–13.
54. Couser WG. Rapidly progressive glomerulonephritis: classification, pathogenetic mechanisms, and therapy. Am J Kidney Dis 1988;11:449–464.
55. Washio M, Oh Y, Okuda S, Yanase T, Miishima C, Fujimi S, Ohchi N, Nanishi F,

Onoyama K, Fujishima M. Clinicopathological study of poststreptococcal glomerulonephritis in the elderly. Clin Nephrol 1994;41:265–270.
56. Koyama A, Kobayashi M, Yamaguchi N, Yamagata K, Takano K, Nakajima M, Irie F, Goto M, Igarashi M, Iitsuka T, Aoki Y, Sakurai H, Sakurayama N, Fukao K. Glomerulonephritis associated with MRSA infection: a possible role of bacterial superantigen. Kidney Int 1995;47:207–216.
57. Neves PL, Anunciada AI, Godinho C, Bexiga I, Amorim JP. Acute renal failure in elderly patients. Geriatr Nephrol Urol 1993;3:133–137.
58. Batlle DC, Arruda JA, Kurtzman NA. Hyperkalemic distal renal tubular acidosis associated with obstructive uropathy. N Engl J Med 1981;304:373–380.
59. Platt JF, Rubin JM, Ellis JH, Di Pietro M. Duplex Doppler ultrasound of the kidney: Differentiation of obstructive from nonobstructive dilatation. Radiology 1989;171: 515–517.
60. Porush JG, Faubert PF. Renal Disease in the Aged. Boston: Little, Brown & Company; 1991.
61. Himmelfarb J, Tolkoff-Rubin N, Chandran P, Parker RA, Wingard RL, Hakim R. A multicenter comparison of dialysis membranes in the treatment of acute renal failure requiring dialysis. J Am Soc Nephrol 1998;9:257–266.
62. Alarabi A, Nystrom SO, Stahle E, Wikstrom B. Acute renal failure and outcome of continuous arteriovenous hemodialysis (CAVHD) and continuous hemofiltration (CAVH) in elderly patients following cardiovascular surgery. Geriatr Nephrol Urol 1997;7:45–49.
63. van Bommel EF, Ponssen HH. Intermittent versus continuous treatment for acute renal failure: where do we stand? Am J Kidney Dis 1997;30(suppl 4):S72–S79.
64. Liano F, Garcia-Martin F, Gallego A, Orte L, Teruel JL, Marcen R, Matesanz R, Ortuno J. Easy and early prognosis in acute tubular necrosis: a forward analysis of 228 cases. Nephron 1989;51:307–313.
65. Liano F, Gallego A, Pascual J, Garcia-Martin F, Teruel JL, Marcen R, Orofino L, Orte L, Rivera M, Gallego N, Quereda C, Ortuno J. Prognosis of acute tubular necrosis: an extended prospectively contrasted study. Nephron 1993;63:21–31.
66. Arora P, Kher V, Kohli HS, Sharma RK, Gupta A, Jha R. Acute renal failure in the elderly: experience from a single centre in India. Nephrol Dial Transplant 1993;8: 827–830.
67. Gentric A, Cledes J. Immediate and long-term prognosis in acute renal failure in the elderly. Nephrol Dial Transplant 1991;6:86–90.
68. Baldyga AP, Paganini EP, Chaff C, Higgins TL. Acute dialytic support of the octogenarian: is it worth it? ASAIO J 1993;39:M805–M808.
69. Parker RA, Himmelfarb J, Tolkoff-Rubin N, Chandran P, Wingard RL, Hakim RM. Prognosis of patients with acute renal failure requiring dialysis: results of a multicenter study. Am J Kidney Dis 1998;32:432–443.
70. Santacruz F, Barreto S, Mayor MM, Cabrera W, Breuer N. Mortality in elderly patients with acute renal failure. Ren Fail 1996;18:601–605.
71. Rodgers H, Staniland JR, Lipkin GW, Turney JH. Acute renal failure: a study of elderly patients. Age Ageing 1990;19:36–42.

16

Alterations in Electrolytes and Acid-Base Homeostasis with Aging

Adebenga Adetola
Charles R. Drew University of Medicine and Science, and Martin Luther King, Jr.–Charles R. Drew Medical Center, Los Angeles, California

Keith C. Norris
Charles R. Drew University of Medicine and Science, Martin Luther King, Jr.–Charles R. Drew Medical Center, and UCLA School of Medicine, Los Angeles, California

I. RENAL PHYSIOLOGY AND AGING

A. Clinical Relevance

The kidney undergoes several age-related anatomical and physiological changes that are associated with a greater susceptibility toward the development of specific electrolyte and acid-base disturbances. In particular, advancing age is associated with a decline in glomerular filtration rate (GFR) and an impaired ability to maintain water, sodium, potassium, and acid-base homeostasis in response to exogenous stimuli. Some of these renal changes are due to degenerative cardiovascular processes and a subsequent functional reduction in renal perfusion, whereas others reflect intrinsic alterations in renal function. It is important that the clinician be aware of not only subtle alterations that may occur in the baseline electrolyte and acid-base settings but also more importantly the blunted response to disease processes, environmental conditions, and commonly used medications. A greater understanding of the alterations in renal physiological and related neurohormonal responses that occur with aging can help guide the clinician toward a more timely and appropriate response to a given disease process.

Under normal circumstances, age has no significant effect on baseline plasma electrolyte concentrations, plasma pH, or the routine maintenance of extracellular fluid (ECF) volume. Because adaptive mechanisms responsible for maintaining the consistency of both the composition and volume status of the ECF are attenuated, the acutely ill elderly are especially vulnerable to the development of severe derangement in fluid and electrolyte balance and systemic pH that delays recovery, prolongs hospitalizations, and adversely affects outcome.

B. Glomerular Number and Function

In 1937, Moore counted the number of glomeruli per kidney in 29 persons ranging from 1 to 70 years of age (1). Between the ages of 1 and 40 he noted each kidney contained between 500,000 and 1.2 million glomeruli. However, a 30% to 50% reduction in the number of glomeruli was noted by the seventh decade. The progressive nature of the aging process in the kidney is demonstrated anatomically in the basement membranes of the glomeruli, renal tubules, and renal arterial tree (2). In the renal arterioles, a gradual age-related development of medial hypertrophy, intimal proliferation, reduplication of elastic tissue, and hyalinization in vessels occurs. When microdissection techniques were used to determine renal tubule length and volume, graduated reductions with age were found in proximal renal tubule volume and glomerular surface area, whereas no gender differences were detected (2) (Figure 1).

C. Glomerular Filtration

Commensurate with the decline in the number of glomeruli is an average decrease in the GFR of about 1%/year or 10%/decade after age 40 (3,4). Despite the fall in

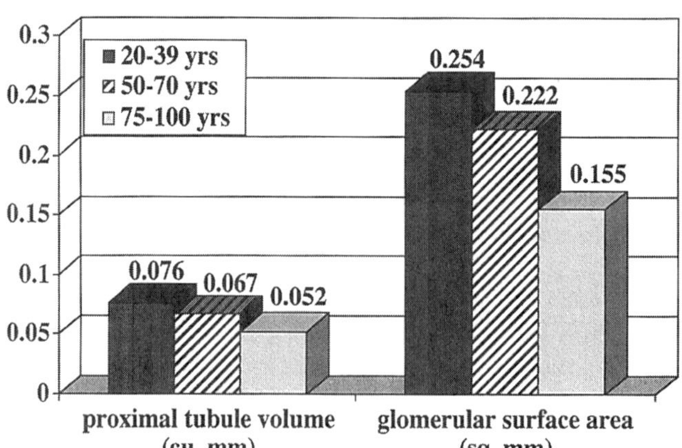

Figure 1 Age-related anatomical changes within the kidney.

GFR, serum creatinine does not increase by 10% per decade and in most instances remains unchanged because of a reduction in muscle mass and proportional decline in endogenous creatinine production (3,5). Thus, the importance of more accurately assessing the GFR in an older patient cannot be overemphasized. Because serum creatinine is commonly used an estimate of renal function, the stability of the serum creatinine value can mislead the clinician into believing the GFR is unaltered in an elderly individual with a ''normal'' serum creatinine. This predisposes to inaccuracies in medication dosing and other therapies that should be modified to compensate for a reduction in renal function. This may lead to multiple iatrogenic complications including, but limited to, acute renal failure, drug toxicities, and a variety of electrolyte abnormalities (6–8).

Cockcroft and Gault (9) have established a formula to estimate changes in GFR adjusting for body mass and age that is now commonly used in clinical practice (Table 1). Thus, a serum creatinine of 1.2 mg/dL in a 20-year-old, 80-kg man reflects a GFR of 111 mL/min, whereas a serum creatinine of 1.2 mg/dL in a 70-year-old, 60-kg woman reflects a GFR of 41 mL/min, highlighting the need to account for the influence of body mass and age, as well as gender, on the serum creatinine.

D. Renal Plasma Flow

A progressive reduction in renal plasma flow from 600 mL/min in young adulthood to as low as 300 mL/min by 80 years of age has been documented (4). Two key factors contributing to this reduction include an age-related decline in the renal fraction of cardiac output and an increase in renovascular arteriolar resistance, the latter caused by a blunted vasodilatory response (10,11). A significant decrease in the cortical component of blood flow occurs with advancing age, a finding consistent with histological studies showing selective loss of cortical vasculature (11). These histological and functional demonstrations of selective decrease in cortical blood flow may explain the observation that the filtration fraction (the fraction of renal plasma flow that is filtered at the glomerulus) actually increases with advancing age because outer cortical nephrons have a lower filtration fraction than juxtamedullary nephrons.

Table 1 Cockcroft and Gault Formula for Estimating Glomerular Filtration Rate

$$\frac{(140 - \text{Age in yr}) \times \text{Lean body weight in kg}}{72 \times \text{Serum creatinine (mg/dL)}} = \text{estimated GFR (mL/min)}^{a}$$

[a] × 0.85 for women.

E. Renal Concentration and Diluting Capacity

With aging urinary concentration and diluting abnormalities occur that reflect diminished tubular function (12). In the healthy young adult, maximum urinary concentrating ability of 1200 mOsm/kg is achievable, whereas a healthy elderly person can only achieve a urine osmolality of 700 to 800 mOsm/kg (13). In addition, the elderly individual cannot dilute urine to less than 100 mOsm/kg compared with 50 mOsm/kg in young adults (14,15). These alterations in concentration and diluting capacity reduce the ability of the elderly to handle sodium or water loads and/or deficits that may occur.

F. Water Metabolism

Regulation of water homeostasis primarily depends on three key factors: (1) an intact thirst mechanism, (2) appropriate renal handling of water and solute, and (3) intact release of arginine vasopressin or antidiuretic hormone (ADH), a nonapeptide produced by the neurohypophysis (16). Derangements in water metabolism are largely reflected as changes in serum sodium concentration. Water is the predominant constituent of the human body and makes up 55% to 65% of healthy adults. With age the proportion of water diminishes, possibly because the ratio of muscle to water-poor tissues such as fat and bone is reduced (17). Between 55% and 75% of water is contained within the intracellular compartment. Plasma constitutes approximately one-quarter of the extracellular space, and ADH closely regulates the water content within this compartment. Although many variables influence the secretion of ADH, the most important mediator under normal physiological conditions is the plasma osmolality (18). By adjusting water content, the body maintains plasma osmolality and its principal determinant, plasma sodium concentration, within an extremely narrow range of 285 to 295 mOsm/L. The sensitivity of the osmoregulatory system appears to increase with age (19,20). By contrast, sensitivity of thirst is diminished in elderly persons, predisposing them to the development of water deficiency and hypernatremia (20–22). In addition, the ability of the elderly to excrete free water is also blunted, likely because of a decline in GFR (15) or reduced tubular responsiveness to ADH (23), predisposing them to hyponatremia. Elderly patients are more likely to consume prescribed or over-the-counter medications for a variety of conditions, and many of these medications can influence ADH secretion and affect water metabolism (Table 2). Other conditions such as the destruction of the neurohypophysis by tumors, granulomatous disease, vascular insults, trauma, and metabolic or other disturbances can lead to ADH deficiency and reduced thirst. This is especially important in elderly persons, in whom even a partial deficiency of ADH may be superimposed on an impaired thirst response and lead to negative free water balance and hypernatremia.

Table 2 Common Medications in the Elderly that Can Influence Antidiuretic Hormone Secretion and Affect Water Metabolism

Nicotine[a]	Alcohol[b]	Lithium[c]
Morphine (high dose)[a]	Morphine (low dose)[b]	Colchicine[c]
Epinephrine[a]	Clonidine[b]	Demclocycline[c]
Cyclophosphamide[a]	Glucocorticoids[b]	Glyburide[c]
Tolbutamide[d]	Haloperidol[b]	Loop diuretics[c]
Chlorpropamide[d]	Cisplatinum[b]	Vinblastine[c]
NSAIDs[d]	Cabamazepine[b]	Methoxyflurane[c]

NSAIDs, Nonsteroidal anti-inflammatory drugs.
[a] Enhances ADH secretion.
[b] Reduces ADH secretion.
[c] Diminishes renal tubular responsiveness.
[d] Increases renal tubular responsiveness.

G. Sodium Metabolism

With aging the ability of the kidney to both conserve sodium in response to sodium deprivation and to excrete sodium in response to sodium loading is impaired. Epstein and Hollenberg noted the half-time for reduction of urinary sodium after salt restriction was 17.6 hours in young subjects and 31 hours in elderly subjects (24). This salt-losing tendency of the senescent kidney is due both to nephron loss that leads to increased osmotic load per nephron and resultant mild osmotic diuresis and possibly to age-related alterations in the renin-aldosterone system. Basal renin and aldosterone levels are diminished by 30% to 50% in the face of a normal level of renin substrate (25–30). An age-related reduction in end organ responsiveness to atrial natriuretic peptide (ANP), a 28 aminoacid peptide, may also occur, which has both a natriuretic and a vasodilatory effect on the kidney (31–34).

II. HYPONATREMIA AND HYPERNATREMIA

A. Hyponatremia

1. Clinical Relevance

Serum sodium is usually maintained within the normal range of 135 to 145 mEq/L. A reduction in serum sodium to less than 130 mEq/L should be considered clinically significant. Hyponatremia is one of the most common electrolyte disorders in the elderly (35). This is due, in part, to the aged kidney's blunted response to sodium deficiency, a diminished diluting capacity and an impaired ability to excrete free water.

2. Clinical Manifestations

Depending on the magnitude and rate of development of hyponatremia, the clinical presentation may range from asymptomatic to overt central nervous system symptoms such as lethargy, confusion, seizures, coma, and death. Subtle findings such as loss of attention may be one of the earliest signs of altered sensorium, and this should be specifically evaluated in the older patient with hyponatremia or other metabolic abnormalities.

3. Immediate Diagnostic Approach

The first step in evaluating a patient with a reduced serum sodium level is to evaluate the plasma osmolality. If the plasma osmolality is low, the patient is classified as being in a true hypo-osmotic state. A useful working classification is to then place the patient into one of three categories on the basis of the clinical assessment: (1) hyponatremia with ECF volume depletion, (2) hyponatremia with normal ECF volume, or (3) hyponatremia with ECF volume excess. In the setting of hyponatremia with overt ECF volume depletion, the baroreceptor stimuli override the osmoreceptors and stimulate ADH release. Likewise, in patients with hyponatremia and a clinical excess of ECF volume (i.e., cirrhosis, congestive heart failure, nephrotic syndrome), the underlying disorder is associated with a reduced effective arterial pressure that initiates the overriding baroreceptor response. The patient with hyponatremia and normal ECF volume will often have either an endocrine abnormality, medication induced, or a true inappropriate secretion of ADH. A more detailed approach to the patient with hyponatremia has been described elsewhere (36). In the elderly patient with hyponatremia and ECF volume depletion, it is particularly important to consider diuretic use or poor oral intake with a predominately liquid diet such as tea or juices (Table 3).

Elderly patients with hyponatremia with normal ECF volume should always be screened for hypothyroidism and glucorticoid deficiency. The incidence of hypothyroidism increases substantially with advancing age. Also medications

Table 3 Common Causes of Hyponatremia in Elderly

Thiazide diuretics (up to 50% of cases)	Hypotonic intravenous fluids
SIADH; pulmonary disorders, CNS disorders, idiopathic	Edematous states: congestive heart failure, cirrhosis of liver, nephrotic syndrome
Low solute intake: tea-toast diet, low osmolar tube feeding, ''beer drinking potomania''	Miscellaneous: hypothyroidism, Addison's disease, psychogenic polydipsia, glucocorticoid deficiency
Drugs affecting vasopressin	

SIADH, Syndrome of inappropriate antidiuretic hormone secretion; CNS, central nervous system.

can lead to an excess secretion of vasopressin or an enhanced renal tubular responsiveness to circulating vasopressin (Table 2). If these possibilities have been excluded, the diagnosis of the syndrome inappropriate ADH secretion (SIADH) is likely, and investigation of a central nervous system disorder, malignancy, or abnormal pulmonary process becomes extremely important, although a cause may not be found in all cases. Indeed, in an ambulatory geriatric population Miller and colleagues reported that 46 of 405 subjects (11%) had hyponatremia, with SIADH the apparent cause in 27 of 46 (59%), of which one-quarter had no apparent underlying cause and were considered to have idiopathic SIADH. This SIADH-like hyponatremia occurred more commonly among the old elderly, suggesting that aging might be a risk factor for the development of a SIADH-like hyponatremia (35).

4. Intervention

Treatment depends on the pathogenesis of the hyponatremia and the severity of symptoms. A low serum sodium level in a symptomatic or hypotensive patient should be corrected by the infusion of normal saline or in rare instances hypertonic saline, depending on the level of severity. The rate of rise of serum sodium should not exceed 0.3–0.4 mmol/h (8 mmol/24 h) because correction of hyponatremia at a rate greater than 0.5 mmol/h has been associated with severe neurological complications (37). Care must be taken not to induce fluid overload and pulmonary vascular congestion. For a serum sodium level of 115 to 125 mEq/L the administration of normal saline at 75 to 100 mL/h for 24 to 48 hours is usually adequate. If any concern of heart disease exits, a rate of 50 to 75 mL/h is advisable. The serum sodium level should be repeated 1–2 times per day and the rate of fluid adjusted as necessary. The quantity of sodium required to increase the plasma sodium concentration by a given amount can be estimated more precisely by multiplying the desired change in plasma sodium by the total body water (e.g., 8 mmol/L change in a 60-kg person over 24 hours is 8 mmol/L $\times$ 36 L = 288 mmol = approx. 1.9 L normal saline or 560 mL 3% NaCl). It should be noted that symptoms related to hyponatremia occur disproportionately throughout the population. Interestingly, both aging and the male sex appear to confer protection against the development of hyponatremia-associated seizures, permanent brain damage, or mortality, although the reason(s) for this is unclear (38,39).

In asymptomatic patients with no evidence of volume depletion, correction of the underlying problem and restriction of free water intake to 1 L/day is usually sufficient to normalize the serum sodium. In patients with clinical evidence of excess total body sodium and water, the estimated total body water excess can be derived from the formula shown in Table 4. Bed rest and increasing water excretion with furosemide (20–40 mg intravenously twice a day), which inhibits

Table 4 Formula for Calculating Excess Free Water in a Patient with Hyponatremia

Excess water = TBW − {(actual pNa/ desired pNa) × TBW}

TBW, Total body water or body weight in kilograms × 0.6; PNa, plasma sodium in milliequivalents per liter.

free water reabsorption by inducing hypotonic urine and generating a negative free water balance, is effective in many patients. In cases of SIADH refractory to free water restriction (i.e., malignancies, other), demeclocylcine, 300 mg orally four times a day for up to 10 days, can be used to blunt the renal tubular response to circulating ADH and stimulate water diuresis.

B. Hypernatremia

1. Clinical Relevance

Hypernatremia is not uncommon at the extremes of age and is particularly prevalent among the elderly (Figure 2). A serum sodium of 150 mEq/L or greater should be considered clinically significant. The prevalence of hypernatremia in the elderly has been reported to be about 1% in both hospitalized patients and in long-term care facility residents (40). Because the percent total body water falls with age, equal volumes of fluid loss in young and old individuals may represent more severe dehydration in the elderly.

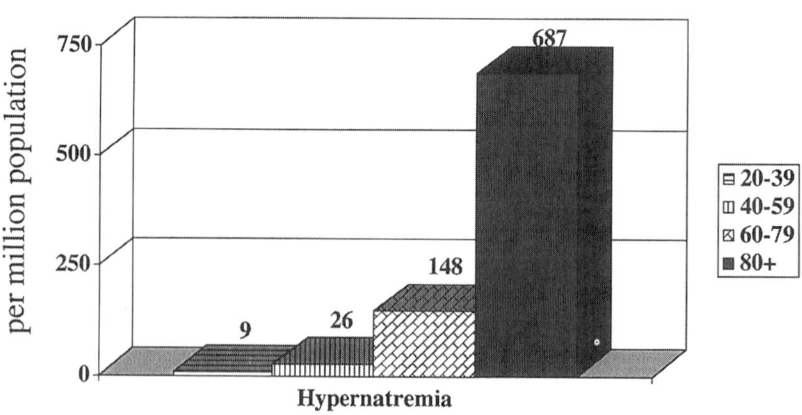

Figure 2 Prevalence of hypernatremia on admission by age group [1995 California hospital discharge database].

The age-related alterations in the physiological responses to water deprivation are important in understanding the pathogenesis of hypernatremia in the elderly (38). In healthy older men compared with younger controls, deficits exist in both the intensity and threshold of the thirst response (19–21). In addition the GFR and the ability to concentrate urine decline with age, and an increased incidence of renal disease exists, which may further contribute to the impaired ability to conserve water. In the elderly, hypernatremia carries a high risk of morbidity and mortality, ranging from 40% to 60% (40,41). Mortality rate was highest in those with a rapid onset and those with serum sodium level >160 mEq/L. Borra and coworkers reported an overall mortality rate of 48.6% among hospitalized elderly patients with hypernatremia and noted that slow correction of serum sodium over a 72-hour period significantly improved recovery of mental functions (40). Several common causes of hypernatremia in the elderly are shown (Table 5).

2. Clinical Manifestations

Nonspecific lethargy and weakness are common. Obtundation, stupor, coma, and seizures may accompany more severe hypernatremia. Clinical signs include decreased skin turgor, dry mouth, orthostatic hypotension, absent sweating, and hemoconcentration. In rare cases, hyperosmolality may lead to shrinkage of brain volume, capillary hemorrhage, or spontaneous subdural hematoma resulting in permanent neurological deficits.

3. Immediate Diagnostic Approach

An assessment should be made to exclude diabetes mellitus, sepsis, diarrhea, vomiting, or inadequate fluid intake, as well as tests for renal function, serum calcium, and osmolality.

Table 5 Etiology of Hypernatremia in Elderly

Decreased water intake	Increased water loss	Increased sodium intake
Febrile illness	Diarrhea, fever	Prolonged infusion of normal saline
Altered mental status	Osmotic diuresis (glycosuria, high-protein tube feeding)	Sodium bicarbonate therapy
Physical impairment	Diabetes insipidus, hypercalcemia, hypokalemia, chronic renal disease	

Table 6 Calculation of Water Deficit in a Patient with Hypernatremia

FWD = [(pNa − 140)/140] × 0.6 BW

FWD, Free water deficit; pNa, plasma sodium in milliequivalents per liter; BW, total body weight in kilograms.

4. Intervention

Correcting hypernatremia usually requires replacing body water deficits with hypotonic fluid. If the patient is alert and cooperative, oral water replacement is preferred. If oral fluids cannot be given, an intravenous infusion of dextrose in water is appropriate. However, if hypotension exists, normal saline is necessary to first improve blood pressure and end organ perfusion. Including projected insensible losses, the estimated water deficit should be replaced over 48 to 72 hours. The calculation of the water deficit is described in Table 6. A serum sodium of 160 mEq/L in an older person can usually be treated with an infusion of 5% dextrose in water at a rate of 100 to 125 mL/h. In general, for each additional 10 mEq rise in serum sodium the rate of fluid should be increased by 50 mL/h. Plasma electrolytes should be monitored at least daily and two to three times a day if the patient is severely ill, so adjustments in therapy can be made accordingly. Serum sodium level should be lowered no more rapidly that 0.5 mEq/L/h. Intranasal desmopressin is the appropriate treatment of central diabetes insipidus. Excessively rapid correction may lead to cerebral edema that can progress to permanent brain insult.

III. POTASSIUM DISORDERS

A. Clinical Relevance

1. Hyperkalemia

Serum plasma levels of potassium are normally maintained within the normal range of 3.5 to 5.0 mEq/L in the older patient. Although the serum potassium level is normal, evidence suggests an age-related reduction in total body potassium exists because of a decline in muscle mass (42,43). Ford and colleagues have reported an increase in plasma potassium after exercise in elderly subjects likely caused by an age-related impairment in the beta-adrenergic mediation of potassium flux into the skeletal muscles (44). However, this could also be related to the reduction in the overall muscle mass. In addition, the susceptibility to the development of hyperkalemia in an older patient may be due to an age-related reduction in the activity of the renin-aldosterone system (45). Indeed, healthy elderly subjects (65–85 years of age) compared with healthy younger subjects (20–35 years of age) had lower basal levels of plasma aldosterone and a blunted aldosterone response to potassium infusion, indicating an age-related increased susceptibility to hyperkalemia (45). The age-related decline in renal plasma flow and GFR further increases the risk of hyperkalemia developing. Concomitant therapy with nonsteroidal anti-inflammatory drugs and other medications that either further reduce aldosterone or otherwise impair potassium excretion (Table 7) must be used with care because this clinical scenario may result in significant hyperkalemia, including cardiac complications such as complete heart block (7,8). Patients with diabetes mellitus or hypertension who may have type IV renal tubular acidosis are at an even greater risk of hyperkalemia developing (46).

2. Hypokalemia

By contrast the development of hypokalemia in the elderly person is of particular concern because the presence of either underlying or overt coronary artery disease may be associated with increased dysrhythmias or sudden death. The prevalent use of diuretic therapy in this population, for states such as hypertension that affect more than 60% of patients older than 60 years of age (47), further increases the risk of the development of significant hypokalemia. In the Berlin Study of Aging hypokalemia accounted for 19% of side effects caused by drug-drug interactions, and this was frequently related to thiazide diuretic use (6). Also, the inability to maintain an adequate dietary potassium intake in a subset of the aging population may further compromise potassium homeostasis.

B. Clinical Manifestations and Immediate Diagnostic Approach

Nonspecific lethargy and weakness are common in both hyperkalemia and hypokalemia. Electrocardiographic changes of hyperkalemia include flattening or absence of P waves, peaked T waves, widened QRS complex, sine waves, and

Table 7 Common Medications Associated with Potassium Disorders in the Elderly

Hyperkalemia	Hypokalemia
Beta-blockers	Thiazide diuretics
Angiotensin-converting enzyme inhibitors	Loop diuretics
Potassium-sparing diuretics	
Nonsteroidal anti-inflammatory drugs	

atrioventricular conduction delay. The latter three findings herald the presence of life-threatening cardiac complications and require emergency treatment. Electrocardiographic changes of hypokalemia include flattening of the T waves and the presence of U waves; severe hypokalemia can cause prolonged PR interval, widening and decreased voltage of QRS complex, and ventricular dysrhythmias.

A careful evaluation of medications, assessment of renal function including urinary electrolytes, and measurement of blood glucose and arterial pH are essential.

C. Intervention

1. Hyperkalemia

The presence of widened QRS complexes or a sine wave pattern mandates therapy with intravenous calcium (one ampule of calcium gluconate, 90 mg calcium per ampule) over 2 to 3 minutes to minimize cardiac membrane depolarization. If the QRS complex is normal but tall peaked T waves are present, treatment with 10 units of regular insulin intravenously followed by 1 ampule (50 mL) of 50% dextrose is usually adequate to drive enough potassium intracellularly to normalize the electrocardiographic changes. At the same time measures to remove potassium from the body should be initiated. Commonly used measures include the oral administration of 25 to 50 g of the potassium-sodium exchange resin sodium polystyrene sulfonate (Kayexalate) with 30 mL of sorbitol every 2 to 4 hours for two to three doses, or 50 g administered as a retention enema. Intravenous furosemide, 20 to 40 mg, can also be used to enhance renal potassium excretion if renal function is normal. If significant renal impairment is present, dialysis treatment may be necessary.

2. Hypokalemia

If the serum potassium level is between 2.5 and 3.5 mEq/L, treatment is usually begun with oral potassium supplements, 30 to 40 mEq every 2 to 4 hours for two to three doses and then the serum potassium level is rechecked. Each 1 mEq fall in potassium below normal is associated with approximately 100 to 150 mEq deficit in total body potassium. If the serum potassium level falls to less than 2.5 mEq/L (or less than 3.0 in patients with cardiac disease), consideration for intravenous replacement is warranted. Intravenous potassium should be administered at a rate not to exceed 10 mEq/h (10 mEq KCl in 100 mL D5W at 100 mL/h) unless the patient is monitored on telemetry.

IV. ACID-BASE DISORDERS

A. Clinical Relevance

Acid-base homeostasis is maintained within a narrow range through a series of reversible chemical buffers and physiological pulmonary and renal responses.

Although the hydrogen ion concentration (pH) of the ECF is maintained between 7.38 and 7.42, evidence suggests this occurs at the expense of a reduced bicarbonate ion (HCO_3^-) reserve. A recent review of age-related acid-base changes noted a significant increase in the steady-state blood hydrogen ion (H^+) and reduction in steady-state plasma HCO_3 from subjects age 20 to 100 years, suggesting a progressive age-related low-level metabolic acidosis. This was associated with the expected respiratory adaptation of a reduced arterial partial pressure of carbon dioxide (P_{CO_2}), indicating a well-maintained pulmonary response (48). Because the body's homeostatic response to these pathological processes is efficient, maintaining serum HCO_3 and blood pH within the ''normal'' range occurs at the expense of an impaired HCO_3 reserve. The homeostatic responses to chronic metabolic acidosis in aging may engender pathological consequences such as nephrolithiasis, bone demineralization, and muscle protein breakdown. Indeed, these maladaptive changes have suggested a ''eubicarbonatemic'' metabolic acidosis may exist in older patients and emphasizes the importance of recognition and treatment of even mild acid loads to prevent these maladaptive homeostatic responses (49).

This apparent ''eubicarbonatemic'' metabolic acidosis with aging appears to be most directly related to a decline of renal function. However, an age-related, low-grade, diet-dependent metabolic acidosis has also been reported, although, again, age could not be dissociated from a reduced GFR. Examining 64 apparently healthy adult humans from 17 to 74 years of age ingesting controlled diets, Frassetto and coworkers noted a rise in steady-state blood hydrogen ion concentration and fall in plasma bicarbonate concentration with an increase in subject age and associated fall in GFR (50). In addition to the normal physiological changes that occur with aging, the increased frequency of comorbid conditions and potential exposure to additional insults that may have a further impact on both pulmonary and renal function increase the susceptibility toward the development of acid-base disturbances. Many common disorders in the elderly such as anemia, congestive heart failure, sepsis, diabetes mellitus, renal disease, and pulmonary disease can more easily overwhelm the acid-base regulatory system in these persons. In addition, many common drugs such as diuretics, nonsteroidal, anti-inflammatory agents, angiotensin-converting enzyme inhibitors, and laxatives can precipitate acid-base disturbances.

B. Immediate Diagnostic Approach

Acidosis is a process that, if left unopposed, results in acidemia (pH <7.38). Likewise, alkalosis is a process that, if left unopposed, results in alkalemia (pH >7.42). The physiological response to changes in pH involves changes in alveolar ventilation (P_{CO_2}) or in renal acid excretion and HCO_3 reclamation. The respiratory response to metabolic acidosis is almost immediate, whereas the renal response usually requires 12 to 48 hours.

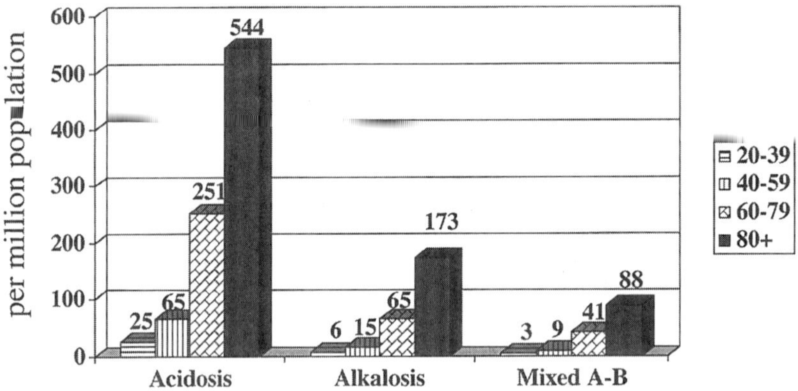

Figure 3 Prevalence of acid-base disturbances on admission by age group [1995 California hospital discharge database].

Thus, evaluating a patient with acid-base disturbance requires assessment of the clinical presentation, renal and pulmonary function status, electrolytes (including anion gap), and arterial blood gas. Urinary electrolyte levels and pH may also be helpful. One commonly used approach is to compare the pH and serum bicarbonate. If they move in the same direction, the primary disturbance is metabolic; if they move in opposite directions, the primary disturbance is respiratory. A normal pH with an increased anion gap reflects a mixed acid-base disorder, which is more common as age increases (Figure 3). A rough guide to determining appropriate responses to a given primary disturbance is shown in Table 8.

C. Metabolic Acidosis

1. Clinical Relevance

Metabolic acidosis is defined as a decrease in plasma HCO_3^- and a decrease in plasma pH or a normal plasma pH with an elevated anion gap. This can occur

Table 8 Simple Guide to Estimating Physiological Response for a Given Primary Acid-Base Disturbance

Primary disturbance		Response
Metabolic acidosis	(10 mEq/L fall HCO_3)	10–12 fall P_{CO_2}
Metabolic alkalosis	(10 mEq/L rise HCO_3)	4–6 rise P_{CO_2}
Respiratory acidosis[a]	(10 mm Hg rise P_{CO_2})	4–6 rise HCO_3
Respiratory alkalosis[a]	(10 mm Hg fall P_{CO_2})	4–6 fall HCO_3

[a] If acute, then 10 mm Hg change P_{CO_2}: 1–2 change HCO_3.

by the addition of a strong acid, direct loss of bicarbonate by the gastrointestinal tract or the kidney, or rapid dilution of the ECF by a nonbicarbonate-containing solution. The physiological response to acidemia is an increase in ventilation that returns pH toward normal. In clinical practice metabolic acidosis is divided into two functional categories, increased anion gap and normal anion gap (Table 9).

2. Clinical Manifestations

The patient with mild acidemia may exhibit no symptoms. With severe acidemia, nausea, vomiting, anorexia, lethargy, hyperventilation, and Kussmaul respirations may develop. Severe acidemia is associated with decreased myocardial contractility, hypotension, pulmonary edema, and tissue hypoxia. Animal studies suggest the extent of acidemia-associated myocardial impairment is more severe with advancing age. Abete and colleagues noted that compared with adult rats, senescent rats exposed to hypercapnic acidosis had a greater decrease in left ventricular pressure, a greater rise in left ventricular end-diastolic pressure, and a greater reduction of contractility, suggesting a greater vulnerability of the aged heart to acidemia-associated myocardial dysfunction (51).

3. Intervention

Initial treatment is directed toward correcting the underlying disease process. Oral bicarbonate or precursors such as citrate can be administered to treat mild and chronic metabolic acidoses. Severe acidemia, pH <7.10, mandates intravenous (IV) sodium bicarbonate to help maintain normal cardiac function and cellular integrity. Caution must be used especially in the elderly to avoid iatrogenic volume and sodium overload that can occur with vigorous HCO_3 replacement. In general, half of the deficit should be replaced over the first 24 hours and half

Table 9 Common Causes of Metabolic Acidosis in the Elderly

High anion gap metabolic acidosis	Normal anion gap metabolic acidosis
L-lactic acid (tissue hypoxia)	Renal tubular acidosis
D-lactic acid (altered GI flora, e.g., blind loop syndromes)	Diarrhea
Ketone body acids (insulin deficiency, alcohol)	Reduced renal function
Renal failure (organic acids)	Uretero-GI fistulas
Acetosalicylic acid	HCl acids
Intoxicants (check osmotic gap)	Dilution
Methanol to formic acid	
Ethylene glycol to glyoxalic acid	
Paraldehyde to acetic acid	

GI, gastrointestinal; HCl, hydrochloric.

over the following 24 to 48 hours. The HCO_3 deficit can be estimated as follows: HCO_3 (mEq/L) deficit = 60% body weight (kg) × [24 − HCO_3 (meq/L) observed]. A serum HCO_3 of 14 in a 60-kg person is 360 mEq acid deficit and to replace 180 mEq in 24 hours one can add two ampules of $NaHCO_3$ (44 mEq/ampule) to 1L 5% dextrose and administer at 83 mL/h (2L/day or 176 mEq/day). The treatment of lactic acidosis remains controversial, but several authorities recommend aggressive treatment with sodium bicarbonate while efforts to correct the underlying problem are initiated (52).

D. Metabolic Alkalosis

1. Clinical Relevance

An increase in plasma bicarbonate concentration and an increase in blood pH characterize metabolic alkalosis. A mixed disturbance of metabolic alkalosis and metabolic acidosis can be diagnosed by a significantly increased anion gap in the presence of a normal plasma pH. Metabolic alkalosis can result from ECF hydrogen ion loss, addition of bicarbonate or bicarbonate precursors to the ECF, or ECF volume contraction. Elderly patients are predisposed to volume depletion that is associated with an increase in proximal tubular bicarbonate reabsorption and the development of metabolic alkalosis. A list of common conditions associated with metabolic alkalosis is presented in Table 10.

2. Clinical Manifestations

Patients may have muscle cramps, weakness, and hypereflexia. Marked increases in serum pH can induce seizures. Alveolar hypoventilation can lead to a reduction in arterial partial pressure of oxygen (Po_2) and signs of hypoxia. Hypochloremia and hypokalemia are almost invariably present, and severe hypokalemia can lead to cardiac dysrhythmias. Volume contraction often leads to increased blood urea nitrogen and serum creatinine levels. Clinically, metabolic alkalosis can be di-

Table 10 Common Causes of Metabolic Alkalosis in the Elderly

Chloride (CL^-) responsive (urine CL^- <10)	Chloride resistant (urine CL^- >10)
Gastric fluid loss	Aldosterone/cortisol excess
Postdiuretic therapy	Bartter's syndrome
Diarrhea	Potassium depletion
Posthypercapnia	

vided into chloride-responsive and chloride-resistant states. Chloride-responsive states are usually associated with volume depletion caused by vomiting or nasogastric suction and characterized by a low urinary chloride concentration, <10 mEq/L. One exception is the active use of diuretics, in which instance urine chloride concentration may be >10 mEq/L. This must always be considered in an older patient with metabolic alkalosis. By contrast, chloride-resistant metabolic alkalosis is usually due to a high aldosterone or aldosterone-like state such as primary hyperaldosteronism or Cushing's syndrome. Chloride-resistant metabolic alkalosis is almost always associated with an increase in sodium retention, hypertension, and a high urinary chloride concentration.

3. Intervention

Initial treatment is directed toward correcting the underlying disease process. Specific therapy for chloride-responsive metabolic alkalosis requires administration of sodium chloride and frequently potassium. In the volume-depleted older patient 100 to 150 mL/h of normal saline for 24 to 48 hours with reassessment of arterial blood gases is adequate in most instances. If hypokalemia is present, 20 to 40 mEq of potassium chloride should be added to each liter of normal saline. In many cases of chloride-resistant states the use of direct or indirect aldosterone antagonists such as spironolactone and amiloride is effective.

E. Respiratory Acidosis

1. Clinical Relevance

Respiratory acidosis is characterized by an increase in P_{CO_2} and a reduction in pH. The increased CO_2 results in an increased carbonic acid concentration. In respiratory acidosis, carbonic acid is buffered by intracellular buffers including hemoglobin and phosphate, resulting in a slight increase in plasma bicarbonate concentration. The kidneys compensate by increasing acid secretion that generates additional bicarbonate. This renal response may take 24 to 48 hours to develop.

A variety of clinical conditions may be associated with respiratory acidosis. In general, abnormalities leading to a reduction in alveolar ventilation such as pulmonary obstruction, primary depression of the respiratory center, mechanical/structural defect, or a neuromuscular disorder can lead to CO_2 retention and acidemia. Salicylate intoxication, which classically is seen as a mixed metabolic acidosis and respiratory alkalosis, may initially present as a respiratory acidosis in the elderly because of the frequent association of other ingested substances, primarily central nervous system depressants (53).

2. Clinical Manifestations

Patients may exhibit respiratory distress, dyspnea, confusion, or lethargy. If severe, the patient may show signs of increased intracranial pressure caused by vasodilatory properties of CO_2, which increases cerebral blood flow.

3. Intervention

The treatment of respiratory acidosis is correction of the underlying disorder and restoration of adequate ventilation. This may necessitate the use of a mechanical ventilator. In addition to the standard clinical assessment, urine drug screening for possible overdose or intoxication is critical, particularly for salicylate toxicity and central nervous system depressants.

F. Respiratory Alkalosis

1. Clinical Relevance

Respiratory alkalosis is a common acid-base disorder encountered among the elderly. It results from increased alveolar ventilation, leading to a reduced P_{CO_2} and an elevated plasma pH. The initial response to alkalemia is buffering with intracellular protons (H+). Renal compensation occurs over several days, with a reduction in both net acid excretion and bicarbonate reclamation, reducing plasma bicarbonate concentration and lowering plasma pH toward normal.

Clinical disorders that increase central nervous system respiratory drive or increase stimulation of chemoreceptor may lead to hyperventilation and reduce systemic P_{CO_2}. In the elderly, it is especially important to consider anxiety and associated hyperventilation, central nervous system infection/infarction, sepsis, pulmonary edema, pulmonary emboli, or medications/drugs, especially salicylate intoxication (53–55).

2. Clinical Manifestations

The patient often manifests hyperventilation and signs of hypocapnia. These may include light-headedness, perioral and extremity paresthesias, muscle cramps, seizures, and cardiac dysrhythmias. In the elderly it may often be a clue to the early state of a serious underlying disorder as described earlier.

3. Intervention

The most effective therapy is to treat the underlying disorder. The transient use of a rebreathing mask, bag, or similar instrument may help resolve the acute symptoms of hypocapnia. Serum salicylate levels should be checked to exclude occult salicylate toxicity. Appropriate cultures and broad-spectrum antibiotics should be instituted if sepsis is suspected.

V. DISORDERS OF SERUM CALCIUM

Calcium balance is impaired with advancing age, although serum calcium values are usually maintained within the normal range. A reduction in intestinal calcium absorption may be related to subnormal levels of vitamin D, increased circulating levels of parathyroid hormone (PTH), or reduced calcium intake (56–61). The renal tubular reabsorption of calcium appears to remain intact with aging, helping to maintain serum calcium within normal limits. However, the age-related reduction in dietary calcium intake associated with impaired intestinal calcium absorption can lead to clinically significant net negative calcium balance with bone calcium loss and in some cases hypocalcemia (62,63). By contrast, hypercalcemia is not uncommonly seen in the older patient because of the higher prevalence of specific hypercalcemic-related disorders.

In the ECF calcium exists in three forms: (1) protein bound, 40%; (2) complexed to several anions, including citrate, sulfate, and phosphate, 15%; and (3) ionized, which is the biologically active component, 45%. Serum calcium is primarily under the regulation of PTH and vitamin D. Calcium is absorbed from the gastrointestinal tract under the influence of vitamin D and its metabolites and is stored primarily in bone. Bone deposition and release of calcium are predominately under the regulation of vitamin D and PTH. The renal excretion of calcium is, in turn, determined mainly by the filtered calcium load and serum PTH level. In clinical practice, total serum calcium levels and not ionized serum calcium levels are measured. The total serum calcium level can be adjusted for a fall in the serum albumin concentration as follows: for every 1 g/dL fall in albumin less than 4 g/dL, total serum calcium falls by 0.8 mg/dL.

A. Hypercalcemia

1. Clinical Relevance

Hypercalcemia is defined as a corrected serum calcium >10.4 mg/dL (2.63 mmol/L) or an ionized calcium >4.8 mg/dL (1.2 mmol/L).

The two most common causes of hypercalcemia are primary hyperparathyroidism and malignancy. Each occurs more commonly with advancing age. Less common causes include vitamin D intoxication, granulomatous diseases, immobilization, hyperthyroidism, adrenal insufficiency, thiazide diuretics, or hypocalciuric hypercalcemia.

Several pathogenic mechanisms are associated with malignant hypercalcemia. Parathyroid hormone–related protein (PTHrP) accounts for the humoral hypercalcemia of malignancy associated with many solid tumors. Metastasis to bone with a local increase in bone-resorbing cytokines or osteoclast-activating factors, including prostaglandin E_2, interleukin 1, and tumor necrosis factor beta, also plays a role in some tumors.

Because of a fall in vitamin D production with age, hyperabsorption of calcium is an uncommon cause of hypercalcemia in the elderly. However, lymphomas and granulomatous diseases can produce hypercalcemia through unregulated synthesis of 1,25 dihydroxyvitamin D_3 by activated macrophages (64). For older populations, it is important to consider tuberculosis, which is highly prevalent among older institutionalized persons (65) and has been reported to be associated with hypercalcemia (66,67), although not as commonly as other granulomatous disorders (64,68). Also, vitamin D intoxication may be seen more commonly with the increasing consumption of vitamins and herbs associated with the expanding use of alternative medicine practices.

2. Clinical Manifestations

Because hypercalcemia is often a manifestation of an underlying disease process, several clinical symptoms and signs are often related to the primary disease process. Symptoms and signs more directly related to hypercalcemia include anorexia, nausea, vomiting, constipation, polyuria, nocturia and polydipsia, hypertension, confusion, nephrolithiasis, metastatic calcifications, peptic ulcer disease, pancreatitis, stupor, and coma.

3. Immediate Diagnostic Approach

Serum intact PTH levels in combination with a comprehensive serum chemistry panel and the overall clinical picture are most likely to yield a definitive answer. In selected cases evaluating urinary calcium excretion or vitamin D metabolites may be necessary. Intact PTH levels can help discriminate between hyperparathyroidism and malignancy. A low serum phosphate level suggests primary hyperparathyroidism but is not diagnostic. An elevated level of 25 (OH) D indicates vitamin D toxicity, whereas high 1,25 $(OH)_2D$ levels with a reduced level of 25 (OH) D suggest the presence of a granulomatous disease, lymphoma, or excess 1,25 $(OH)_2D$ ingestion.

4. Intervention

Hypercalcemia in the older patient requires immediate therapy when central nervous system symptoms are present, the total serum calcium level exceeds 12 mg/dL, or the Ca/P product is >70 (risk of metastatic calcification is high). Intravenous saline is effective in most cases. However, close monitoring of fluids and urine output is crucial to avoid fluid overall. The administration of 100 to 125 mL/h of normal saline for the first 24 to 48 hours is safe and effective for most older patients. Once the patient has been volume repleted, the addition of 20 to 40 mg of furosemide twice daily can further reduce serum calcium by enhancing urinary calcium excretion. In some instances a more aggressive therapeutic approach with up to 200 mL/h of normal saline is necessary. The addition of subcutaneous salmon calcitonin (4 units/kg subcutaneously every 12 hours for 2 days), which acts rapidly, and IV biphosphonate therapy (pamidronate, 60 mg in 1 L normal saline IV over 24 hours), which acts more slowly, are both potent inhibitors of bone resorption and are effective in normalizing serum calcium in most instances of hypercalcemia of malignancy.

B. Hypocalcemia

1. Clinical Relevance

Hypocalcemia is defined as a corrected serum calcium level <8.8 mg/dL (2.2 mmol) or an ionized calcium level <4.4 mg/dL (1.1 mmol).

Long-term negative calcium balance contributes to the high incidence of osteoporosis that occurs in older persons, although serum calcium levels are usually normal. Aging alters the metabolism of calcium and vitamin D in a number of ways. Intake of calcium and vitamin D, exposure to sunlight, cutaneous production of vitamin D_3, renal production of 1,25-dihydroxyvitamin D, intestinal absorption of calcium, and circulating vitamin D levels may all be reduced in elderly subjects (56–59,69–73). Less common causes of hypocalcemia include vitamin D deficiency, accelerated loss of 25 vitamin D_3 in patients with the nephrotic syndrome, hypoparathyroidism (i.e., tumor, idiopathic, hypomagnesemia), postparathyroidectomy (''hungry bone'' syndrome), secondary hyperparathyroidism caused by renal failure (more than 50% of newly diagnosed cases of end-stage renal disease occur in persons aged 65 and older), chronic hyperphosphatemia, osteoblastic metastases (prostate and breast cancer), and pancreatitis.

2. Clinical Manifestations

Manifestations of hypocalcemia range from acute, dramatic, and life threatening to the subtle. Tetany muscle spasms, cramps, carpal pedal spasm, seizures, myopathy, psychiatric disturbances, cataracts, congestive heart failure, and dysrhythmias (prolonged QT interval on electrocardiogram) may occur. Latent tetany can be detected by a light tap over the facial nerve resulting in ipsilateral facial twitch (Chvostek's sign) or by inflation of a sphygmomanometer above the systolic pressure for more than 3 minutes resulting in carpal spasm (Trousseau's sign).

3. Immediate Diagnostic Approach

The first step is verification of true hypocalcemia (reduction of ionized calcium). In clinical practice, this is most commonly done by adjusting the total serum calcium for any reduction in the serum albumin concentration. For every 1 g/dL reduction in serum albumin below normal, total serum calcium falls by 0.8 mg/dL. The next step is measurement of serum magnesium, which, if deficient, can cause hypocalcemia. Serum phosphate and intact PTH levels are also helpful information in many instances. Further investigation may necessitate the evaluation of vitamin D metabolites, although this is only done in rare circumstances.

4. Intervention

Immediate treatment of severe hypocalcemia with tetany or other overt clinical symptoms consists of the IV infusion of 1 ampule of 10% calcium gluconate (90 mg elemental calcium per 10-mL ampule) over 5 to 10 minutes. A continuous infusion of calcium can be administered as 3 ampules of 10% calcium chloride (360 mg elemental calcium per 10 mL) in 1 L 5% dextrose at 50 mL/h (54 mg/h) and titrated according to serum levels. A continuous infusion is most commonly necessary after parathyoridectomy when patients may experience severe prolonged hypocalcemia. Magnesium supplementation should be instituted if the serum magnesium level is low. Often 1.0 to 1.5 g of daily elemental calcium supplementation restores calcium balance and serum calcium levels to normal. Several studies suggest 400 to 800 IU of vitamin D per day is effective in maintaining normal serum 25(OH)D concentrations and preventing hypocalcemia and vitamin D deficiency (62,74,75), often with daily calcium supplementation (56,76,77). In cases of hypocalcemia not response to vitamin D or 25-hydroxyvitamin D therapy, the active form of vitamin D, (calcitriol or 1,25 dihydroxyvitamin D3) should be administered at 0.5 to 2.0 μg/day while continuing oral calcium supplementation.

VI. PHOSPHORUS BALANCE

A. Clinical Relevance

Hypophosphatemia occurs much more commonly than hyperphosphatemia. Hyperphosphatemia is uncommon in the absence of renal failure. Like calcium, there is reduction in intestinal phosphorus absorption with aging, which is also related, at least in part, to the subnormal levels of circulating 1,25 dihydroxy vitamin D3 (78). In addition, an age-related decrement in the renal tubular reabsorption of phosphorus appears to exist (79,80). Serum levels and renal handling of phosphorus may be affected by an age-related increase in serum PTH (73). However, Mulroney and co-workers demonstrated in rats that aging is associated with a

PTH-independent decrease in renal phosphate reabsorption (81). Impaired intestinal absorption or reduced intake, increased renal excretion, or redistribution of phosphate into cells may cause hypophosphatemia. Clinically, a low serum phosphate level in combination with hypercalcemia suggests primary hyperparathyroidism that occurs more commonly in aging populations. Other causes of hypophosphatemia include diabetic ketoacidosis, chronic alcoholism, dietary vitamin D deficiency, malabsorption, and malnutrition, which are common in some elderly populations. Hyperphosphatemia occurs most commonly in patients with renal failure. Other causes of hyperphosphatemia include hypoparathyroidism, rhabdomyolysis, tumor lysis syndrome, or excess phosphate administration but are uncommon if renal function is not impaired.

B. Immediate Diagnostic Approach

In addition to serum phosphorus and calcium levels, a complete chemical panel including renal function; serum PTH, vitamin D, electrolytes, and albumin; and liver function tests should be obtained. Serum phosphorus levels are normally maintained between 3.0 and 4.5 mEq/L. Clinically significant hyperphosphatemia occurs when serum phosphate exceeds 6.5 to 7.0 mEq/L, and significant hypophosphatemia occurs when serum phosphate falls to less than 2.0 to 2.5 mEq/L.

C. Clinical Manifestations

1. Hypophosphatemia

Symptoms and signs of hypophosphatemia typically occur only if total body phosphate is depleted and the serum phosphorus level is less than 1 mg/dL. Muscular abnormalities include rhabdomyolysis, generalized weakness, impaired diaphragmatic function, respiratory failure, and heart failure. Neurological abnormalities include paresthesias, dysarthria, confusion, stupor, seizures, and coma. Hematological findings, such as intravascular hemolysis and platelet and leukocyte dysfunction, occur in some instances. Chronic hypophosphatemia may cause osteomalacia in adults.

2. Hyperphosphatemia

Symptoms and signs of hyperphosphatemia are those attributable to hypocalcemia, such as tetany. When the calcium × phosphate product is greater than 70, a markedly increased risk of ectopic vascular and soft tissue calcifications, including smaller blood vessels, cornea, skin, kidney, and periarticular tissue, exists. In patients with renal failure, chronic hyperphosphatemia contributes to renal osteodystrophy.

D. Intervention

1. Hypophosphatemia

Severe hypophosphatemia (<1 mg/dL) may require IV phosphate therapy when associated with serious clinical manifestations. Infuse 20 mmol of phosphate in 1 L 0.45% saline over 12 hours (83 mL/h) and repeat if necessary until the serum phosphorus level exceeds 1.5 mg/dL or when symptoms resolve, and simultaneously administer oral therapy if possible. Extreme care must be used to avoid hyperphosphatemia, especially in the presence of renal impairment.

Mild acute hypophosphatemia (1.0 to 2.5 mg/dL) is usually asymptomatic and requires no therapy except correction of the underlying cause. Persistent hypophosphatemia should be treated with oral phosphate supplements, 0.5 to 1.0 g of elemental phosphorus two to three times daily (Neutra-Phos, 250 mg elemental phosphorus and 7 mEq each of sodium and potassium per capsule in water). Serum phosphorus, calcium, and creatinine should be measured daily as the dose is adjusted. Side effects include diarrhea, which is often dose limiting, and nausea.

2. Hyperphosphatemia

Restriction of dietary phosphate to 0.6 to 0.9 g/day and administration of oral phosphate binders (calcium carbonate or acetate) at an initial dosage of 0.5 to 1.0 g elemental calcium orally three times a day with meals are recommended for patients with renal impairment. Saline diuresis can acutely reduce hyperphosphatemia in patients who have normal renal function. If severe renal failure is present, dialysis may also be required to treat hyperphosphatemia.

VII. SERUM MAGNESIUM

A. Clinical Relevance

Magnesium plays an important role in neuromuscular function. Approximately 60% of body magnesium is in bone, and most of the remainder is within cells. Only 1% is in the ECF. Serum magnesium levels often do not reflect total body magnesium content. Magnesium deficit originates primarily from two etiological mechanisms, deficient intake or malabsorption or renal losses. However, serum magnesium handling appears to remain normal with aging. A higher prevalence of hypomagnesemia has been reported and is suggested to be related to a reduction in dietary magnesium intake (82). The decline in urinary magnesium concentration with advancing age reported by Simeckova et al is consistent with a fall in dietary magnesium intake (83). Among the elderly, primary magnesium deficiency caused by insufficient magnesium intake is more pronounced in institutionalized groups (84). Secondary magnesium deficiency caused by non-insulin-dependent diabetes mellitus and use of hypermagnesuric diuretics or other factors has also been noted in elderly populations (84). Moreover, significant subclinical total body magnesium deficit, not detected by serum magnesium, may be present in healthy elderly subjects (85). Hypermagnesemia is uncommon, but the use of magnesium-containing laxatives or antacids, especially in the presence of renal insufficiency, may be associated with hypermagnesemia.

B. Immediate Diagnostic Approach

Serum magnesium levels are normally maintained between 1.3 and 2.2 mEq/L. Clinically significant hypermagnesemia is often associated with serum magnesium values greater than 4 mEq/L, and clinically significant hypomagnesemia is often associated with serum magnesium values less than 1 mEq/L. Serum calcium and phosphorus and renal function tests and an electrocardiogram should be obtained immediately.

C. Clinical Manifestations

1. Hypermagnesemia

Symptoms and signs of hypermagnesemia are usually associated with serum magnesium levels greater than 4 mEq/L. Neuromuscular abnormalities include areflexia, lethargy, weakness, and in severe instances paralysis or respiratory failure. Cardiac findings may include hypotension, bradycardia, prolonged PR, QRS, and QT intervals, complete heart block, and asystole.

2. Hypomagnesemia

Symptoms and signs of hypomagnesemia are usually associated with serum magnesium levels less than 0.8 mEq/L. Neurological abnormalities include lethargy, confusion, tremor, fasciculations, ataxia, nystagmus, tetany, and seizures. Electrocardiographic abnormalities include prolonged PR and QT intervals, and patients receiving digoxin are at a greater risk for atrial and ventricular dysrhythmias.

D. Intervention

1. Hypermagnesemia

Elevated levels of serum magnesium are almost always related to excess magnesium intake in the presence of renal impairment. Asymptomatic hypermagnesemia requires only discontinuation of magnesium therapies. Severe, symptomatic hypermagnesemia should be treated with 10% calcium gluconate, 10 mL (1 ampule) IV over 10 minutes, to temporarily antagonize the cardiac effects of magnesium. Supportive therapy may include mechanical ventilation for respiratory failure and a temporary pacemaker for dysrhythmias. In the absence of severe renal failure, diuresis with 0.9% saline and 1 g calcium gluconate/L (10–11 ampules 10% calcium gluconate) can be administered at 150 mL/h to enhance urinary magnesium excretion. If renal failure is present, hemodialysis is required.

2. Hypomagnesemia

Mild hypomagnesemia can be treated with 250 mg magnesium oxide (12.5 mEq) given orally 2 to 4 times a day. For severe, symptomatic hypomagnesemia, treatment includes an infusion of 10 mL of 50% magnesium sulfate (40 mEq) per liter of IV fluids at 100 mL/h over 24 hours on day 1 and then 40 mEq/day thereafter until serum magnesium levels normalize. In more severe cases, an initial bolus of 4 mL of 50% magnesium sulfate in 100 mL 5% dextrose should be given over 30 minutes.

ACKNOWLEDGMENTS

This chapter was supported in part by P20-RR11145-03 NIH/RCMI Clinical Research Center Grant and G12-RR03026-11 Biomedical Infrastructure Development Grant.

REFERENCES

1. Moore RA. The total number of glomeruli in the normal human kidney. Anat Rec 1958;48:153–168.
2. Darmady EM, Offer J, Woodhouse MA. The parameters of the aging kidney. J Pathol 1973;109:195–200.
3. Rowe JW, Andres R, Tobin JD, Norris AH, Shock NW. The effect of age on creatinine clearance in men: A cross-sectional and longitudinal study. J Gerontol 1976; 31:155–163.
4. Davies D, Shock N. Age changes in glomerular filtration rate, effective renal plasma flow, and tubular excretory capacity in adult males. J Clin Invest 1950;29:496–507.
5. Walser M. Creatinine excretion as a measure of protein nutrition in adults of varying age. J Parenteral Enteral Nutr 1987:11;73S–78S.
6. Borchelt M. Potential side-effects and interactions in multiple medication in elderly patients: methodology and results of the Berlin Study of Aging. Z Gerontol Geriatr 1995;28(6):420–428.
7. Weir MR. Non-diuretic-based antihypertensive therapy and potassium homeostasis in elderly patients. Coron Artery Dis 1997;8(8–9):499–504.
8. Perazella MA, Mahnensmith RL. Hyperkalemia in the elderly: drugs exacerbate impaired potassium homeostasis. J Gen Intern Med 1997;12(10):646–656.

9. Cockcroft DW, Gault MH. Prediction of creatinine clearance from serum creatinine. Nephron 1976;16:31–41.
10. Brandfonbrener M, Landsdowne M, Shock NW. Changes in cardiac output with age. Circulation 1955;12:557–565.
11. Hollenberg NK, Adams DF, Solomon HS, Rashid A, Abrams HL, Merrill JP. Senescence and the renal vasculature in normal man. Circ Res 1974;34:309–316.
12. Lewis W, Alving A. Changes with age in the renal function in adult men. Am J Physiol 1938;123:500–515.
13. Rowe J, Shock N, DeFronzo R. The influence of age on the renal response to water deprivation in man. Nephron 1976;17:270–278.
14. Arieff A, Guisado R. Effects on the central nervous system of hypernatremic and hyponatremic states. Kidney Int 1976;10:104–116.
15. Crowe MJ, Forsling ML, Rolls BJ, Phillips PA, Ledingham JG, Smith RF. Altered water excretion in healthy elderly man. Age Ageing 1987;16:285–293.
16. Schmale H, Fehr S, Richter D. Vasopressin biosynthesis—from gene to peptide hormone. Kidney Int 1987;32:S8–S13.
17. Edelman IS, Leibman J. Anatomy of body water and electrolytes. Am J Med 1959; 27:256–277.
18. Robertson GL. Thirst and vasopressin function in normal and disordered states of water balance. J Lab Clin Med 1983;101(3):351–371.
19. Helderman JH, Vestal RE, Rowe JW, Tobin JD, Andres R, Robertson GL. The response of arginine vasopressin to intravenous ethanol and hypertonic saline in man: The impact of aging. J Gerontol 1978;33:39–47.
20. Ledingham JG, Crowe MJ, Forsling ML, Phillips PA, Rolls BJ. Effects of aging on vasopressin secretion, water secretion, and thirst in man. Kidney Int 1987;32(suppl. 21):S90–S92.
21. Phillips PA, Rolls BJ, Ledingham JG, Forsling ML, Morton JJ, Crowe MJ, Wollner L. Reduced thirst after water deprivation in healthy elderly men. N Engl J Med 1984; 311:753–759.
22. Miller P, Krebs R, Neal B, McIntyre D. Hypodipsia in geriatric patients. Am J Med 1982;73:354–356.
23. Miller JH, Shock NW. Age differences in the renal tubular response to antidiuretic hormone. J Gerontol 1953;8:446–450.
24. Epstein M, Hollenberg N. Age as a determinant of renal sodium conservation in normal man. J Lab Clin Med 1976;87:411–417.
25. Crane MG, Harris JJ. Effect of aging on renin activity and aldosterone excretion. J Lab Clin Med 1976;87:947–959.
26. Hall JE, Coleman TG, Guyton AC. The renin-angiotensin system normal physiology and changes in older hypertensives. J Am Geriatr Soc 1989;37:801–813.
27. Noth RH, Lassman MN, Tan SY, Fernandez-Cruz A Jr, Mulrow PJ. Age and the renin-aldosterone system. Arch Intern Med 1977;137:1414–1417.
28. Tsunoda K, Abe K, Goto T, Yasujima M, Sato M, Omata K, Seino M, Yoshinaga K. Effect of age on the renin-angiotensin-aldosterone system in normal subjects: Simultaneous measurement of active and inactive renin, renin substrate, and aldosterone in plasma. J Clin Endocrinol Metab 1986;62:384–389.
29. Weidmann P, de Chatel R, Schiffmann A, Bachmann E, Beretta-Piccoli C, Reubi FC, Ziegler WH, Vetter W. Interrelations between age and plasma renin, aldosterone

and cortisol, urinary catecholamines, and the body sodium/volume state in normal man. Klin Wochenschr 1977;55:725–733.
30. Weidmann P, De Myttenaere-Bursztein S, Maxwell M, De Lima J. Effect of aging on plasma renin and aldosterone in normal man. Kidney Int 1975;8:325–333.
31. Tan AC, Hoefnagels WH, Swinkels LM, Kloppenborg PW, Benraad TJ. The effect of volume expansion on atrial natriuretic peptide and cyclic guanosine monophosphate levels in young and aged subjects. J Am Geriatr Soc 1990;38:1215–1219.
32. Jansen TL, Tan AC, Smits P, de Boo T, Benraad TJ, Thien T. Hemodynamic effects of atrial natriuretic factor in young and elderly subjects. Clin Pharmacol Ther 1990; 48:179–188.
33. Clark BA, Elahi D, Shannon RP, Wei JY, Epstein FH. Influence of age and dose on the end-organ responses to atrial natriuretic peptide in humans. Am J Hypertens 1991;4:500–507.
34. Or K, Richards AM, Espiner EA, Yandle T, Gilchrist N, Sainsbury R. Effect of low dose infusions of ile-atrial natriuretic peptide in healthy elderly males: Evidence for a postreceptor defect. J Clin Endocrinol Metab 1993;76:1271–1274.
35. Miller M, Carter JM, Friedlander DA, Hecker MS. Apparent idiopathic hyponatremia in an ambulatory geriatric population. J Am Geriatr Soc 1996;44(4):404–408.
36. Cogan M. Fluid and Electrolytes. Norwalk, CT: Appleton & Lange, 1991, pp. 77–100.
37. Sterns RH. Severe symptomatic hyponatremia: Treatment and outcome. Ann Intern Med 1987;107:656–664.
38. Ayus JC, Arieff AI. Abnormalities of water metabolism in the elderly. Semin Nephrol 1996;16(4):277–288.
39. Arieff AI, Kucharczyk J, Ayus JC, Vexler ZS, Roberts TP, Kozniewska E. Age, gender, and vasopressin affect survival and brain adaptation in rats with metabolic encephalopathy. Am J Physiol 1995;268(5 Pt 2):R1143–1152.
40. Borra SI, Kleinfeld M, Beredo R. Hypernatremia in the aging: causes, manifestations, and outcome. J Natl Med Assoc 1995;87(3):220–224.
41. Palevsky PM. Hypernatremia. Semin Nephrol 1998;18(1):20–30.
42. Allen TH, Anderson EC, Langham WH. Total body potassium and gross body composition in relation to age. J Gerontol 1960;15:348–357.
43. Sagild U. Total exchangeable potassium in normal subjects with special reference to changes with age. Scand J Clin Lab Invest 1956;8:44–50.
44. Ford GA, Blaschke T, Wiswell R, Hoffman B. Effect of aging on changes in plasma potassium during exercise. J Gerontol 1993;48:M140–M145.
45. Mulkerrin E, Clark BA, Epstein FH. Aldosterone responses to hyperkalemia in healthy elderly humans. J Am Soc Nephrol 1995;6(5):1459–1462.
46. Perazella MA. Hyperkalemia in the elderly: a group at high risk. Conn Med 1996; 60(4):195–198.
47. Burt VL, Whelton P, Roccella EJ, Brown C, Cutler JA, Higgins M, Horan MJ, Labarthe D. Prevalence of hypertension in the US adult population: results from the third National Health and Nutrition Examination Survey, 1988–1991. Hypertension 1995;25:305–313.
48. Frassetto L, Sebastian A. Age and systemic acid-base equilibrium: analysis of published data. J Gerontol (Biol Sci Med Sci) 1996;51(1):B91–99.

49. Alpern RJ, Sakhaee K. The clinical spectrum of chronic metabolic acidosis: homeostatic mechanisms produce significant morbidity. Am J Kidney Dis 1997;29(2):291–302.
50. Frassetto LA, Sebastian A, Morris RC Jr. Effect of age on blood acid-base composition in adult humans: role of age-related renal functional decline. Am J Physiol 1996; 271(6 Pt 2):F1114–1122.
51. Abete P, Rengo F, Ferrara N, Cacciatore F, Napoli C, Calabrese C, Bianco S, Ferrara P. Age-related effects of acidosis in isolated cardiac muscle. J Gerontol (Biol Sci Med Sci) 1998;53(1):B42–48.
52. Narins RG, Cohen JJ. Bicarbonate therapy for organic acidosis: the case for its continued use. Ann Intern Med 1987;106(4):615–618.
53. Gabow PA, Anderson RJ, Potts DE, Schrier RW. Acid-base disturbances in the salicylate-intoxicated adult. Arch Intern Med 1978;138(10):1481–1484.
54. Durnas C, Cusack BJ. Salicylate intoxication in the elderly. Recognition and recommendations on how to prevent it. Drugs Aging 1992;2(1):20–34.
55. Anderson RJ, Potts DE, Gabow PA, Rumack BH, Schrier RW. Unrecognized adult salicylate intoxication. Ann Intern Med 1976;85(6):745–748.
56. Bouillon R, Carmeliet G, Boonen S. Ageing and calcium metabolism. Baillieres Clin Endocrinol Metab 1997;11(2):341–365.
57. Saltzman JR, Russell RM. The aging gut. Nutritional issues. Gastroenterol Clin North Am 1998;27(2):309–324.
58. Jacques PF, Felson DT, Tucker KL, Mahnken B, Wilson PW, Rosenberg IH, Rush D. Plasma 25-hydroxyvitamin D and its determinants in an elderly population sample. Am J Clin Nutr 1997;66(4):929–936.
59. Delvin EE, Imbach A, Copti M. Vitamin D nutritional status and related biochemical indices in an autonomous elderly population. Am J Clin Nutr 1988;48(2):373–378.
60. Chapuy MC, Chapuy P, Meunier PJ. Calcium and vitamin D supplements: effects on calcium metabolism in elderly people. Am J Clin Nutr 1987;46(2):324–328.
61. McKane WR, Khosla S, Egan KS, Robins SP, Burritt MF, Riggs BL. Role of calcium intake in modulating age-related increases in parathyroid function and bone resorption. J Clin Endocrinol Metab 1996;81(5):1699–1703.
62. Gloth FM III, Tobin JD. Vitamin D deficiency in older people [see comments]. J Am Geriatr Soc 1995;43(7):822–828.
63. Rosen CJ, Morrison A, Zhou H, Storm D, Hunter SJ, Musgrave K, Chen T, Wei W, Holick MF. Elderly women in northern New England exhibit seasonal changes in bone mineral density and calciotropic hormones. Bone Miner 1994;25(2):83–92.
64. Fuss M, Pepersack T, Gillet C, Karmali R, Corvilain J. Calcium and vitamin D metabolism in granulomatous diseases. Clin Rheumatol 1992;11(1):28–36.
65. Yoshikawa TT. Tuberculosis in aging adults. J Am Geriatr Soc 1992;40(2):178–187.
66. Epstein S, Stern PH, Bell NH, Dowdeswell I, Turner RT. Evidence for abnormal regulation of circulating 1 alpha, 25-dihydroxyvitamin D in patients with pulmonary tuberculosis and normal calcium metabolism. Calcif Tissue Int 1984;36(5):541–544.
67. Chan TY, Chan CH, Shek CC. The prevalence of hypercalcaemia in pulmonary and miliary tuberculosis—a longitudinal study. Singapore Med J 1994;35(6):613–615.

68. Kelestimur F, Guven M, Ozesmi M, Pasaoglu H. Does tuberculosis really cause hypercalcemia? J Endocrinol Invest 1996;19(10):678–681.
69. Webb AR, Pilbeam C, Hanafin N, Holick MF. An evaluation of the relative contributions of exposure to sunlight and of diet to the circulating concentrations of 25-hydroxyvitamin D in an elderly nursing home population in Boston. Am J Clin Nutr 1990;51(6):1075–1081.
70. Egsmose C, Lund B, McNair P, Lund B, Storm T, Sorensen OH. Low serum levels of 25-hydroxyvitamin D and 1,25-dihydroxyvitamin D in institutionalized old people: influence of solar exposure and vitamin D supplementation. Age Ageing 1987;16(1): 35–40.
71. MacLaughlin J, Holick MF. Aging decreases the capacity of human skin to produce vitamin D3. J Clin Invest 1985;76(4):1536–1538.
72. Armbrecht HJ, Forte LR, Halloran BP. Effect of age and dietary calcium on renal 25(OH)D metabolism, serum 1,25(OH)2D, and PTH. Am J Physiol 1984;246(3 Pt 1):E266–270.
73. Kinyamu HK, Gallagher JC, Balhorn KE, Petranick KM, Rafferty KA. Serum vitamin D metabolites and calcium absorption in normal young and elderly free-living women and in women living in nursing homes. Am J Clin Nutr 1997;65(3):790–797.
74. Parfitt AM, Gallagher JC, Heaney RP, Johnston CC, Neer R, Whedon GD. Vitamin D and bone health in the elderly. Am J Clin Nutr 1982;36(5 Suppl):1014–1031.
75. Byrne PM, Freaney R, McKenna MJ. Vitamin D supplementation in the elderly: review of safety and effectiveness of different regimes. Calcif Tissue Int 1995;56(6): 518–520.
76. Hoffman N. Diet in the elderly. Needs and risks. Med Clin North Am 1993;77(4): 745–756.
77. Delvin EE, Imbach A, Copti M. Vitamin D nutritional status and related biochemical indices in an autonomous elderly population. Am J Clin Nutr 1988;48(2):373–378.
78. Portale AA, Halloran BP, Morris RC Jr, Lonergan ET. Effect of aging on the metabolism of phosphorus and 1,25-dihydroxyvitamin D in healthy men. Am J Physiol 1996;270(3 Pt 1):E483–490.
79. Kiebzak GM, Sacktor B. Effect of age on renal conservation of phosphate in the rat. Am J Physiol 1986;251:F399–F407.
80. Lee DBN, Yanagawa N, Jo O. Phosphaturia of aging: Studies on mechanisms. Adv Exp Med Biol 1984;178:103–108.
81. Mulroney SE, Woda C, Haramati A. Changes in renal phosphate reabsorption in the aged rat. Proc Soc Exp Biol Med 1998;218(1):62–67.
82. Singh RB, Postiglione A, Moshir M, Singh NK, Aslam M, Srivastav S, Niaz MA, Singh R, Rastogi V. Magnesium and antioxidant vitamin status and risk of complications of ageing in an elderly urban population. Magnes Res 1996;9(4):299–306.
83. Simeckova A, Zamrazil V, Cerovska J. Calciuria, magnesiuria and creatininuria—relation to age. Physiol Res 1998;47(1):35–40.
84. Durlach J, Bac P, Durlach V, Rayssiguier Y, Bara M. Guiet-Bara A. Magnesium status and ageing: an update. Magnes Res 1998;11(1):25–42.
85. Gullestad L, Nes M, Ronneberg R, Midtvedt K, Falch D, Kjekshus J. Magnesium status in healthy free-living elderly Norwegians. J Am Coll Nutr 1994;13(1):45–50.

17

Hyperosmolar Hyperglycemia and Diabetic Ketoacidosis

Robert V. Hogikyan and Jeffrey B. Halter
University of Michigan, Ann Arbor, Michigan

I. CLINICAL RELEVANCE

Diabetes mellitus, uncontrolled to the extent that diabetic ketoacidosis (DKA) or hyperglycemic hyperosmolar nonketotic syndrome (HHNS) develops, is a life-threatening complication for a patient of any age. When that individual is an older adult, there are additional challenges to the diagnosis and management of these two states, in part by virtue of age-related physiological changes but also because of comorbidity. Functional and social factors may also contribute to the development of DKA and HHNS or play a role in the management of these serious complications. Although some objective data exist on which to base recommendations in older adults with these serious acute complications of diabetes, a need for ongoing investigation exists.

A. Definitions and Criteria

DKA and HHNS are points along a spectrum of severe hyperglycemia in patients with poorly controlled diabetes (1,2). For the purpose of this discussion, the standard definitions for DKA and HHNS will be used because no rationale has been established for different criteria for older adults. The hallmarks of DKA include hyperglycemia (glucose level >250 mg/dL), presence of ketosis, and acidosis (arterial pH <7.3 and serum bicarbonate <15 mEq/L). Criteria for HHNS are somewhat less defined, but the usually accepted features include severe hyperglycemia (serum glucose >600 mg/dL), elevated serum osmolality (usually >350 mOsm/kg), and absence of significant ketosis. Thus, the key differentiating feature is the ketosis and metabolic acidosis of DKA versus profound volume depletion and associated severe hyperglycemia in the absence of ketoacidosis in HHNS. Of course, some patients with DKA also have profound volume depletion and severe hyperglycemia. Patients with HHNS may also have a metabolic acidosis, usually caused by accumulation of lactic acid rather than ketoacids. Insulin deficiency is a key factor in the pathophysiology of both DKA and HHNS (3).

In the older adult, sometimes challenges exist in making diagnoses of DKA or HHNS and sometimes in treating them once identified. These considerations will be discussed in this chapter. In this discussion, the patients may come from a variety of settings, including independent living, assisted living, community nursing home, or an interim situation such as a shelter.

B. Epidemiology

Both DKA and HHNS are relatively uncommon complications of diabetes mellitus in older adults. As increasing numbers of people with type 1 diabetes survive until old age, however, the incidence of DKA may increase proportionately. Although type 1 diabetes usually begins earlier in life, new onset of type 1 diabetes can occur in older adults and thus some older individuals are seen with DKA. Some of these individuals do not have evidence of cell-mediated autoimmunity, usually present in younger people with type 1 diabetes, and therefore have idiopathic type 1 diabetes. As with HHNS, morbidity and mortality related to DKA is generally the result of co-existing medical conditions that may have precipitated the development of DKA rather than a direct consequence of DKA itself.

In contrast to DKA, HHNS is predominantly found in older people with type 2 diabetes or no previous diabetes history at all. The high mortality rate associated with HHNS (10%–45%) reflects the severity of the precipitating condition rather than direct consequences of the metabolic disturbance itself. Morbidity associated with HHNS may also reflect the relatively long time course for the development of this condition, often in a setting in which the patient has been isolated and unable to obtain assistance.

C. Pathogenesis

DKA is a direct result of severe insulin deficiency leading to massive lipolysis, release of free fatty acids into the circulation and their metabolism to ketones, and ketoacids leading to metabolic acidosis, which can be severe and life threatening. Lack of insulin also markedly impairs glucose use by insulin-dependent tissues and causes inability to suppress hepatic glucose production, thereby leading to substantial hyperglycemia. The degree of hyperglycemia depends primarily on the degree to which renal excretion of glucose can compensate for the impairments of glucose metabolism. Thus, underlying renal function and the degree to which renal perfusion is maintained in the face of hyperglycemia-induced osmotic diuresis become key determinants of the resulting degree of hyperglycemia. Older individuals with impaired renal function, reduced ability to increase renal perfusion caused by atherosclerotic disease, and impaired ability to maintain large amounts of fluid intake (because of co-existing illness or limited self-care capability) are more likely to have severe hyperglycemia and hyperosmolality develop in this setting. However, in general, the predominant clinical feature is the metabolic acidosis.

In contrast, HHNS, by definition has minimal or no ketoacidosis. Insulin deficiency is the predominant pathogenetic feature, which in the presence of often severe co-existing illness and impaired self-care capabilities leads to profound hyperglycemia, hyperosmolality, and extracellular volume depletion. Metabolic acidosis may be present but is due to accumulation of lactic acid rather than ketoacids. At present, no clear explanation exists for the lack of development of ketoacidosis by such individuals. Insulin levels are no higher in patients with HHNS than in patients with DKA. Co-existing insulin resistance at the level of the fat cells, often present in patients with type 2 diabetes, should even further enhance susceptibility to lipolysis and release of free fatty acids under these conditions. Elevation of stress hormones such as catecholamines, which have also been demonstrated in these patients, should further increase the likelihood of lipolysis. Thus, some antilipolytic factors may prevent these patients from having DKA develop. Alternately, conversion of free fatty acids to ketone bodies may be limited, but at present little evidence exists for this. As with DKA, older patients may be especially susceptible to marked hyperglycemia and hyperosmolality developing because of underlying impairments of renal function, renal perfusion, or ability to maintain fluid intake.

D. Precipitating Factors

Particularly in an older patient, the presence of DKA or HHNS should be viewed as a symptom or manifestation of an underlying major illness rather than a diagnostic endpoint in itself. Although a major precipitating illness is not always identified, the presence of such a condition is the major factor influencing the patient's outcome. Of course, withdrawal of insulin therapy, or an inappropriate reduction in insulin dose, can lead to DKA in an older patient with type 1 diabetes just as it would in a younger individual. However, withdrawal of antihyperglycemic therapy alone rarely leads to the development of HHNS.

Acute infection is the most common precipitating factor for the development of DKA or HHNS. In a retrospective study covering admissions over 11 years, female gender, newly diagnosed diabetes, and acute infection were independent predictors of HHNS developing. Residing in a nursing home and having dementia were seen more commonly in the study subjects but did not enter the multivariate model (4). The most common infections to precipitate HHNS include pneumonia, urinary tract infection, and sepsis (5,6).

Older adults with diabetes may be more susceptible to infection as a result of their diabetes (7) and possibly age (8). Such patients may not manifest infection in typical fashion, and so it is necessary to approach these individuals with a high degree of suspicion to identify infection if it is present. In the institutional long-term care setting, a resident with diabetes may be predisposed to infection as a result of stroke, which in some cases increases aspiration risk and may result in a neurogenic bladder necessitating catheterization at least intermittently.

Serious infection can contribute to severe metabolic decompensation leading to DKA or HHNS in several ways. Activation of stress hormones and cytokine mediators can impair insulin secretion, interfere with insulin-mediated glucose use, and directly stimulate endogenous glucose production and accelerate lipolysis in susceptible individuals. Fever associated with infection can accelerate loss of water and electrolytes, thereby contributing to the profound volume depletion associated with these metabolic syndromes. Finally, the debilitation associated with major acute infection can substantially limit patient self-care activities, particularly maintenance of adequate fluid and electrolyte intake.

A wide range of other acute medical illnesses can also precipitate metabolic decompensation because of activation of stress hormones and impaired self-care capability. These conditions include acute myocardial infarction, acute stroke, and a fall-related injury leading to loss of mobility or impaired consciousness. Patients with underlying renal disease are particularly susceptible to HHNS. Furthermore, any cause of acute renal insufficiency will heighten this risk. Impaired thirst mechanisms can contribute to the risk of volume depletion, resulting both from age-related changes in thirst mechanisms and especially in patients with a cognitive or motor deficit that limits their ability to recognize thirst signals to elicit an appropriate behavioral response. Patients with such deficits who depend on caregivers for maintenance of appropriate fluid and electrolyte intake can have metabolic decompensation develop if the caregiving system breaks down. This situation most frequently occurs for patients living alone with marginal self-care capabilities or in a setting where one or more other people may be living, but either through inattention or neglect are unable to meet caregiving needs. Decompensation can also occur in the institutional long-term care setting if the patient's needs are not adequately recognized or are exacerbated by an unrecognized change in the patient's status such as occult infection, new stroke, aspiration pneumonia, or acute renal insufficiency.

Both DKA and HHNS are potentially preventable conditions. Given the morbidity and mortality associated with these conditions in older patients, particularly for HHNS, prevention should receive attention. Because many patients with HHNS are seen with previously undiagnosed type 2 diabetes, attention to earlier diagnosis and appropriate intervention and follow-up could reduce risk for this adverse outcome. Patient and family education efforts that could also reduce risk include training in home glucose monitoring to detect early increases of glucose levels, recognition of signs of a major illness such as pneumonia with a clear protocol for contact with health care providers, and ongoing review of the living situation and caregiver support mechanisms. In particular, strengthening communication systems between patients and their caregiver support structure and in turn between them and their health care providers, including a lifeline type system, could have a substantial impact given the usual length of time for HHNS development before the patient actually is seen by health care providers.

II. CLINICAL MANIFESTATIONS

A. History

The patient may have a spectrum of consciousness from completely clear thought through coma, with most patients having at least some alteration in consciousness. This may compromise the ability to obtain a history from the patient. Whether the patient can render a history or not, it is important to obtain historical information from the family or caregivers, because a key focus of the initial evaluation should be a search for an underlying illness that precipitated DKA or HHNS. If the patient is known to have diabetes, a recent history of level of glucose control and medication intake should also be pursued.

Typically DKA develops over a day or two, whereas HHNS develops insidiously over days or weeks. During the time before DKA or HHNS reaches clinical attention, the community-dwelling older diabetic patient may experience classical polyuria and polydipsia, lethargy, and weakness. Some patients, particularly those living in institutional long-term care, may manifest an altered set of symptoms and signs. These may include decreased appetite, abdominal discomfort, nausea and sometimes vomiting, and decreased participation in usual activities. Initially, more frequent episodes of urinary incontinence may be observed followed by fewer episodes as intravascular depletion develops after polyuria in a patient who does not or cannot take adequate fluids. In the older adult whose existing general functional level is low, becoming more lethargic and functioning less well may not be as noticeable to family or other caregivers. The patient may progress through stages of altered consciousness, including delirium ultimately leading to coma. In the patient with diabetes, the serum osmolarity needs to be greater than 340 mOsm/L to attribute coma to hyperosmolarity (6).

Social history information about the support that is available to the patient will be critical for hospital discharge planning. An occupational therapist can assist the clinician with assessing the extent to which the older patient with diabetes needs assistance with performing activities of daily living.

Table 1 Clinical Features of DKA and HHNS in Older Adults

Volume depletion
Metabolic acidosis[a]
Hyperosmolality
Hyperglycemia
Cognitive impairment
Impaired renal function

DKA, Diabetic ketoacidosis; HHNS, hyperglycemia hyperosmolar nonketotic syndrome.
[a] Ketoacidosis in DKA. Lactic acidosis in HHNS (rare).

B. Physical Findings

Body weight can provide an important clue to the degree of fluid deficit if historical information is available. On examination the patient will appear quite ill. The skin will appear dry with poor turgor and the oral cavity will also be dry. Vital signs can be difficult to interpret in the older adult with diabetes who has DKA or HHNS. The presence of fever would suggest a precipitating infection, although in the older adult with infection temperature may not be elevated and in fact may be low. The pulse will likely be rapid and weak with a blood pressure that is normal or low. Historical information (e.g., history of hypertension) may help with interpretation of the blood pressure. Postural change in blood pressure, although a crude test, is still the best noninvasive test for the degree of volume depletion. Particular respiratory patterns are not characteristic of HHNS. In DKA the respiratory rate will likely be increased, but might not be classical Kussmaul's respirations if the patient has underlying cardiac or pulmonary disease. The remaining physical examination will not likely be specific to DKA or HHNS but rather may lend insight to other potentially precipitating causes. Signs of a precipitating stroke would be important to identify (Table 1).

III. IMMEDIATE DIAGNOSTIC APPROACH

A. Hyperglycemia and Ketosis

Beside testing of the blood glucose level can provide the first confirmation of the presence of DKA or HHNS. Further confirmation should come from measurement of serum electrolytes, glucose, ketones and arterial pH. Effective serum osmolality should also be calculated (S_{osm} = 2[NA^+ + K^+] + serum glucose [mg/dL]/18). These tests will differentiate DKA from HHNS. Although the definition of DKA varies somewhat, diagnostic findings include a metabolic acidosis with arterial blood pH <7.3 and an increase in circulating total blood ketone concentrations to >5 mmol/L. The ketonemia will result in an anion gap acidosis. Laboratory results can help to distinguish between DKA and other ketoacidoses versus other causes of anion gap acidosis and hyperchloremic acidosis. In addition, the clinician needs to be looking for the possibility of a mixed acid-base disorder in the older patient with diabetes. Calculation of the anion gap and the delta gap can be useful in differentiating mixed acid-base disorders (9).

As the patient loses ketoanions in the urine, these are replaced with chloride giving a component of hyperchloremic acidosis. To the extent that the patient is intravascularly depleted, the associated decrease in renal function may limit the urinary loss of ketone bodies leading to a purer anion gap acidosis (10).

B. Other Causes of Metabolic Acidosis

DKA is one type of ketoacidosis that is one of four causes of anion gap acidosis, and the others must be considered when evaluating the patient suspected of having DKA. The causes of anion gap acidoses include ketoacidosis, lactic acidosis, chronic renal failure, and drugs. If the ketostix registers <2+ or nitroprusside reaction is negative at 1:8 dilution, the causes of anion gap acidosis other than DKA need to be considered. Lactic acidosis can be diagnosed with measurement of the serum lactate concentration. In this setting, the anion gap might be quite large (>40 mEq/L) (10). Renal insufficiency may contribute to retained acid anions if the insufficiency is significant enough. To the extent that renal function may rapidly undergo significant change in these patients, renal function needs to be monitored throughout the treatment phase. Finally, ingestion of certain compounds can lead to the development of metabolic acidosis. Some of these compounds include salicylate, methanol, and ethylene glycol through differing mechanisms.

The causes of ketosis other than DKA include starvation and alcoholism (10). Alcoholic ketoacidosis usually occurs in the setting of heavy alcohol use with co-existing poor caloric intake, leading to mobilization of free fatty acids. It might be suspected in the older adult who has a mild elevation in serum glucose and a low bicarbonate, although the individual may also have hypoglycemia and lactic acidosis. Ketosis caused by starvation is also a state that older adults are at risk for, especially those who are functionally impaired enough to be dependent on others for assistance with nourishment. However, starvation alone rarely causes significant systemic acidosis.

Table 2 Precipitating Causes of DKA/HHNS

Acute infection
Pneumonia
Urinary tract infection
Septicemia
Stroke
Myocardial infarction
Congestive heart failure
Pancreatitis
Pulmonary embolism
Trauma
Alcohol abuse
Emotional stress
Corticosteroid use

DKA, Diabetic ketoacidosis; HHNS, hyperglycemia hyperosmolar nonketotic syndrome.

C. Precipitating Factors

Together with the initial treatment of a patient in either DKA or HHNS attention needs to be aimed at diagnosing a precipitating cause for the older patient manifesting such severely uncontrolled hyperglycemia. Some common precipitating events are listed in Table 2. It is critical that these be considered early in the management process because early identification of an acute myocardial infarction, for example, may prevent unnecessary morbidity with prompt monitoring and treatment. A thorough history and physical examination, chest x-ray film, electrocardiogram, pulse oximetry, urinalysis, and a screening battery of laboratory testing should assist in identifying a precipitating cause.

IV. INTERVENTION

A. General Approach for Therapy

Because the therapeutic approach to both DKA and HHNS should be similar in an older patient, management of these conditions will be discussed together (Table 3). In treating an older patient with diabetes who has DKA or HHNS, an overall concern is that this individual may have less reserve function to call on while correcting the hyperglycemic crisis. Reduced reserve capacity may also affect the capacity of an older adult with diabetes to tolerate iatrogenic problems

Table 3 Management of DKA and HHNS in Older Adults

Fluid and electrolyte replacement
Insulin
Monitoring
Cardiovascular
Serum glucose/electrolytes
Renal function
Evaluation for underlying/precipitating illness
Delirium/bed rest precautions

DKA, Diabetic ketoacidosis; HHNS, hyperglycemia hyperosmolar nonketotic syndrome.

such as treatment-induced hypoglycemia. Therapy needs to be directed at (1) correction of volume deficits; (2) lowering of serum glucose/hyperosmolality; (3) for DKA, reversing the metabolic acidosis by clearing ketonemia; (4) correction of other electrolyte abnormalities; and (5) seeking a precipitating cause (Table 2). While targeting therapies to bring about these corrections, the older adult with diabetes needs to be monitored frequently and carefully both from clinical and laboratory standpoints.

B. Fluid Replacement

Whether one begins with correcting volume deficits alone or adds insulin therapy initially is determined primarily by how hemodynamically compromised the patient is on presentation. If the patient is severely volume depleted and manifesting marked hyperglycemia, insulin administration should be withheld until the patient is more hemodynamically stable. The rapid movement of intravascular glucose into cells with insulin administration could significantly worsen the intravascular fluid deficit, resulting in worsening hypotension (11). This consideration needs to be balanced against the importance of immediate insulin administration for a DKA patient with severe acidosis. Initially, fluid should be replaced with isotonic saline. A typical deficit would be 4 to 6 L in DKA and 6 to 10 L in HHNS, with 2 to 4 L of fluid needing to be replaced with isotonic saline, depending on the severity of the volume depletion. The rate of initial fluid replacement can range from 1 L/h to 4 L/h in a severely volume-depleted older adult with DKA or HHNS. In the patient with hypoalbuminemia and significant hypotension, consideration should be given to use of a colloid expander or albumin in conjunction with the crystalloids.

The clinical examination should guide the rate of fluid replacement. Throughout the replacement process it is of critical importance that cardiovascular and renal function are closely monitored. Noninvasive monitoring of orthostatic blood pressure responses and urine output will suffice for some patients. However, invasive cardiovascular monitoring should be considered in patients with known cardiac dysfunction or if signs of cardiac decompensation develop. Bladder catheterization may be necessary to accurately follow urine output. If the patient is unable to maintain an adequate blood pressure with fluids, pressors may be necessary for a limited time. If pressors are necessary, it should trigger consideration of sepsis as contributing to the inability to maintain an adequate blood pressure.

After the initial fluid resuscitation, the fluid composition should be changed to 0.45% normal saline to address the replacement of free water. The remaining free water deficit (140 $\times$ [0.6 $\times$ Usual body wt in kg]/Measured serum Na^+ = Current total body water; body water deficit = 0.6 $\times$ Usual body weight in kg $-$ Current total body water) should be corrected over 24 to 48 hours. The suggestion for a gradual correction of the remaining deficit is in part due to concern about rapid shifts of fluids potentially resulting in brain edema. Also of importance in preventing rapid shift of fluids is gradual lowering serum glucose to achieve a plateau of approximately 200 to 250 mg/dL during this acute phase.

C. Insulin Therapy

Once fluid resuscitation has been initiated and hemodynamic stability achieved, insulin therapy should be initiated. Current recommendations are for a bolus of insulin intravenously (IV) of 0.1 U/kg body weight followed by an IV infusion of 0.1 U/kg/h. Some protocols suggest this could be administered intramuscularly (IM). We suggest IV should be used in older adults with DKA or HHNS in part because of the loss of lean muscle mass with age; but also because of comorbidities that may affect the response to IM insulin. Some such situations might include the patient who is anticoagulated as a result of a previous stroke or in the presence of atrial fibrillation. The potential for variable absorption of the insulin if given IM is also a factor to consider in the older patient with diabetes.

In the past much larger doses of insulin were sometimes recommended. However, the currently recommended doses are adequate because the insulin levels achieved suppress lipolysis and ketogenesis while stimulating glucose uptake by insulin-sensitive tissues. Slightly higher doses of insulin may be required during the initial period of treatment when insulin resistance is exacerbated by the associated counterregulatory hormone and catecholamine responses. It is desirable to achieve a rate of serum glucose reduction of approximately 75 to 100 mg/dL/h. The rate of plasma glucose fall will depend on both the insulin effect, which is time dependent, and renal excretion of glucose, which can be immediate if fluid status is corrected and kidney function is within the normal range. If the plasma glucose is not falling at the expected rate, consideration should be given to increasing the rate of insulin infusion to approximately double the initial rate. For the patient with DKA the insulin infusion should continue until ketonemia clears. For both DKA and HHNS, when the plasma glucose drops into the 250 to 300 mg/dL range, intravenous glucose should be added to keep the plasma glucose greater than 200 mg/dL. Careful monitoring of glucose levels is key to avoidance of iatrogenic hypoglycemia because the glucose level may fall precipitously once tissues are adequately insulinized and volume repletion restores renal perfusion, thereby enhancing renal glucose excretion.

D. Electrolyte Replacement

Electrolyte replacement is important in the older adult with DKA or HHNS. After consideration of sodium during the choice of IV fluids, potassium is particularly important. Total body potassium stores may be depleted because of osmotic diuresis, gastrointestinal losses in some patients, and in patients with DKA acidosis-mediated loss of intracellular potassium. However, initially the patient may have a high serum potassium, caused by systemic acidosis, co-existing acute renal failure, or co-existing tissue injury. In this situation, no potassium should be added to the initial fluids. If the potassium level is normal initially, 20 to 40 mEq/L of potassium should be added to the fluid being infused to begin to replace the total body deficit. If the serum potassium level is low initially, total body stores of potassium are likely to be depleted. For example, an older patient may have been taking a diuretic for hypertension or congestive heart failure with inadequate potassium supplementation, exacerbating DKA- or HHNS-induced potassium loss. In this situation potassium needs to be supplemented more aggressively because the deficit could be as high as 600 to 800 mEq. The presence of initial hypokalemia is another indication to delay insulin administration because insulin-mediated cellular uptake of potassium would further exacerbate the hypokalemia.

E. Phosphate Loss

Phosphate loss can also occur with DKA or HHNS through osmotic diuresis and other tubular mechanisms. When treatment is instituted with insulin, extracellular phosphate also shifts into cells (10), thus exacerbating the risk for hypophosphatemia. The most significant risk of hypophosphatemia is the "phosphate depletion syndrome," which can result in impaired myocardial, respiratory, and skeletal muscle contraction; central nervous system depression; and acute renal insufficiency. Whether patients with DKA or HHNS benefit from parenteral supplementation of phosphate is controversial because most studies do not support a benefit from parenteral supplementation. Supplementation would be indicated if the plasma level drops particularly low, in the range of <1.5 mg/dL. One of the risks of parenteral phosphate is hypocalcemia. Thus serum calcium should be monitored throughout phosphate administration.

F. Acidosis

Bicarbonate supplementation is sometimes considered for patients with severe metabolic acidosis. This may be appropriate in a patient with lactic acidosis complicating DKA or HHNS. Studies in DKA have not demonstrated benefit from adding bicarbonate to reverse ketoacidosis. The key to ketoacidosis reversal is insulin replacement.

G. Complications

Because of multiple comorbidities that may be present in an older patient, multiple complications from the extreme metabolic, renal, and hemodynamic stress of DKA or HHNS may be present. One potential complication is drug toxicity. For example, the patient taking digoxin may be at increased risk for dysrhythmia during periods of rapidly changing renal function, potassium, and fluid shifts. Others include complications from immobility such as deconditioning to the point where a previously independent individual is unable to perform the basic activities of daily living. Prolonged bed rest, often present as HHNS develops, predisposes the patient to pressure ulcers that can be particularly difficult to heal in the diabetic patient. Delirium is another potential complication that the older adult is predisposed to, both as a result of comorbidities and of treatments (e.g., hypoglycemia). Baseline cognitive or memory deficits may predispose the older adult with DKA or HHNS to delirium, a problem that may complicate treatment and lengthen time to recovery and discharge.

The complication of cerebral edema has been observed in both DKA and HHNS, however, only rarely in adults. If cerebral edema does occur, it will most likely occur within the first 12 to 16 hours after initiating treatment. Other complications are seen in the management of older patients with DKA and HHNS, including acute respiratory distress syndrome, arterial and venous thrombosis, hyperchloremic metabolic acidosis (in DKA), aspiration pneumonia, rhabdomyolysis, and sometimes pancreatitis.

REFERENCES

1. Carroll P, Matz R. Uncontrolled diabetes mellitus in adults: experience in treating diabetic ketoacidosis and hyperosmolar nonketotic coma with low-dose insulin and a uniform treatment regimen. Diabetes Care 1983;6(6):579–585.

2. Wachtel TJ, Tetu-Mouradjian LM, Goldman DL, Ellis SE, O'Sullivan PS. Hyperosmolarity and acidosis in diabetes mellitus: a three-year experience in Rhode Island. J Gen Intern Med 1991;6:495–502.
3. Ennis ED, Stahl EJvB, Kreisberg RA. The hyperosmolar hyperglycemic syndrome. Diabetes Rev 1994;2(1):115–126.
4. Wachtel TJ, Silliman RA, Lamberton P. Predisposing factors for the diabetic hyperosmolar state. Arch Intern Med 1987;147:499–501.
5. Wachtel TJ. The diabetic hyperosmolar state. Clin Geriatr Med 1990;6(4):797–806.
6. Siperstein MD. Diabetic ketoacidosis and hyperosmolar coma. Endocrinol Metab Clin North Am 1992;21(2):415–432.
7. Marhoffer W, Stein M, Maeser E, Federlin K. Impairment of polymorphonuclear leukocyte function and metabolic control of diabetes. Diabetes Care 1992;15:256–260.
8. Yoshikawa TT. Aging and infectious diseases: state of the art. Gerontology 1984; 30(5):275–278.
9. Salem MM, Mujais SK. Gaps in the anion gap. Arch Intern Med 1992;152:1625–1629.
10. DeFronzo RA, Matsuma M, Barrett EJ. Diabetic ketoacidosis: a combined metabolic-nephrologic approach to therapy. Diabetes Rev 1994;2(2):209–238.
11. McCurdy DK. Hyperosmolar hyperglycemic nonketotic diabetic coma. Med Clin North Am 1970;54:683–699.

18
Infectious Disease Emergencies

Shobita Rajagopalan
Charles R. Drew University of Medicine and Science, and Martin Luther King, Jr.–Charles R. Drew Medical Center, Los Angeles, California

Deborah Moran
Department of Veterans Affairs Medical Center, Brooklyn, New York

Concomitant with the process of aging of the United States population, health care professionals and emergency departments can expect to encounter steady increases in the numbers of acutely ill older persons. Among other geriatric emergencies, serious infections result in significant morbidity and mortality in elderly individuals (1). Infectious diseases account for one of the five leading causes of death and one of the top 10 indications for hospitalization in persons aged 65 years or older (2). Pneumonia and influenza represent the fifth leading cause of death in the elderly (3) and meet the most frequent admission criteria for hospitalization in the frail elderly (4). Chronic medical conditions and functional disability are associated with a heightened risk for serious infection in the elderly. Treatment is often delayed because of atypical presentations and the scarcity of classic clinical clues that are frequently masked and confounded by co-existing and comorbid conditions, as well as age-related changes (4,5). Associated factors, such as malnutrition, alcoholism, immobility, institutionalization, and urinary incontinence, superimposed on underlying illness (e.g., diabetes mellitus, cerebrovascular accidents (CVAs), malignancies) and altered immune function with senescence further contribute to this enhanced risk for severe infections with aging (6).

This chapter will briefly review only the most important and common infectious disease emergencies in the elderly (i.e., sepsis, pneumonia, urinary tract infection (UTI), necrotizing soft tissue infection, complicated herpes zoster infection, meningitis, malignant external otitis, and infective endocarditis). Further detailed analyses and descriptive readings on these and other particular infections in the elderly can be found in a variety of textbooks.

I. SEPSIS AND SEPTIC SHOCK

A. Clinical Relevance

Despite numerous advances in the therapy, sepsis (the clinical manifestations of systemic response to infection) remains an entity with extremely high mortality (7). An estimated 20% to 50% of all patients with sepsis and its sequelae die (8). With the exception of the acquired immunodeficiency syndrome (AIDS), the predisposing factors for sepsis and septic shock (sepsis with hypotension, defined as systolic blood pressure of less than 90 mm Hg or a 40 mm Hg or greater decrease below the baseline systolic blood pressure) are found predominantly in older persons (9). Sepsis now ranks as the thirteenth leading cause of death in the United States and accounts for approximately \$5 to \$10 billion in annual health care costs (10,11).

Sepsis and its sequelae are generally caused by bacteremic infections; in aging individuals, pneumonia, UTIs, cellulitis, and gastrointestinal pathological conditions are frequently implicated (12). Septic shock is most often associated with gram-negative bacteremic infections (i.e., *Klebsiella* spp, *Escherichia coli*, and *Serratia* spp) (12,13). Shock can also result from gram-positive infections or be associated with toxemia from localized infections (e.g., toxic shock syndrome). Septic shock is an increasingly common infectious disease emergency in the elderly (14,15). The definitions of sepsis and its sequelae are outlined in Table 1 (16).

B. Pathophysiology and Clinical Manifestations

The pathophysiological cascade that results from gram-negative sepsis is attributed to the lipopolysaccharide component (endotoxin) of the bacterial cell wall (17). Endotoxin is believed to trigger Hageman factor activation and endothelial cell damage, leading to disseminated intravascular coagulation (DIC), complement consumption, kinin activation, and prostaglandin release. Activation of the these systems may result not only from exposure to endotoxin, but also tumor necrosis factor α, interleukin 1, or other endogenous mediator, or through a more specific agent, such as vascular permeability factor. An initial increase in the cardiac output (CO) resulting from tachycardia in response to a decrease in arterial blood pressure is followed by venous pooling with a concomitant fall in CO and hypotension. Pulmonary hypertension and adult respiratory distress syndrome that develop in 20% of cases are thought to be a consequence of thrombi-induced plugging of the capillary beds. Failure to perfuse tissues leads to oliguria,

Table 1 Defining Sepsis and Its Sequelae

Disorder	Requirement(s) for diagnosis	Values
Bacteremia	Positive blood cultures	
Sepsis	Clinical evidence suggestive of infection plus	
	Signs of systemic response to the infection (all of the following)	
	Tachypnea	>20 breaths/min[a]
	Tachycardia	>90 beats/min
	Hyperthermia or hypothermia	>38.4°C (101°F) or <35.6°C (96.1°F)
	Positive blood cultures are not required	
Sepsis syndrome (may also be considered incipient septic shock in patients who later become hypotensive)	Clinical diagnosis of sepsis as outlined above plus evidence of altered organ perfusion (one or more of the following)	
	Hypoxia	O_2 saturation <95%
	Increased plasma lactate	>normal upper limit
	Oliguria	<0.5 mL/kg for at least 1 h
	Altered mental status	
Early septic shock	Clinical diagnosis of sepsis syndrome as outlined above plus hypotension	<90 mm Hg (or a 40 mm Hg decrease below baseline) that lasts for <1 h and is responsive to conventional therapy
Refractory septic shock	Clinical diagnosis of sepsis syndrome as outlined above plus hypotension	<90 mm Hg (or a 40 mm Hg decrease below baseline) that lasts for >1 h despite adequate therapy

[a] If patient is mechanically ventilated, >10 L/min.
Source: Modified from Ref. 16.

lactic acidosis, hypoxia, and mental obtundation referred to as the sepsis syndrome shown in Table 1. Sepsis in aging persons represents an ominous medical dilemma because of lack of early clinical clues to its recognition and initiation of appropriate therapy (7). Elderly persons with altered mental status, hypothermia or hyperthermia, dyspnea, oliguria, thrombocytopenia, and DIC, should arouse clinical suspicion for sepsis and septic shock.

C. Immediate Diagnostic Approach

Sepsis and septic shock cause death in a significant number of elderly persons. Prompt recognition of clinical clues to sepsis is thus imperative for the initiation of appropriate therapeutic measures. In addition to a careful history and physical examination, basic laboratory investigation (i.e., complete blood count [CBC], chemistries, and electrolytes), coagulation parameters, arterial blood gases, electrocardiogram, blood and urine cultures, chest radiography, and other studies directed by clinical findings should be obtained.

D. Intervention

Management should include sufficient fluid resuscitation, pressor support when necessary, adequate oxygenation, pulmonary artery and capillary wedge pressure measurements when indicated, and broad-spectrum antibiotics as dictated by the likely site of infection. Extended-spectrum antibiotic combination agents that provide adequate gram-positive, gram-negative, and anaerobic coverage are often required (Table 2) (6). Trials with corticosteroids and several immune modulators in sepsis have yielded equivocal results (16). Details on the management of shock, including that caused by sepsis, have also been discussed in another section of this text. (See Chapter 11.)

II. PNEUMONIA

A. Clinical Relevance

Pneumonia may manifest as an important and common infectious disease emergency in elderly individuals residing both in the community and in nursing homes (1). Disproportionate mortality associated with pneumonia in this population results from co-existing chronic and debilitating conditions (cigarette smoking, chronic obstructive pulmonary disease, congestive heart failure [CHF], CVA, dementia, seizure disorder, alcoholism, diabetes mellitus, the use of corticosteroids or other immunosuppressive agents, and lung cancer), delay in diagnosis and treatment because of atypical presentations, and a higher prevalence of bacteremia and its complications, such as empyema, infective endocarditis, and men-

Table 2 Empiric Antibiotic Therapy by Source and Setting

Infection source	Modifying circumstances	Predominant organism	Suggested regimen[a]
Systemic infection without obvious source (bacteremia/sepsis)	Adult, nonimmunocompromised	Enterobacteriaceae, group A or D streptococci, *Streptococcus pneumoniae, Bacteroides*, *Staphyloccous aureus*, coagulase-negative staphylococci, *Escherichia coli*, *Klebsiella* spp	Ceftazidime ± aminoglycoside; or ampicillin + aminoglycoside + clindamycin; or imipenem/cilastatin
Pneumonia	Community-acquired (hospitalized)	*S. pneumoniae*, *Haemophilus influenzae*, group A streptococcus, *S. aureus*, *Legionella pneumoniae*, *Mycoplasma*, polymicrobial, and anaerobic bacteria	Erythromycin + second- or third-generation cephalosporin (may add quinolone for severe infections)
	Nosocomial (hospital-acquired)	*Klebsiella pneumoniae*, *Pseudomonas* species, *E. coli*, *S. pneumoniae*, ? anaerobic bacteria	Ceftazidime; antipseudomonal pencillin + aminoglycoside; or quinolone
	Nursing home–acquired	*S. pneumoniae*, *K. pneumoniae*, *E. coli*, ? anaerobic bacteria	Second-or third-generation cephalosporin; ticarcillin-clavulanate; or ampicillin-sulbactam
Urinary tract (not sepsis)	Community-acquired	*E. coli*, *Proteus* spp, *Klebsiella* spp	Trimethoprim-sulfamethoxazole; cephalosporins; or quinolones
	Recurrent, indwelling catheter	*E. coli*, *Proteus* spp, *Klebsiella* spp, *Pseudomonas*, spp, *Citrobacter* spp, *Providencia* spp, *Enterococcus* spp	Third-generation cephalosporin ± ampicillin; ampicillin-sulbactam; quinolone; or aminoglycoside
Skin	Cellulitis/erysipelas	Group A streptococci, *S. aureus*	Nafcillin; oxacillin; methicillin; or cefazolin
	Pressure ulcers with systemic infection	Polymicrobial: anaerobic streptococci, Enterobacteriaceae, *Bacteroides*	Augmentin, cefoxitin + aminoglycoside, imipenem, or ampicillin-sulbactam

[a] All drugs administered intravenously or intramuscularly.

ingitis, particularly with pneumococcal pneumonia (18,19). Pneumonia in the elderly results from colonization of the oropharynx and microaspiration of pathogens that overwhelm and evade the normal host defenses, such as cough reflex, ciliary clearance, and macrophage phagocytosis. Colonization with gram-negative flora occurs more often with debility, esophageal motility disorders, lack of cough reflex or gag reflex, neoplasms, CVA, malnutrition, incontinence, institutionalization, and the use of broad-spectrum antibiotics; pneumonia caused by gram-negative colonizing bacteria results as a consequence of aspiration (20). High mortality rates with pneumonia are associated with admission from long-term care facilities, advanced age, tachypnea, confusion, increased blood urea nitrogen, leukocytosis or leukopenia, hypothermia, and cyanosis (21).

B. Clinical Manifestations

Pneumonia in the elderly may present in an insidious manner and without the classic symptoms of fever, rigors, pleuritic chest pain, and productive cough (21). Cognitive impairment exhibited as malaise, confusion, or delirium may be the only initial symptom, and tachycardia or tachypnea may be the only sign that heralds the onset of pneumonia. Delirium is present in approximately 45% of elderly people with pneumonia and is found in 65% of those who die from this infection (22). Dullness to percussion over the involved lung fields, when elicited, may be a helpful clinical clue (23). Absence of a fever response to pneumonia in the elderly is seen in 40% to 65% of cases and is associated with a poor outcome, particularly in cases of pneumococcal pneumonia (22). The recognition of pneumonia in the elderly is thus often problematic, resulting in a later presentation with serious and emergent sequelae (i.e., hypoxemia and sepsis).

C. Immediate Diagnostic Approach

In addition to the chest radiograph, the diagnostic evaluation of elderly patients with severe pneumonia necessitating hospitalization includes a CBC, serum chemistries, and arterial blood gas measurements guided by clinical criteria such as respiratory rate and mental status. Two-step skin testing for tuberculosis with the standard 5 tuberculin unit strength purified protein derivative is also recommended in such patients. Although tuberculous pneumonia characteristically is first seen in an insidious manner, elderly patients, as alluded to earlier, can frequently have atypical symptoms and signs of infection. Thus, because of the high morbidity and mortality associated with tuberculosis (TB) in the elderly and the public health implications with respect to its communicability, it is of immense importance that health care professionals suspect TB in older persons with a pneumonic process accompanied by hemoptysis, weight loss, night sweats, and fevers (24).

Microbiological diagnosis of pneumonia is often problematic when sputum samples are difficult to obtain. Although the value of sputum cultures has been debated, most infectious disease specialists still recommend this test be performed (23,25). Sputum specimens may also be sent for direct fluorescent antibody tests for *Legionella* spp and Ziehl-Neelsen or fluorescent stains and cultures for mycobacteria. Transtracheal aspiration, bronchoscopy with protected brush, or bronchoalveolar lavage specimens can be obtained for severe pneumonia associated with treatment failures (26,27). Blood cultures are an important diagnostic tool (28). Ideally, a minimum of two separate blood cultures should be obtained before antibiotic therapy is begun. Although chest radiography can be a useful tool in the diagnosis of pneumonia, lung consolidation may often not be evident initially or may not correlate with the clinical severity of the illness (26). This false-negative finding is not because of dehydration, per se, but rather is observed in the early stages of pneumonia and in cases of pneumonia in neutropenic hosts (29). In addition, infiltrates, when present, often characteristically do not improve until 8 to 10 weeks after clinical resolution (26). *Streptococcus pneumoniae* is the most common cause of community-acquired and nursing home–acquired pneumonia in the elderly, but in 35% to 58% of cases, no pathogen is identified (27). The incidence of *Staphylococcus aureus* pneumonia in the elderly increases 10 to 20 times during influenza epidemics (30). *Klebsiella pneumoniae* is the most common gram-negative bacterial agent associated with pneumonia acquired in nursing homes (27). Among other common bacterial pathogens associated with severe pneumonia in the elderly, nontypable *Haemophilus influenzae*, *E. coli*, *Acinetobacter* spp, *Moraxella catarrhalis*, *Legionella* spp, and *Pseudomonas* spp, have been implicated (26,27). The role of anaerobic bacteria, although suspected to be important in aspiration pneumonia, has not been documented in the elderly (19).

D. Intervention

Hospitalization for the treatment of pneumonia in the elderly is often necessary because of associated factors i.e., marked debility, comorbid conditions, respiratory compromise, dehydration, delirium, electrolyte abnormalities, secondary complications of bacteremic illness [empyemas, meningitis, and endocarditis], and septic shock may be present. Pleural effusions require diagnostic evaluation because empyemas may develop that require tube thoracostomy drainage. Parenteral antibiotics are required for the treatment of severe pneumonia in the elderly. The appropriate choice of antibiotics is guided by organisms seen on Gram's stain of adequate specimens (sputum or pleural fluid) or initiated empirically on the basis of the patient's clinical status, environment, and co-existent conditions. Table 2 provides recommendations for antimicrobial therapy for community-acquired, nosocomial (hospital-acquired), and nursing home–acquired pneumonia in the elderly. Many effective regimens are available in the therapeutic armamentarium for pneumonia and include penicillins, cephalosporins, macrolides, and the newer quinolones (31) (Table 2). The duration of therapy generally ranges from 14 to 21 days. Information on prevention of pneumococcal pneumonia can be obtained from the Advisory Council for Immunization guidelines published by the Centers for Disease Control and Prevention (32).

III. URINARY TRACT INFECTION

A. Clinical Relevance

Urinary tract infection and its serious complications (i.e., sepsis, shock, abscess formation, and emphysematous pyelonephritis) represent an important infectious disease emergency in the elderly. Urinary tract infection is the most common bacterial infection in the elderly, occurring with almost equal frequency in older men and women (33). The overall occurrence by age 70 is 20% in the community and 50% in long-term care facilities (34). In men, the incidence of UTI increases dramatically with age, from 2% to 4% for those 65 to 70 years of age to more than 22% for those older than 81 (35). The reasons for this increase include decreased prostatic secretions and impaired bladder emptying from outlet obstruction. The increased incidence in elderly women is a consequence of ineffective micturition, previous instrumentation, or underlying disease (36).

B. Clinical Manifestations

In older persons, UTI, including its emergency complications, can first be seen in an insidious manner with nonspecific evidence for clinical deterioration (i.e., mental status changes or as a new onset of urinary incontinence); the classic symptoms of dysuria, urgency, and frequency are often absent. The differentiation of upper from lower UTI is challenging in elderly persons. The most frequent complication of UTI in the elderly is bacteremia; 26% of these progress to generalized sepsis (37). Urinary tract infection can lead to sepsis in approximately 22% of older women with pyelonephritis (33). Urosepsis or UTI accompanied by bacteremia and signs of sepsis, such as fever and hypotension, is associated with a particularly high mortality (38), and all patients require hospitalization.

C. Immediate Diagnostic Approach

The clinical diagnosis of UTI even in the context of an infectious disease emergency in older patients requires confirmation by a careful urinalysis and culture (from a clean-catch midstream sample or a sterile straight catheterized specimen). Indwelling bladder catheters should ideally be replaced before collecting samples for urinalysis and urine cultures. Blood cultures should be obtained in elderly patients as should CBC, electrolytes, and renal function. After clinical stabilization of the patient, further evaluation of the urinary tract and prostate, including ultrasonography, intravenous pyelography, and cystoscopy, is indicated for elderly patients with UTI complicated by sepsis, pyelonephritis, or renal abscess. *E. coli* is the most common etiological agent for UTI in the elderly, but other gram-negative organisms are also important. Residents of nursing homes and patients with chronic indwelling bladder catheters or outlet obstruction are more likely to have UTIs from more resistant bacteria, particularly in the setting of recurrent UTIs and prolonged antibiotic use (39). Common bacterial pathogens implicated in such cases include *Proteus mirabilis*, *K. pneumoniae*, *Pseudomonas* spp, *Enterococcus* spp, and coagulase-negative staphylococci.

D. Intervention

Empiric therapy initiated in such patients should thus be directed toward these organisms. Parenteral trimethoprim-sulfamethoxazole is a good and inexpensive initial choice; however, its coverage against *Pseudomonas* spp is limited; the second-generation cephalosporins or quinolones are excellent alternatives. Table 2 provides recommendations for antibiotics for urosepsis.

IV. SKIN AND SOFT TISSUE INFECTIONS

The skin and soft tissue represent the third most common site of infection, preceded only by urinary tract and respiratory tract infections, respectively, as a recognizable focus for sepsis in the elderly (40). In addition to their common occurrence in elderly patients, some skin and soft tissue infections are unique to aging, either by their distinct manifestations or by their occurrence. Thus, elderly patients have cellulitis with varying degrees of severity, toxic forms of erysipelas or a toxic necrotizing fasciitis, chronic *Pseudomonas* folliculitis, diabetic foot infection, infected pressure ulcers with recurrent sepsis, or herpes zoster infections associated with unrelenting and severe postherpetic neuralgia (PHN). This section will focus on necrotizing fasciitis, an important infectious disease emergency of the skin and soft tissue, and briefly review herpes zoster infection from the perspective of an infectious disease emergency in the elderly. Empiric antimicrobial therapy for cellulitis/erysipelas and infected pressure ulcers with systemic infection is outlined in Table 2.

A. Necrotizing Fasciitis

Necrotizing fasciitis is the most frequently overlooked infectious disease emergency of the skin and soft tissue (40). Clinically, necrotizing fasciitis is characterized by acute pain at the site of involvement. The sites are primarily the lower extremities, abdominal wall, and inguinal region. Physical findings demonstrate varying degrees of erythema and edema but often appear misleadingly normal in appearance. Severe pain and toxicity out of proportion to the clinical findings are hallmarks of necrotizing fasciitis. Local skin changes of tenseness with shiny and smooth texture progress rapidly to purplish discoloration and necrosis, with occasional development of bullae. Lymphadenitis and lymphangitis are uncommon, and marked gangrene may develop in the terminal stages. Associated with toxicity and toxic encephalopathy are consumption of platelets and fibrinogen and marked white blood cell elevation with a left shift; severe dehydration and electrolyte abnormalities and eventual cardiovascular collapse are characteristic of this infection. Gas in the soft tissue is rarely seen. The microbial causes of necrotizing fasciitis in the elderly are anaerobes, *E. coli*, *Pseudomonas* spp, and streptococci. With the exception of narcotic addiction, diabetes mellitus, and trauma, other predisposing factors are not known. The differential diagnosis includes erysipelas and gas gangrene, both clostridial and nonclostridial. Aggressive surgical debridement particularly in the initial stages is key to success. Concomitant diabetes mellitus and atherosclerosis increase overall mortality from this serious infectious disease emergency; venous thrombosis is a common complication. Fournier's gangrene may represent an anaerobic variant of necrotizing fasciitis involving the scrotum, characterized by profound foul odor associated with testicular and adjacent wall necrosis; *Bacteroides* spp is isolated in 50% of cases. Early aggressive surgery is imperative for survival, with antibiotics playing a lesser role. Antibiotic coverage must include anaerobic organisms such as *B. fragilis* and drugs effective against gram-negative bacilli; the average duration of therapy is 2 to 3 weeks (41,42).

B. Herpes Zoster Infection

Herpes zoster infection (shingles) is exceedingly common in the elderly, with a peak age incidence of 50 and 70 years (6). Precipitating factors for this infection unique to older persons include stress, trauma, underlying malignancy, alcoholism, immunosuppressive therapy, and age-related diminished cell-mediated immune responses (43). Although these infections are usually self-limiting, life-threatening or serious complications from this infection are dissemination and ocular involvement (i.e., keratitis, uveitis, and glaucoma). Prolonged severe PHN, motor neuropathies, otitis, Bell's palsy and other cranial nerve palsies, myelitis, encephalitis, meningitis, and secondary bacterial infection are other complications.

Intravenous antiviral therapy should be administered immediately for disseminated disease and extensive ocular involvement. Acyclovir, famciclovir, and valacyclovir are the currently available antiviral agents active against herpes zoster infections; the latter two agents are particularly effective in healing lesions and alleviating of pain (44). Ocular involvement warrants careful ophthalmological evaluation because of the potential for permanent visual loss. Symptomatic therapeutic modalities for PHN include drying lotions (i.e., calamine lotion or Burrow's solution); the local application of capsaicin (a topical analgesic that depletes stores of substance P) (45); nonsteroidal anti-inflammatory agents, acetaminophen, or aspirin; and in recalcitrant cases, tricyclic antidepressant agents or narcotic analgesics (46). Recent studies suggest that corticosteroids, acyclovir, and sympathetic nerve blocks have inconsistently been reported to curtail PHN (47). Secondary bacterial superinfection of herpes zoster lesions necessitates prompt institution of antibacterial agents effective against skin flora (staphylococci and streptococci).

V. MENINGITIS

A. Clinical Relevance

Meningitis in the elderly remains a formidable disease with significant mortality rates (in some studies ranging from 40%–80%) despite appropriate antibiotics (48). Meningitis can be caused by a variety of organisms, including bacteria, viruses, and fungi, or mycobacteria; in one study, among various causes of meningitis in the elderly, 75% were bacterial, 3% granulomatous, and 11% aseptic in nature (49). As with many other infections and potential infectious disease emergencies in the elderly, the initial symptoms and signs of meningitis can be vague and nonspecific. When meningitis is suspected, the diagnosis must be confirmed by lumbar puncture (LP) and cerebrospinal fluid (CSF) analysis.

B. Clinical Manifestations

Although elderly patients with meningitis can be first seen with the classic symptoms of abrupt onset of fever, headache, and meningismus, alteration in mental status with obtundation and coma may occur in about 50% of patients with pneumococcal meningitis (49). Other common symptoms include nausea, vomiting, rigors, photophobia, malaise, and seizures. The finding of nuchal rigidity in the elderly is often misleading and can be a result of chronic conditions (i.e., cervical spine spondyloarthropathies or parkinsonism). Nevertheless, spinal fluid analysis is warranted in elderly persons with a stiff neck suspected to have an infection without an obvious source.

Bacterial meningitis may be caused by bacteremia from a distant infection (e.g., pneumonia or UTI); contiguous spread from sinusitis, otitis media, or mastoiditis; or by direct inoculation from head trauma or neurosurgery. *S. pneumoniae* is the most common cause of bacterial meningitis and accounts for 24% to 54% of all cases in elderly persons (50). Underlying comorbid conditions (i.e., alcoholism, hepatic cirrhosis, asplenia, plasma cell dyscrasias, and chronic lymphocytic leukemia) are frequently associated with fulminant pneumococcal bacteremia, meningitis, pneumonia, and otitis media. Aerobic gram-negative bacilli are the next most frequent bacterial causes of meningitis in the elderly; hematogenous seeding of the meninges is believed to be the likely pathophysiological mechanism. These organisms include *E. coli*, *K. pneumoniae*, *P. aeruginosa*, *Proteus* spp, and *Enterobacter* spp, which are rare causes of bacterial meningitis in healthy younger adults. *Listeria monocytogenes*, a gram-positive bacillus associated with meningitis in persons with altered host defenses, is also common in the elderly (50). *Neisseria meningitidis* has been associated with meningitis in 20% of the elderly; *H. influenzae*, *S. aureus*, and group B streptococci can also occasionally cause meningitis in this population.

C. Immediate Diagnostic Approach

Analysis of routine CSF parameters (cell count, differential, protein and glucose, Gram stain, acid fast stain, cultures, and bacterial antigens) is required to confirm the diagnosis of bacterial meningitis and to identify the specific microbiological cause. As in younger patients, seizures, altered consciousness, focal neurological findings, and presence of papilledema require a brain imaging study before CSF analysis to exclude intracranial hypertension and avoid brain herniation after LP; blood cultures must preferably be drawn before initiation of antibiotics (1,51).

D. Intervention

Treatment of specific causes of bacterial meningitis should be initiated with bactericidal antibiotics as outlined in Table 3. However, if empiric therapy is warranted, treatment should be initiated with penicillin and ceftriaxone or cefotaxime. If penicillin-resistant *S. pneumoniae* is suspected, vancomycin should replace penicillin until culture and sensitivity results become available.

VI. MALIGNANT EXTERNAL OTITIS

A. Clinical Relevance

A virulent form of external otitis, malignant otitis externa, has a particular predilection for elderly diabetic patients. This is a necrotizing vasculitic infection most often caused by *P. aeruginosa*, with a mean age of onset of 60 years (52,53).

Table 3 Antimicrobial Agents of Choice in Treatment of Bacterial Meningitis in the Elderly

Pathogens	Antimicrobial agents preferred[a]	Alternate choice
Streptococcus pneumoniae	Pencillin G, 20–24 million units daily in divided doses every 3–4 h[b]	Ceftriaxone (2–4 g q day) or cefotaxime (2 g q 4–6); chloramphenicol IV, 4–6 g daily in 4 divided doses
Neisseria meningitidis	Penicillin G, 20–24 million units daily in divided doses every 3–4 h	Cefotaxime (2–4 g/day) or ceftriaxone (2 g q 4–6); chloramphenicol 4–6 g daily
Haemophilus influenzae	Ampicillin, 12 g daily in 6 divided doses (in beta-lactam-negative *H. influenzae*); chloramphenicol 4–6 g daily in divided doses (beta lactamase-positive *H. influenzae*)	Cefotaxime (2–4 g/day) or ceftriaxone (2 g q 4–6)
Listeria monocytogenes	Ampicillin 12 g daily in 6 divided doses	Trimethoprim (10 mg/kg/day); sulfamethoxazole (50 mg/kg/day)
Staphylococcus aureus	Nafcillin or oxacillin, 12 g daily in 6 divided doses	Vancomycin, 2 g daily in 4 divided doses
Enterobacteriaceae (*Escherichia coli*, *Klebsiella pneumoniae*)	Cefotaxime, 12 g daily, in 6 divided doses	Trimethoprim (10 mg/kg/day), sulfamethoxazole (50 mg/kg/day); ofloxacin, 400 mg q12
Pseudomonas aeruginosa	Gentamicin 5 mg/kg/day + gentamicin (intrathecal) 2–4 mg/day	Piperacillin or azlocillin, 18–24 g daily in 6 divided doses; ceftazidime, 12 g in 4 doses; or ofloxacin, 400 mg q12h

[a] All drugs administered intravenously.
[b] Replace with vancomycin if penicillin-resistant *S. pneumoniae* is suspected.

Most patients have diabetes mellitus usually of prolonged duration, with evidence of local or systemic diabetic or atherosclerotic microvascular disease (54). Impaired cellular immunity has been demonstrated concomitant with this infection (54). The combination of poor local perfusion and impaired immunity is believed to create an optimal environment for proliferation of organisms indigenous to the canal (i.e., *S. aureus*, coagulase-negative staphylococci, diphtheroids, and anaerobic gram-positive cocci, as well as gram-negative bacilli—*P. aeruginosa*, in particular). The decreased water content of aging skin, increased epithelial sloughing, and increased production of thicker, drier cerumen with age may increase local debris and the potential for obstruction and development of subsequent ear infection. The involved ear may be pruritic, erythematous, edematous, and increasingly painful, often associated with purulent drainage necessitating treatment with local antibiotic-containing otic solutions (i.e., polymixin or gentamicin combined with a corticosteroid preparation).

B. Clinical Manifestations

Clinically, patients have otalgia, external ear drainage, swelling, and erythema of the external ear canal or surrounding structures. Granulation tissue may be visible in the canal. The tympanic membrane is generally not involved. Neurological deficits ranging from isolated facial nerve palsies to multiple cranial nerve deficits, basilar meningitis, or central nervous system suppuration have been reported.

C. Immediate Diagnostic Approach

Culture of purulent drainage from the ear canal frequently reveals *P. aeruginosa* in nearly all cases (55). Useful diagnostic studies include computed tomography scanning, which may best delineate the extent of soft tissue, cartilage, and bone damage (56). Bone and gallium scanning may help define the presence of bony involvement and inflammation early in the course of the disease (57). Computed tomography scanning is also useful in following the progression of disease and gallium scanning to follow the efficacy of therapy.

D. Intervention

Therapy usually requires the combination of an antipseudomonal penicillin and aminoglycoside often in addition to extensive surgical debridement and adjuvant hyperbaric oxygen therapy (55). Third-generation antipseudomonal cephalosporins or the newer quinolones (generally in combination with another agent active against *P. aeruginosa*) may also be considered in the treatment regimen for malignant external otitis (58). The duration of anti-infective therapy for this serious condition requires 6 to 8 weeks. Mortality rates depend on the extent of disease and the degree of cranial nerve involvement at the time of recognition and the institution of appropriate therapy. The overall mortality ranges from 15% to 35% and rises to 50% in the presence of cranial nerve involvement (52).

VII. INFECTIVE ENDOCARDITIS

A. Clinical Relevance

Infective endocarditis (IE) can represent a significant infectious disease emergency in elderly persons, with a mortality rate of 40% to 70% (1,58). The increase in the longevity of patients with rheumatic or congenital valvular disease and age-related degenerative disease (e.g., aortic stenosis) inevitably contributes to this increased risk. Older persons are also at a higher risk for nosocomial endocarditis as a result of infection of pacemakers, intravascular catheters, dialysis shunts, and prosthetic valves (59,60). In vitro, experimental models have suggested that the enhanced progression and dissemination of *S. aureus* endocarditis have been associated with resistance to thrombin-induced platelet microbicidal protein (61).

B. Clinical Manifestations

The classic symptoms and signs of IE (i.e., fever, constitutional symptoms, changing cardiac murmurs, splenomegaly, and embolic phenomena) are frequently but not consistently found in elderly patients. Neurological manifestations (i.e., confusion, delirium, focal findings, aphasia, and coma) are not uncommon (62). As is the case of many infectious diseases in the elderly, clinical features can be somewhat atypical, presenting as a subacute illness with vague and nonspecific symptoms to malaise, fatigue, or unexplained weight loss (63).

The bacteriology of IE in the elderly is no different than for younger adults but deserves brief mention (1). The viridans streptococci group remains the most common cause of native valve endocarditis particularly after dental manipulation; IE resulting from *Streptococcus bovis* and *Enterococcus* spp occurs in association with colorectal disease and genitourinary or biliary tract disease, respectively. *S. aureus* is cultured in 20% to 30% of hospital-acquired cases. Prosthetic-valve endocarditis in the elderly as in younger adults is seen in association with *S. aureus*, coagulase-negative staphylococci, streptococci, gram-negative bacilli, and fungi, in that order.

C. Immediate Diagnostic Approach

The diagnostic clinical and pathological criteria for IE in the elderly is similar to that for younger adults (64). Demonstration of continuous bacteremia is an important and definitive diagnostic criterion for IE and can be achieved by obtaining three sets of blood cultures at different times during a 24-hour period. When an acutely ill older person requires rapid initiation of antibiotic therapy, three sets of blood cultures can be drawn every 15 minutes. The two-dimensional echocardiogram can be used as an adjunct to substantiate the presence of valve vegetations; however, valvular vegetations may not be demonstrable in 40% to 80% of suspected cases with conventional transthoracic technique (60). Transesophageal echocardiography in such cases is likely to improve the sensitivity and diagnostic accuracy of this study, particularly in the presence of ''breakthrough'' bacteremia and the suspicion for valve-ring abscess formation that may necessitate valve replacement. In addition to routine laboratory tests (i.e., a CBC, routine chemistries, and urinalysis), a chest roentgenogram and electrocardiogram must be part of the diagnostic evaluation of IE in the elderly; the latter is of particular importance because cardiac dysrhythmias and CHF are common complicating factors in this population (1).

D. Intervention

Antibiotic treatment should be initiated in the presence of new regurgitant murmurs, embolic phenomena, significant CHF, or sepsis (60). Empiric therapy for native-valve endocarditis can be initiated with benzyl penicillin or an antistaphylococcal penicillin (nafcillin or oxacillin) plus an aminoglycoside. Vancomycin is recommended for patients with a history of a penicillin allergy; infections caused by *Enterococcus* spp and *S. aureus* resistant to ampicillin and methicillin, respectively; and empiric therapy for prosthetic valve, nosocomial, or culture-negative endocarditis (1). The recommended duration of antibiotic therapy ranges from 4 to 6 weeks; close monitoring of serum antibiotic levels and renal function in addition to a regular physical examination follow-up and electrocardiography are imperative. Surgical treatment indications both for native and prosthetic valve IE include progressive CHF, repeated septic embolization, persistently positive blood cultures despite appropriate antibiotics (breakthrough bacteremia), development of myocardial abscesses, or fungal endocarditis (65).

REFERENCES

1. Jacobs LG. Infectious disease emergencies in the geriatric population. Clin Geriatr Med 1993;9(3):559–575.
2. Norman DC, Toledo SD. Infections in the elderly persons: An altered clinical presentation. Clin Geriatr Med 1992;8:713–719.
3. Gardner P, Judson BL. Advance report of final mortality statistics. 1993 Monthly Vital Statistics Report 1996;44(7) suppl).

4. Jones SR. Infection in frail and vulnerable elderly patients. Am J Med 1990;88(suppl 3C):30S–33S.
5. Garibaldi RA. Infections in the elderly. Am J Med 1986;81(suppl 1A):53–58.
6. Rhyne RL, Roche RJ. Infection in the elderly. In:Brillman JC, Quenzer RW, eds. Infectious Disease in Emergency Medicine. Philadelphia: Lippincot-Raven, 1997, pp 291–316.
7. Bender BS. Sepsis. Clin Geriatr Med 1992;8:913–924.
8. Bone RC, Fisher CJ, Clemmer TP, Slotman GJ, Metz CA, Balk RA. A controlled clinical trial of high-dose methylprednisolone in the treatment of severe sepsis and septic shock. N Engl J Med 1987;317:853–858.
9. Koscove EM. Sepsis and septic shock. In: Brillman JC, Quenzer RW, eds. Infectious Disease in Emergency Medicine. Lippincot-Raven: Philadelphia, 1997, pp 129–152.
10. Centers for Disease Control and Prevention, National Center for Health Statistics. Mortality Patterns—United States, 1990. Monthly Vital Statistics Report 1993;41: 5.
11. Centers for Disease Control. Increase in National Hospital Discharge Survey rates for septicemia—United States, 1979–87. MMWR 1990;39:31–34.
12. Plewa M. Altered host response and special infections in the elderly. Emerg Med Clin North Am 1990;8:193–206.
13. Rackow EC, Astiz ME. Pathophysiology and treatment of septic shock. JAMA 1991; 266:548–554.
14. Myers BR, Sherman E, Mendeson MH, Velasquez G, Srulevitch-Chin E, Hubbard M, Hirschman SZ. Bloodstream infections in the elderly. Am J Med 1989;86:379–384.
15. Sasse KC, Nauenberg E, Long A, Anton B, Tucker HJ, Hu TW. Long term survival after intensive care unit admissions with sepsis. Crit Care Med 1995;23:1040–1047.
16. Bone RC. Sepsis syndrome. New insights into its pathogenesis and treatment. Infect Dis Clin North Am 1995;5:793–805.
17. Waage A, Brandtzaeg P, Espevik T, Halstensen A. Current understanding of the pathogenesis of gram-negative shock. Infect Dis Clin North Am 1991;5:781–791.
18. Marrie TJ, Haldane EV, Faulkner RS, Durant H, Kwan C. Community-acquired pneumonia requiring hospitalization. It is different in the elderly? J Am Geriatr Soc 1985;33:671–680.
19. Verghese A, Berk S. Bacterial pneumonia in the elderly. Medicine 1983;62:271–285.
20. Niederman MS, Fein AM. Pneumonia in the elderly. Clin Geriatr Med 1986;2:241–268.
21. Fein AM, Neiderman AS. Severe pneumonia in the elderly. Clin Geriatr Med 1994; 10:121–143.
22. Yoshikawa TT, Norman DC. Treatment of infections in elderly patients. Med Clin North Am 1995;79:651–666.
23. Bentley D. Diagnosis and management of pneumonia in the elderly patient. Mod Med 1987;55:68–82.
24. Yoshikawa TT. Tuberculosis in aging adults. J Am Geriatr Soc 1992;40:178–185.
25. Niederman MS, Bass JB Jr. Campbell GD, Fein AM, Grossman RF, Mandell LA, Marrie TJ, Sarosi GA, Torres A, Yu VL. Guidelines for the initial management of

adults with community-acquired pneumonia: diagnosis, assessment of severity, and initial antimicrobial therapy. Am Rev Respir Dis 1993;148:1418–1426.
26. Marrie TJ. Pneumonia. Clin Geriatr Med 1992;8:721–731.
27. Leeper KV Jr, Torres A. Community acquired pneumonia in the intensive care unit. Clin Chest Med 1995;16:155–171.
28. Berk SL. Justifying the use of blood cultures when diagnosing community-acquired pneumonia. Chest 1995;108:891–892.
29. Caldwell A, Glauser FL, Smith WR, Hoshiko M, Morton ME. The effects of dehydration on the radiologic and pathologic appearance of experimental canine segmental pneumonia. Am Rev Respir Dis 1975;112:651–656.
30. Mostow SR. Infectious complications in the elderly COPD patient. Geriatrics 1993; 38(10):42–48.
31. Bartlett JG. Community-acquired pneumonia in adults: guidelines for the management, Infectious Disease Society of America. Clin Infect Dis 1998;26(4):81–83.
32. CDC. Prevention of Pneumococcal Disease. Recommendations of the Advisory Committee on Immunization Practices (ACIP). MMWR 1997;46(RR-08):1–24.
33. Gleckman RA. Urinary tract infection. Clin Geriatr Med 1992;8:793–803.
34. Zilkoski MW, Smucker DR, Mayhew HE. Urinary tract infections in elderly patients. Postgrad Med J 1988;84(3):191–206.
35. Bertakis KD, Ross JL. Office evaluation of urinary tract infection in elderly women. J Fam Pract 1987;24(1):72–75.
36. Flournay DJ, Bernard MA. Problems in diagnosing infections in the elderly. J Natl Med Assoc 1993;85:835–840.
37. Roberts JA. Pyelonephritis, cortical abscess and perinephric abscess. Urol Clin North Am 1986;13(4):637–645.
38. Johnson R. Urosepsis. Urol Clin North Am 1986;13(4):637–647.
39. Warren JW. Catheter associated bacteriuria. Clin Geriatr Med 1992;8:805–819.
40. Smith LG, Sensakovic JW. Skin and soft tissue infections. In: Cunha BA, ed. Infectious Diseases in the Elderly. Massachusetts: PSG Publishing Co Inc, 1988;145: 243–253.
41. Majeski JA, Alexander JW. Early diagnosis, nutritional support, and immediate extensive debridement improve survival in necrotizing fasciitis. Am J Surg 1983;145: 784–787.
42. Brenner Be, Vitullo M, Simon RR. Necrotizing fasciitis. Ann Emerg Med 1982;11: 384–386.
43. Weksler ME. Immune senescence. Ann Neurol 1994;35 (suppl): S35–S37.
44. Lancaster T, Silagy C, Gray S. Primary care management of acute herpes zoster: Systematic review of evidence from randomized controlled trials. Br J Gen Pract 1995;45(390):39–45.
45. Post BT, Philbrick JT. Do corticosteroids prevent post herpetic neuralgia: a review of the evidence. J Am Acad Dermatol 1988;18:605–610.
46. Bowshen D. Post-herpertic neuralgia in older persons: Incidence and optimal treatment. Drugs Aging 1994;6(6): 411–418.
47. Choo PW, Galil K, Donahue JG, Walker AM, Speigelman D, Platt R. Risk factors for postherpetic neuralgia. Arch Intern Med 1997;147:1217–1224.
48. Yoshikawa TT, Norman DC. Central nervous system infections. In: Aging and Clini-

cal Practice: Infectious Diseases, Diagnosis and Treatment. New York: Igaku-Shoin, 1987, pp 90–93.
49. Gorse GJ, Thrupp LD, Nudleman KL, Wyle FA, Hawkins B, Cesario TC. Bacterial meningitis in the elderly. Arch Intern Med 1984;144:1603–1607.
50. Miller LG, Choi C. Meningitis in older patients: how to diagnose and treat a deadly infection. Geriatrics 1997; 52:43–55.
51. Choi C. Bacterial meningitis. Clin Geriatr Med 1992;8:889–902.
52. Yoshikawa TT. Infections in the diabetic patient. In: Cunha BA, ed. Infectious Diseases in the Elderly. Massachusetts: PSG Publishing Co Inc, 1988, pp 312–323.
53. Zaky DA, Bentley DW, Lowy K, Betts RF, Douglas RG Jr. Malignant external otitis: a severe form of otitis in diabetic patients. Am J Med 1976;61:298–302.
54. Rubin JR, Yu VL. Malignant external otitis: Insights into pathogenesis, clinical manifestations, diagnosis, and therapy. Am J Med 1988;85:391–398.
55. Hickham M, Amedee RG. Malignant otitis externa. J La State Med Soc 1996;148: 511–513.
56. Gold S, Som PM, Lucente FE, Lawson W, Mendelson M, Parisier SC. Radiographic findings in progressive necrotizing ''malignant'' external otitis. Laryngoscope 1984; 94:363–366.
57. Marcel PM, Stokkel MD, Ina CN, van Eck-Smt BL. SPECT gallium scintigraphy in malignant external otitis; initial staging and follow-up. Case reports. Laryngoscope 1996;105:338–340.
58. Applefeld MM, Hornick RB. Infective endocarditis in patients over 60. Am Heart J 1974;88:90–94.
59. Cantrell M, Yoshikawa TT. Aging and infective endocarditis. J Am Geriatr Soc 1983;31:216–222.
60. Yoshikawa TT, Norman DC. Infective endocarditis. In: Aging and Clinical Practice: Infectious Diseases, Diagnosis and Treatment. New York: Igaku-Shoin, 1987, pp 185–189.
61. Dhawan VK, Bayer AS, Yeaman MR. In vitro resistance to thrombin-induced platelet microbicidal protein is associated with enhanced progression and hematogenous dissemination in experimental *Staphylococcus aureus* infective endocarditis. Infect Immun 1998;66:3476–3479.
62. Thell R, Martin FH, Edward JE. Bacterial endocarditis in subjects 60 years of age and older. Circulation 1975;51:174–182.
63. Berk SL, Smith JR. Infectious diseases in the elderly. Med Clin North Am 1983; 67(2):273–293.
64. Durack DT, Lukes AS, Bright DK, Duke Endocarditis Service. New criteria for the diagnosis of infective endocarditis: utilization of specific echocardiographic findings. Am J Med 1994;96:200–209.
65. Terpening MS. Infective endocarditis. Clin Geriatr Med 1992;8:903–912.

19
Gastrointestinal Hemorrhage

Abbasi J. Akhtar
Charles R. Drew University of Medicine and Science, and Martin Luther King, Jr.–Charles R. Drew Medical Center, Los Angeles, California

I. CLINICAL RELEVANCE

Gastrointestinal hemorrhage (GIH) is a common and serious condition first seen as a medical emergency. It may prove to be potentially life threatening among the elderly. Among all cases of active upper gastrointestinal hemorrhage (UGIH), 35% to 45% occur in patients older than age 60 (1). The magnitude of the problem is expected to greatly increase, given that the elderly are the most rapidly growing segment of the U.S. population. It is predicted that by the year 2040, 68 million Americans will be age 65 and older, with 12.2 million older than 85 years of age (2). Although the overall cause of GIH is not much different in the elderly compared with younger patients, certain lesions, such as gastrointestinal malignancies, angiodysplasias, and diverticular bleeding, are more common in the elderly. Elderly patients, however, do not tolerate gastrointestinal bleeding as well as younger patients. The elderly bleed more intensively and continue to bleed; bleeding tends to recur, and they require more blood transfusions and surgical interventions and tend to die more frequently compared with younger patients. In half of the elderly patients with peptic ulcer or nonsteroidal anti-inflammatory drug (NSAID)–induced ulcer, gastrointestinal bleeding may be the first sign. Deaths caused by gastrointestinal bleeding in general, and bleeding peptic ulcers in particular, are rare in younger patients, but in the elderly, the mortality may reach as great as 30% or more. Associated diseases, particularly cerebrovascular and cardiovascular conditions, malignancies, increased frailty of the elderly, polypharmacy, and use of NSAIDs, are factors responsible for the increased morbidity and mortality of elderly patients with GIH. Initial poor prognostic indicators at the time of admission include bright red color bleeding (rather than melena or ''coffee-ground'' gastric contents by emesis or by nasogastric aspirate), presence of shock, orthostatic changes, presence of varices, actively bleeding vessel, or visible vessel with adherent clot on endoscopy. Recurrence of bleeding in the hospital is a serious prognostic sign and may require surgical intervention, should medical and endoscopic therapy fail to arrest the bleeding.

Clinically, GIH may be considered under two broad headings according to the site of origin: upper (proximal to the ligament of Treitz of the duodenum) and lower (distal to it). One-third to one-half of the bleeding episodes in the elderly may not be preceded by gastrointestinal complaints such as pain or dyspepsia (3). A significant number of elderly patients may have one or more of the extraintestinal manifestations rather than hematemesis, melena, or hematochezia (4).

Significant causes of UGIH in the elderly include gastric and duodenal ulcers, esophagitis, gastritis, duodenitis, Mallory-Weiss tears, esophageal and gastric varices, esophageal and gastric neoplasms, and vascular malformations, including Dieulafoy's ulcer (Table 1). The incidence of some lesions depends on the population studied. For example, patients from Veterans Affairs medical centers and inner-city hospitals with high alcohol consumption have increased incidence of gastrointestinal varices, gastric erosions, and portal hypertensive gastropathy compared with the general population. Overall, peptic ulcer disease, along with esophageal, gastric and duodenal erosions, and NSAID-induced lesions, remains the most common cause of UGIH in the elderly, accounting for more than 75% of cases. In the younger population, peptic ulcer disease accounts

Table 1 Etiology of Upper Gastrointestinal Hemorrhage in 200 Elderly Patients

Lesion	Number	%
Gastric ulcer	48	24
Duodenal ulcer	42	21
Esophageal/gastric/duodenal erosions	40	20
Varices	28	14
Mallory-Weiss tear	20	10
Angiodysplasia	14	7
Portal hypertensive gastropathy	10	5
Dieulafoy's ulcer	9	4.5
Esophageal cancer with bleeding	6	3
Gastric cancer with bleeding	6	3

Note: Total number exceeds 200 and 100% because 23 patients (11.5%) had more than one lesion.

for more then 50% of cases, and NSAID-induced bleeding is less common than in elderly patients.

Although exact data on the epidemiology and outcome of lower gastrointestinal hemorrhage (LGIH) in the elderly is not clear, LGIH accounts for approximately one-third of all cases of acute GIH in the elderly. One in 10 (10%) patients with LGIH will be bleeding from a source in the upper gastrointestinal tract. In the elderly, this pattern may be more frequent—up to 15%.

Other common causes of LGIH in elderly patients in the order of frequency include diverticular bleeding, vascular anomalies (angiodysplasias, arteriovenous malformations), colorectal neoplasms, ischemic colitis, and hemorrhoids. The culprit lesion is usually colonic in location in approximately 75% of cases of LGIH (Table 2). In contrast to younger patients, *diverticular bleeding and vascular ectasia* are responsible for almost 60% of cases of LGIH in the elderly. These bleeding diverticulae are located in the right side of the colon. In contrast, diverticulitis is located more commonly in the left side of the colon. Diverticular bleeding is arterial in origin and is characterized by sudden onset of painless bright red profuse rectal bleeding. It may be accompanied by symptoms and signs of hypovolemia and shock. Sometimes the elderly patient may not notice bleeding and may be initially seen with extraintestinal manifestations, such as altered mental status and shock. Diverticular bleeding stops spontaneously in most cases; however, it may recur in 25% to 50% of cases. *Vascular anomalies* include angiodysplasias, which may occur sporadically or in association with chronic renal failure, von Willebrand's disease, telangiectasia, occurring de novo, or as a part

Table 2 Endoscopic Findings in 100 Elderly Patients with Lower Gastrointestinal Hemorrhage

Lesion	Number	%
Internal hemorrhoids (evidence of bleeding in 10)	40	40
Angiodysplasias	26	26
Diverticular bleeding	18	18
Polyps	15	15
Cancer	10	10
Ischemic colitis	5	5
Drugs (NSAIDs and/or anticoagulants)	5	5
Solitary rectal ulcer	3	3
Ulcerative colitis	3	3
Colonic varices	3	3

NOTE: Total number exceeds 100 and 100% because 28 patients (28%) had more than one lesion.
NSAIDS: nonsteroidal anti-inflammatory drugs.

of Rendu-Osler-Weber syndrome, hemangioma, and arteriovenous malformation. Dieulafoy's ulcer, which is a small-caliber persistent submucosal artery, may be found anywhere in the gut but more often in the gastric fundus. These lesions may bleed slowly and may cause anemia or profuse bleeding. The bleeding is usually painless. The color of blood may vary from bright red to maroon or even melenic, depending on the site of the lesion (5). *Solitary rectal ulcer syndrome* and *stercoral ulcer* (caused by a retained fecal mass resulting in pressure necrosis of distal colonic mucosa) occur more often in the elderly and may be the cause of LGIH. Both of these conditions are associated with constipation and strained defection. *Hemorrhoids and anal fissures* are more common in the elderly and usually are the cause of trivial blood loss but may be a source of significant bleeding when accompanied by constipation. *Ischemic lesions* of the bowel are also much more frequent causes of LGIH in the elderly than in younger patients. Their spectrum includes mesenteric arterial occlusion, mesenteric venous thrombosis, vasculitis, and ischemic colitis. *Miscellaneous causes of LGIH* include colonic varices, vasculitis, small bowel ulceration and tumors, inflammatory bowel disease (Crohn's disease and ulcerative colitis), and infectious diarrhea caused by *Shigella*, *Salmonella*, *Campylobacter jejuni*, *Clostridium difficile*, enteroinvasive *Escherichia coli*, and some intestinal parasites. Nonsteroidal drug–induced bowel injury and anticoagulants are infrequent but important causes of LGIH. Although more common in children and young adults, Meckel's diverticulum may also be a source of LGIH in the elderly.

II. IMMEDIATE DIAGNOSTIC APPROACH

Initial assessment includes a quick but relevant history and physical examination. Hemodynamic resuscitation of the elderly patient with significant GIH should be initiated simultaneously.

The approach to the bleeding elderly patient should be a custom-tailored one, depending on the site of bleeding, intensity of bleeding, and presence or absence of concomitant comorbid conditions. A quick history and physical examination are integral parts of initial assessment. The hemodynamic status should be assessed rapidly. Orthostatic changes should be recorded. A fall of blood pressure of more than 20 mm Hg systolic and 10 mm Hg diastolic or a rise of more than 20 beats/min in the pulse rate between supine and upright positions indicates loss of more than 20% of the blood volume. Hypovolemic shock in active GIH may indicate loss of more than 40% of blood volume. Stabilization of hemodynamics and maintaining vital signs and vital organ perfusion are priorities in elderly bleeding patients. Because the elderly tolerate shock poorly compared with younger patients, the presence of comorbid illness, especially cardiovascular disease, may make the situation much worse. It should be kept in mind that elderly patients with GIH may simultaneously have one or more diseases that may prove to be as serious as GIH or even more so, such as myocardial infarction, stroke, diabetic complications, and sepsis. Alternately, GIH in the elderly may manifest with extraintestinal presentations such as stroke, myocardial infarction, altered level of consciousness, and syncope in absence of hematemesis or hematochezia (4).

A nasogastric tube should be inserted. The color of the aspirate (clear, coffee ground, or frank blood) may give useful diagnostic and prognostic clues. A clear aspirate should be tested for occult blood and bile. Absence of blood and presence of bile indicates no active bleeding in the stomach or duodenum at the time of examination, whereas coffee-ground aspirate is suggestive of recent bleeding, and red blood signifies active bleeding and mandates urgent therapy. A negative nasogastric aspirate does not always exclude upper GIH. If a high index of suspicion persists, a more definitive test, such as endoscopy, should be performed. Continuous high-grade suction is not recommended because it may cause suction artifacts and even mucosal lesions, which may become a source of bleeding themselves. Should gastric lavage be necessary before endoscopy, a wide-lumen tube, such as an Ewald tube, should be inserted and lavage carried out with tap water at room temperature. No advantage exists to the use of iced saline, which is expensive and even may be harmful at times. Saline solution, with its high sodium content, may be detrimental in the elderly patients, especially those with co-existent cirrhosis, hypertension, and congestive heart failure. Freezing temperatures may compromise viability of gastric mucosa. Gentle digital rectal examination should be done, even if rectal bleeding is obvious because it may provide useful diagnostic information.

Intravenous access should be established by placing large-bore (18- or 16-gauge) lines, preferably at two sites. Blood samples should be sent for typing and cross-match, hemoglobin, hematocrit, and electrolytes. Blood should also be sent for serum folate and vitamin B_{12} levels because many elderly patients may have these deficiencies as a cause or contributory factor of their anemia. Liver chemistry and a coagulation profile should also be obtained. It should be noted that changes in hemoglobin and hematocrit lag behind actual hemodynamic and circulatory status. Occasionally, the initial hematocrit may be greater in acute GIH than at baseline and may convey erroneous information about the severity of bleeding. Changes in vital signs and overall status of vital organ perfusion are more precise measures for acute blood loss. Clinical clues for vital organ perfusion may be obtained by assessment of level of consciousness, urinary output, and skin turgor. Altered level of consciousness suggests inadequate cerebral perfusion, and oliguria suggests renal hypoperfusion. Laboratory findings, such as ischemic changes on electrocardiogram, suggest myocardial hypoperfusion. Nonspecific ST- segment changes may be associated with upper gastrointestinal bleeding and are not clinically significant in the absence of shock or cardiac symptoms, such as angina or dyspnea. Rarely, however, myocardial infarction is associated with GIH (6). Therefore, an electrocardiogram should always be obtained in all cases of GIH, particularly in the elderly. In cases of profuse upper GIH, endotracheal intubation may be required to protect the airway, provide adequate oxygenation, prevent aspiration, and facilitate endoscopy. A chest radiograph should also be obtained because it will provide useful information about cardiopulmonary diseases, aspiration, and the position of inserted tubes and catheters.

Until packed red blood cells are available for transfusion, normal saline infusion should be started. Contrary to younger patients with GIH, in whom large amounts of crystalloid and colloid solutions may safely be given to replace the intravascular volume loss, elderly patients may or may not tolerate such a generous fluid replacement and may quickly have fluid overload and even congestive heart failure develop. Therefore, careful observations and close monitoring is necessary, including frequent chest auscultation and examination for neck vein engorgement. In the elderly patients with shock caused by GIH, monitoring central venous pressure is advisable.

Once hemodynamic resuscitation and stability have been achieved, a rapid but more comprehensive history should be obtained. The elderly patient may not be as good a historian as the younger patient because of impaired memory, confusion, dementia, or apprehension. If this is the case, relatives, caretakers, nursing home personnel, the patient's family physician, or pharmacist may be useful resources for valuable information. Special attention should be given to previous gastrointestinal symptoms and diagnoses, such as abdominal pain and dyspepsia. Previous GIH may be suggestive of peptic ulcer disease. History of hepatitis or alcohol abuse may indicate the possibility of variceal bleeding. Retching and forceful vomiting may indicate a Mallory-Weiss tear, although such a typical history is available only in 50% of cases of Mallory-Weiss tears. The patient should be queried for prior gastrointestinal symptoms and diagnoses, such as peptic ulcer, inflammatory bowel disease, colonic polyps, diverticulosis, hemorrhoids, previous gastrointestinal surgery, arterial bypass graft surgery, radiation therapy, previous episodes of GIH, and associated evaluation and family history of bleeding disorders. A recent change in bowel habits or weight loss should also be determined. Medication use should be carefully questioned, both prescription and nonprescription. Often the elderly do not consider over-the-counter remedies as medications; however, these may contain aspirin and ibuprofen and thus be the etiological factors of GIH. Other NSAIDs and anticoagulants should also be investigated.

After hemodynamic stabilization and obtaining a comprehensive history, a complete physical examination should be undertaken. Oral and nasal cavities should be examined because bleeding from the oral cavity and epistaxis may result in swallowing of blood and subsequent hematemesis or melena, which may give a false impression of upper GIH and may result in misdiagnosis and delay of appropriate treatment. Skin examination may reveal useful markers of underlying diseases, which may be a culprit for GIH. Examples include spider angiomata, palmar erythema, dilated superficial veins and caput medusa of chronic liver disease, pigmentation of lips and oral mucosa in Peutz-Jeghers syndrome, cafe au lait spots of neurofibromatosis, loose skin of pseudoxanthoma elasticum and telangiectasia of the lips and buccal mucosa in Rendu-Osler-Weber-disease. Acanthosis nigricans and tylosis, may indicate underlying gastrointestinal malignancy. Pyoderma gangrenosum is associated with ulcerative colitis. Ascites, splenomegaly, parotid enlargement, testicular atrophy, and white lines on the nails (leukonychia) may be markers of portal hypertension and suggest variceal bleeding. Of note, alcohol and hepatitis do not represent the sole etiological factors for varices. In the elderly, in contrast to younger patients, varices may result from neoplasms such as carcinoma of the head of the pancreas or hepatocellular carcinoma, esophageal cancer infiltrating the portal venous system, or extensive hepatic metastases interfering with portal venous drainage. Sometimes variceal bleeding may be the presenting sign of these tumors. As mentioned earlier, a digital rectal examination and guaiac test are integral parts of physical examination that should never be deferred. Available literature and our own study suggest that recent cardiac events, such as myocardial infarction or cardiac dysrhythmias in a stable patient, are not contraindications for performing gentle digital rectal examination (7).

Except for the trivial GIH in a hemodynamically stable patient, all elderly patients with significant GIH should be admitted to an intensive care unit. A medical gastroenterologist, gastrointestinal surgeon, and interventional radiologist should be informed in all but trivial cases of GIH. The concept of a ''bleeding team'' in some medical centers, especially in Europe, can often be beneficial. One such team involves a medical gastroenterologist, gastrointestinal surgeon, and interventional radiologist, in addition to the primary care physician or geriatrician. They are routinely informed as soon as any patient with gastrointestinal bleeding is admitted, and all members of the team offer their services in a timely manner (8).

Frail elderly patients with severe GIH and comorbid conditions, such as cardiopulmonary disease, may require placement of a central venous (e.g., Swan-Ganz) catheter for monitoring capillary wedge pressure. A pulse oximeter should be placed and supplemental oxygen should be given if evidence of hypoxia exists. This will increase the oxygen-carrying capacity of blood and improve tissue perfusion. Arterial blood gases may be tested in this high-risk group of patients, and the presence of metabolic acidosis may be suggestive of inadequate tissue perfusion or other co-existing conditions (e.g., renal failure). Unless the patient has evidence of congestive heart failure, normal saline infusion may be started to maintain intravascular volume pending availability of blood for transfusion. Packed red blood cells are an adequate form of blood transfusion unless the patient requires large amounts of blood because of continued massive bleeding. In the latter scenario, coagulation factors, platelets, and calcium supplementation may be needed as well. The younger and healthier patients with GIH may tolerate a lower level of hemoglobin/hematocrit without significant compromise in tissue perfusion. In the elderly, a low hemoglobin/hematocrit may be detrimental, therefore, a hematocrit greater than 30% is desirable. In addition, frail elderly bleeders are more prone to hypothermia if multiple transfusions are given without warming of the blood in a short time.

III. THERAPEUTIC INTERVENTIONS

Interventions should be modified according to the site, severity of bleeding, and presence of any comorbid conditions and overall clinical status of the elderly patient with GIH.

In cases of *UGIH* (Fig. 1), upper gastrointestinal endoscopy is the study of choice and serves as the "gold standard" as far as diagnosis and endoscopic therapy are concerned. Endoscopy may also provide useful information about

ALGORITHM FOR UPPER GASTROINTESTINAL HEMORRHAGE

↓

Resuscitation and urgent clinical assessment

↙ ↘

Bleeding continues
↓
Continue volume replacement and stabilize the patient
↓
Bleeding continues
↓
Attempt upper endoscopy-diagnostic/therapeutic after gastric lavage and endotracheal intubation. If successful → → → **Medical therapy as indicated (H2 blockers, vasopressin/ octreotide)**

If unsuccessful
↓
Angiography/Red blood cell scan
↓
Bleeding continues
↓
Surgery

Bleeding stops
↓
Patient stable
↓
Early endoscopy diagnostic/therapeutic
↓
Medical therapy as indicated (H2 blockers, vasopressin/ octreotide)

Figure 1 Algorithm for management of UGIH.

high-risk patients who must be admitted to intensive care units or who will need endoscopic therapy, large amounts of blood transfusions, or surgery. Such endoscopic findings may include active arterial bleeding or oozing, visible vessel(s), sentinel clot, or evidence of recent bleeding from varices in the form of ''red wale'' marks or cherry red spots. Endoscopic biopsies may help in the diagnosis of an underlying disease process, malignancy, or *Helicobacter pylori* infection.

Endoscopic hemostasis may be attempted with injection therapy, heater probe, and multipolar electrocoagulation or laser photocoagulation of the bleeding vessels. Gastroesophageal variceal bleeding is associated with significant mortality in all patients and particularly in the elderly, in whom mortality for the first admission may be as high as 30% to 60%, depending on the cause of varices and the presence of comorbid illnesses. Sclerotherapy or banding is the standard endoscopic therapy for esophageal varices. Other measures to control variceal bleeding include pharmacological therapy to lower portal venous pressure by infusion of vasopressin and nitroglycerin. Vasopressin infusion may result in coronary, renal, and intestinal ischemia. Therefore, careful monitoring is mandatory throughout the duration of therapy. Vasopressin should not be used in patients with coronary artery disease or renal insufficiency. Octreotide, a somatostatin analogue without the side effects of vasopressin, also lowers portal pressure and may be used to stop variceal bleeding. Should endoscopic and pharmacological measures fail to arrest variceal bleeding, temporary hemostasis may be attempted through the use of a balloon tamponade with a Sengstaken-Blakemore or Linton tube placed locally at the site of bleeding. These tubes may stop bleeding but are only temporary measures and are associated with serious side effects, including rupture of the esophagus, aspiration pneumonia and airway obstruction. They do not improve survival, and if the balloon is kept inflated for more than 48 hours, it may result in pressure necrosis of the mucosa, creating a new source of bleeding. A more viable therapeutic option is transjugular intrahepatic portosystemic shunt (TIPS). It usually controls bleeding and ascites but may worsen encephalopathy. Other problems with TIPS include subsequent shunt occlusion, infection, and bleeding.

If the bleeding is so profuse that adequate endoscopic diagnosis and therapy are not possible, angiography may help to localize the site of bleeding. Sometimes angiographic embolization of bleeding vessels may be therapeutic. Surgical intervention may ultimately be required in some cases; however, all attempts should be made to avoid emergency surgery, which may be associated with increased morbidity and mortality in elderly patients, especially those with associated comorbid illnesses. Nevertheless, surgery, when strongly indicated, should not be avoided just because of increased age alone. The elderly patient has a reasonably good outcome of surgery under optimal circumstances.

For *LGIH* (Fig. 2), initial management, including resuscitation of the patient and hemodynamic stabilization, is the same as in cases of UGIH. In 10%

ALGORITHM FOR LOWER GASTROINTESTINAL HEMORRHAGE

Resuscitation and urgent clinical assessment
↓
Nasogastric tube aspiration
↙ ↘

Bloody or coffee ground aspirate
↓
Management as upper GI Bleeding

Blood absent, but bile present
↓
Urgent flexible sigmoidoscopy
↙ ↓

Bleeding lesion found on sigmoidoscopy
↓
Management as indicated

Blood seen coming from above splenic flexure
↓
Colonoscopy → Lesion found on colonoscopy
↓
Management as indicated

Colonoscopy
↓
No definite lesion found or bleeding too brisk to be located endoscopically → Angiography/Tagged red blood cell scan
↓
Bleeding site located
↓
Embolization if possible → → Bleeding continues
↓
Surgery

Embolization if possible
↓
Bleeding stops
↓
Repeat colonoscopy and if negative
↓
Consider small bowel studies (Enteroscopy)

Figure 2 Algorithm for management of LGIH.

to 15% cases of LGIH, the bleeding site is likely to be located in the upper gastrointestinal tract. A nasogastric tube should be inserted and if evidence of bleeding is found, upper endoscopy should be done. However, if blood is absent and bile is present in the nasogastric aspirate, a search for lower gastrointestinal lesions should be undertaken. Digital rectal examination should be done, as well as flexible proctosigmoidoscopy. Bleeding from hemorrhoids and anorectal lesions such as solitary rectal ulcer, stercoraceous ulcer, or neoplasms will thus be diagnosed. This procedure will also make the diagnosis of ulcerative colitis, revealing diffuse inflammation and ulceration of mucosa, ischemic colitis, and volvulus.

A negative proctosigmoidoscopy, or bleeding from above the splenic flexure, should alert the clinician to initiate patient preparation for full colonoscopy by administering oral polyethylene glycol electrolyte or phosphosoda solutions for colonic lavage. Endoscopic therapy, such as cauterization of any bleeding vessel or angiodysplasias, removal of polyps, or injecting a bleeding site, should be done in addition to obtaining a mucosal biopsy specimen. Failure of colonoscopy to reveal the bleeding site will necessitate a nuclear medicine study, such as tagged red blood cell scan, which may provide useful clues to the bleeding site. If bleeding is too profuse to perform a satisfactory colonoscopy, angiography should be done because it may reveal bleeding vessels. Angiographic therapy, such as embolization or intrarterial infusion of vasopressin, may achieve hemostasis. Every attempt should be made to avoid surgery altogether or at least to postpone emergency surgery to elective surgery. However, if endoscopic, pharmacological, and angiographic measures fail to arrest the bleeding, emergency surgery should be performed. If the bleeding site has not been located before surgery, intraoperative endoscopy, including examination of the small bowel, may reveal the bleeding lesion and direct the surgeon.

IV. FOLLOW-UP MANAGEMENT

Once the acute episode of GIH has been controlled, the patient is hemodynamically stable, and initial pharmacological or endoscopic therapy is started, the patient's overall clinical status should be re-evaluated. Some conditions will need special attention (e.g., gastroesophageal variceal bleeding after initial endoscopic therapy may require measures to prevent hepatic encephalopathy, such as administration of lactulose and avoidance of electrolyte imbalance and hepatotoxic drugs). Counseling for abstinence from alcohol should also be recommended. After initial endoscopy and sclerotherapy, repeated endoscopic sclerotherapy should be carried out every 4 to 6 weeks until all the varices are obliterated. Although not absolutely contraindicated, beta-blocker drugs used in younger patients for prevention of variceal bleeding should be used with great caution because elderly patients are more prone to congestive heart failure and chronic obstructive lung disease.

In cases of bleeding from *H. pylori*–positive peptic ulcers, eradication of the organism should be undertaken by use of an appropriate treatment regimen. Repeating endoscopy to confirm *H. pylori* eradication is not necessary. A urea breath test can confirm *H. pylori* eradication. However, in cases of bleeding from a gastric ulcer and if biopsy was not done at the time of the initial endoscopy, a biopsy must be done to rule out the possibility of malignancy. *H. pylori* status may be determined at that time as well. If the bleeding was NSAID-induced, the need for such medications should be re-evaluated and, if possible, NSAIDs should be replaced by medications that are nontoxic for gastrointestinal mucosa, such as paracetamol. However, if NSAID therapy is mandatory, cytoprotective medications, such as misoprostol, should be simultaneously administered. Likewise, in cases of anticoagulant-induced GIH, risks and benefits of anticoagulant therapy should be carefully reassessed. Definitive therapy of any isolated bleeding gastrointestinal lesion and an alternative to anticoagulation should be considered when possible, such as placement of an inferior venacaval umbrella catheter to prevent pulmonary embolism in patients with deep vein thrombosis (9).

REFERENCES

1. Reinus JF, Brandt LJ. Upper and lower gastrointestinal bleeding in the elderly. Gastroenterol Clin North Am 1990;19:293–318.
2. Schneider EL, Guralnik JM. The aging of America. Impact on health care costs. JAMA 1990;263:2335–2340.
3. Wilcox CM, Clark WS. Features associated with painless peptic ulcer bleeding. Am J Gastroenterol 1997;92;1289–1292.
4. Akhtar AJ, Boyapalli RR, Yoshikawa TT. Extraintestinal presentations of gastrointestinal hemorrhage in elderly patients of a minority population. Nurs Home Med 1997; 5:299–301.
5. Reilly HF, al-Kawas FH. Dieulafoy's lesion. Diagnosis and management. Dig Dis Sci 1991;36:1702–1707.
6. Cappell MS. A study of the syndrome of simultaneous acute upper gastrointestinal bleeding and myocardial infarction in 36 patients. Am J Gastroenterol 1995;90:1444–1449.
7. Lee JR, Fred HL. Digital rectal examination during early acute MI. Hosp Pract 1997; Sep 15, 32(9):15–16.
8. Gostout CJ, Wang KK, Ahlquist DA, Clain JE, Hughes RW, Larson MV, Petersen BT, Schroeder KW, Tremaine WJ, Viggiano TR. Acute gastrointestinal bleeding. Experience of a specialized management team. J Clin Gasteroenterol 1992;14:260–267.
9. Choudari CP, Palmer KR. Acute gastrointestinal haemorrhage in patients treated with anticoagulant drugs. Gut 1995;36:483–484.

20
Neurological Emergencies

Michael E. Mahler
UCLA School of Medicine, Los Angeles, California

This chapter will cover four neurological emergencies: altered mental status, strokes, seizures, and spinal cord compression. The emergency department physician or primary care geriatrician needs to initiate emergency management of these conditions, but in most cases consultation with neurologists and other specialists will be necessary also.

I. ALTERED MENTAL STATUS

A. Clinical Relevance

Altered mental status refers to a disorder in the quality or level of consciousness. The spectrum of severity ranges from mild confusion to deep coma, depending on the underlying cause and severity of the neurological dysfunction. Altered mental status results from systemic or neurological conditions that affect the brain diffusely or that have a more selective impact on the upper brain stem and diencephalic structures that regulate attention and arousal (Table 1). Because a wide variety of disorders result in altered mental status in the elderly, it presents a diagnostic challenge to the clinician. Because many of these conditions can be fatal, an acute or subacute alteration in mental status represents a medical emergency.

Overall, more than 5% of hospital admissions are due to conditions causing a disorder of consciousness (1). These conditions are more frequent in the elderly, who are also more vulnerable to the effects of these conditions on mental status (2). As a result, 20% of those aged 65 and older on medical and surgical wards have some degree of acute confusion.

Table 1 Common Causes of Altered Mental Status

- Systemic illness
  - Anemia
  - Cardiac dysfunction and systemic hypoperfusion
  - Electrolyte imbalance
  - Endocrinopathy
    - Adrenal insufficiency
    - Thyroid deficiency/excess
    - Abnormal glucose levels
  - Fluid imbalance
  - Infection
  - Liver disease
  - Pulmonary disease
  - Renal insufficiency
  - Vitamin deficiency
- Intoxication and withdrawal syndromes
  - Prescription drugs and polypharmacy
  - Substance abuse
  - Industrial exposures
- Neurological
  - Mass lesions
    - Tumor
    - Hematoma
    - Hydrocephalus
  - Head trauma
  - Vascular lesions
    - Acute stroke
    - Cerebral hypoperfusion/hypoxia
  - Infections
    - Abscess
    - Meningitis
    - Encephalitis
  - Seizure disorder
- Psychiatric
  - Depression
  - Mania
  - Schizophrenia

B. Clinical Manifestations and Immediate Diagnostic Approach

1. Mental Status Evaluation

Usually little difficulty exists in identifying the presence of a deep stupor or coma. For patients with milder delirium or acute confusional state (ACS), it is necessary to distinguish this from other types of confused behavior, especially that associated with a dementia syndrome. Dementia syndromes typically have an insidious onset and more stable course. In acute confusional states, the course may fluctuate rapidly. Attention and level of arousal are affected in ACS but not in the dementia syndrome.

An accurate mental status examination is necessary. For the patient in a stupor, this consists of assessing the degree of stimulation necessary to arouse a patient and the quality of responsiveness. This includes the response to verbal stimulation, eye movements and pupillary reflexes, and the nature of motor responses, whether spontaneous or reactive to various levels of stimulation.

A patient with lesser degrees of drowsiness or confusion may be characterized as having delirium or encephalopathy. Patients usually have difficulty focusing or sustaining attention. This can be manifest by confusion, distractibility, or lapses of attention. Thought processes appear incoherent, and associated memory difficulties or problems with complex cognition may be present. Patients often experience hallucinations or delusions and emotional distress or agitation. The level of alertness and arousal is reduced and may fluctuate.

2. Physical Examination

A thorough physical and neurological examination is necessary to identify possible structural lesions of the central nervous system. Hyperventilation or hypoventilation is associated with metabolic abnormalities, whereas abnormal breathing patterns such as Cheyne-Stokes respirations, cluster breathing, or apneustic breathing are associated with damage to the midbrain. Fever indicates either systemic or central nervous system infection, although serious infection can occur in the absence of fever in the elderly. The general physical examination provides clues to the presence of trauma or systemic diseases that could affect metabolic function, cardiac status, and pulmonary status. Abnormalities of pupillary function and eye movements associated with reduced consciousness usually indicate a lesion in the upper brain stem, midbrain, or diencephalon. Signs that localize to one hemisphere (unilateral sensory-motor deficits, for example) indicate a focal cerebral lesion such as stroke, subdural hematoma, tumor, or abscess.

3. Medications and Substances

The physician must also ask the patient and family about all the medications used by the patient and the use of alcohol or other psychoactive substances. Because elderly patients often use multiple medications for chronic illnesses, iatrogenic intoxication and drug interactions are frequent causes of altered mental status in this population. Psychiatric illness such as depression, mania, or schizophrenia may also cause abnormal responsiveness or apparently confused behavior, but these do not cause lapses of consciousness.

4. Laboratory and Radiological Tests

The laboratory evaluation must include a complete blood count (CBC) and white blood cell differential count; serum electrolytes, glucose, creatinine, and blood urea nitrogen (BUN); serum calcium and phosphate; and tests for liver and thyroid functions. Chest x-ray films (CXR), electrocardiogram (ECG), and urinalysis are necessary. Arterial blood gas determination and various cultures for microbiological and toxicological analyses are frequently necessary. These studies must be done immediately, and when a plausible cause for the altered mental status is not immediately apparent, additional studies are necessary. Brain imaging, either with computed tomography (CT) scan or magnetic resonance imaging (MRI) scan is necessary to diagnose structural brain lesions. Electroencephalography helps to diagnose diffuse encephalopathy and seizure disorders. Whenever meningitis is suspected, cerebrospinal fluid (CSF) must be obtained and analyzed.

C. Therapeutic Intervention

For patients in deep stupor or coma, the goals of therapy are to prevent further damage to the nervous system while correcting the underlying cause (1). Maintenance of systemic and cerebral perfusion is critical, as is protection of the airway and ventilation. Metabolic imbalances must be corrected quickly. If increased intracranial pressure (ICP) is present, determined by the clinical findings or imaging tests, it must be lowered rapidly to avoid permanent damage from brain herniation or cerebral hypoperfusion. Hypotonic fluids must be avoided, and hyperosmolar agents such as mannitol can be administered. Hyperventilation after intubation will also quickly reduce ICP. A neurosurgeon may be required to insert an ICP monitoring device to assist in the management of ICP. If the elevated ICP results from an intracranial mass (e.g., hematoma, obstructive hydrocephalus, or neoplasm), neurosurgery will be necessary.

Treatment is directed toward the underlying cause of the acute confusional state. General measures for ACS include keeping the patient in a safe and comfortable environment. If a patient is ambulatory, it is preferable to allow the individual to walk in a protected and controlled area rather than to implement restriction or restraint. To assist with sleep, low doses of short-acting hypnotics such as lorazepam or chloral hydrate are effective but should be prescribed for only a few days. If more severe agitation is present, haloperidol, 1 to 2 mg, may be used.

D. Follow-up Management

For patients in a deep stupor or coma, the prognosis depends on whether the underlying condition is corrected rapidly and when consciousness, eye movements, and reactive or spontaneous limb movements return. When these are seen within a few days, the prognosis is generally good. However, if unresponsiveness persists for as long as a week, the prognosis is unfavorable, with recovery generally associated with severe disability or persistent vegetative state. If the pupils are not reactive, corneal reflexes are absent, and oculovestibular responses are absent at 24 hours, the prognosis is also poor (1).

As long as the patient remains unresponsive, all body functions must be supported. The airway must be protected by proper positioning of the patient, frequent suctioning of secretions, and, if necessary, endotracheal intubation. Patients will need fluid management and, if the condition persists, nutrition through nasogastric or gastric tube feeding. An external or internal bladder catheter may be required to monitor urine output. The patient will need frequent turning to avoid pressure ulcers; specialized mattresses will add further protection for the skin.

Patients with ACSs generally recover after identification and correction of the underlying cause. Because the underlying cause is often a life-threatening illness, 25% to 30% of patients do not survive. Among survivors, recovery to baseline function occurs in most cases, although this may take several weeks in older patients.

II. STROKE

A. Clinical Relevance

A stroke is an acute neurological syndrome resulting from cerebrovascular disease. *Ischemic* strokes result from thrombotic occlusion of large cerebral arteries, from emboli from the heart or from atheromatous plaques in extracranial arteries, or from hypertensive vascular disease occluding small, penetrating blood vessels. *Hemorrhagic* stroke is associated with hypertension. Ruptured cerebral aneurysms and arteriovenous malformations also cause hemorrhagic stroke. In many cases, a *transient ischemic attack* (TIA) may precede a stroke by weeks or days. By definition, the manifestations of a TIA resolve completely within 24 hours or, more typically, sooner. A TIA is often a forerunner of a possible impending stroke that may be averted by appropriate and timely intervention. Whatever the type of stroke, it must be treated as a ''brain attack'' with the same urgency as one approaches a ''heart attack.''

Stroke is one of the most common causes of morbidity and mortality in the elderly. It is the third leading cause of death in the United States, with approximately 150,000 fatalities affecting 500,000 stroke patients each year. Many of the survivors have long-term impairments of neurological function. The incidence of stroke rises rapidly with increasing age, doubling in each decade (3). By the ninth decade of life, the annual incidence of stroke is approximately 1% to 2%.

B. Clinical Manifestations

Rapid determination that a stroke has occurred and quick assessment of the type of stroke is crucial because treatment to prevent permanent neuronal damage is available only within a critical window from the time of onset. Specific treatment depends on the type of stroke (3,4) as portrayed schematically in Figure 1. Two events indicate a stroke. First, the symptoms develop rapidly, within seconds or minutes. Second, the symptoms localize to an area of brain within the distribution of one of the major cerebral arteries or their branches. With a massive brain hemorrhage, additional symptoms and signs may result from increased ICP, including headache, nausea and vomiting, and depressed consciousness. For example, aphasia or right arm and leg weakness would indicate a left middle cerebral artery distribution stroke. Loss of vision in half of the visual field would suggest a contralateral posterior cerebral artery stroke. Strokes in the distribution of the vertebrobasilar system cause combinations of slurred speech, ataxia, double vision and eye movement abnormalities, cranial nerve dysfunction on one side of the face, and limb weakness on the opposite side of the body.

Dizziness in the absence of other focal neurological symptoms or signs is usually not a stroke. Similarly, a brief loss of consciousness without focal neurological symptoms or signs is not a stroke, although it may result from systemic hypotension or reduced cardiac output with an associated decrease in brain perfusion. Seizures (described later) must be differentiated from strokes, although a seizure will herald 5% to 10% of acute strokes (5). Focal neurological symptoms that develop more slowly over a period of days or weeks are more likely caused by a mass lesion.

C. Immediate Diagnostic Approach

Once a stroke is suspected on the basis of the history and physical examination, the next diagnostic steps should be to assess the type and extent of stroke with a brain imaging study, the cardiovascular status for contributing causes, and systemic and metabolic status for complicating conditions (4). These assessments must proceed rapidly in the emergency department. Tests to be done include ECG with rhythm tracing; serum electrolytes, glucose, creatinine, and BUN; arterial blood gases and CXR; CBC; prothrombin time; and partial thromboplastin time. Either a brain CT or MRI scan should be obtained as soon as possible. Both are sensitive in detecting intracranial hemorrhages or cerebral masses. The MRI scan

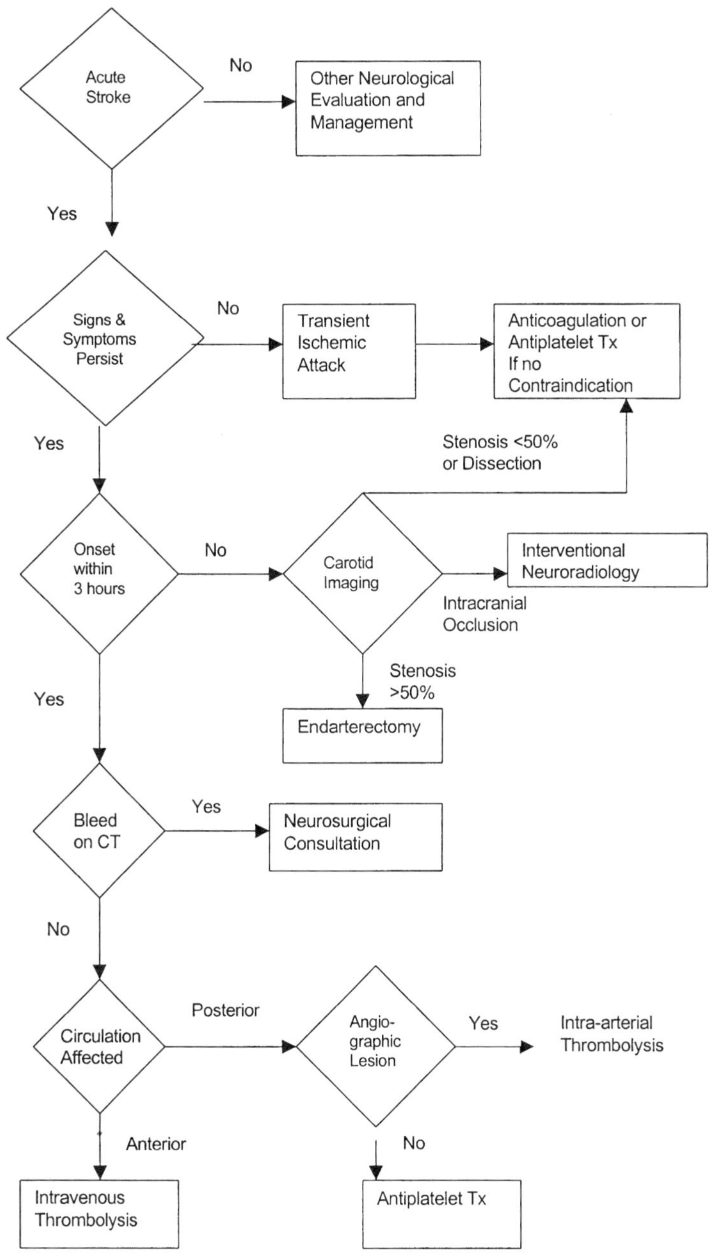

Figure 1 Ischemic flow chart. Tx, Therapy; CT, computed tomography.

is more sensitive to early changes from ischemic strokes, but both CT and MRI scans may not show the presence or full extent of a lesion for 24 hours. Brain imaging is usually sufficient to detect subarachnoid hemorrhage from a cerebral aneurysm, but CSF examination may be necessary at times.

D. Therapeutic Intervention

The airway must be protected to prevent aspiration in patients who are deeply obtunded or have impaired swallowing because of a massive cerebral infarct or hemorrhage or because of a brain stem stroke. Hypertension should be controlled carefully without too rapid a decrease in blood pressure because this may exacerbate hypoperfusion in an ischemic brain. Aggressive efforts to lower the systolic pressure to less than 140 or the diastolic pressure to less than 100 should be avoided in the immediate poststroke period.

If an ischemic (nonhemorrhagic) stroke in the territory of the anterior or middle cerebral arteries is confirmed within 3 hours of onset by clinical evaluation and cerebral imaging, intravenous thrombolytic therapy with recombinant tissue-type plasminogen activator (rTPA) leads to significant improvement in outcome (4,6). If the ischemic event affects the posterior cerebral circulation, selective intra-arterial angiography and intra-arterial thrombolysis may be considered. Because the critical time between onset and treatment is so short, relatively few patients qualify for rTPA therapy. The availability of specialized stroke teams on call to the emergency department would increase the percentage of patients qualifying for rTPA therapy.

If more than 3 hours have elapsed, other specific treatments are appropriate, depending on the type and cause of the stroke (4). Carotid Doppler ultrasonography studies of the carotid arteries may reveal atheromatous plaques that may occlude the artery or may be a source of emboli. If the artery has >50% stenosis, this should be confirmed by intra-arterial angiography or magnetic resonance angiography (MRA). Endarterectomy may be indicated for high-grade stenosis. If <50% stenosis is associated with repeated, recent TIAs (without a completed stroke) or evidence of dissection of the arterial wall, anticoagulation is indicated. However, with lower grade stenosis and a completed stroke, aspirin is the treatment of choice. If angiography or MRA reveals a tight stenosis in the posterior circulation or in the intracranial portion of the internal carotid artery, dilation by special neurororadiology techniques may be possible.

For patients with evidence of cardiac disease, echocardiography and Holter monitoring should be done to assess for a structural cardiac lesion or dysrhythmia associated with the formation of emboli. Anticoagulation may be indicated. In all cases in which anticoagulation is considered, it should not proceed if a cerebral hemorrhage, bacterial emboli from endocarditis, active peptic ulcer disease or other source of gastrointestinal bleeding, or uncontrolled and severe hypertension is present. Long-term anticoagulation is also contraindicated for patients with a tendency to fall or those who are unable to comply with a strictly supervised regimen of anticoagulant medication.

If a subarachnoid or large intracerebral hemorrhage occurs, neurosurgical consultation is essential to manage the patient. The details of surgical management are beyond the scope of this chapter but include control of cerebral edema and ICP, management of blood pressure and arterial vasospasm, and possibly surgery.

E. Follow-up Management

Two themes are important in the follow-up management of patients with stroke. One is to initiate rehabilitation to maximize neurological and functional recovery. The second is to prevent further strokes by identifying and controlling risk factors. As soon as the patient is stable, efforts should be made to mobilize the patient. With more severe strokes and paralysis, this means passive range of motion to avoid limb contractures and frequent turning of the patient to avoid skin breakdown. Although some degree of spontaneous recovery often begins within weeks, physical, occupational, and speech therapy facilitate this. Many stroke patients experience mood disturbances, particularly depression associated with left hemisphere strokes. This can be treated with counseling and antidepressant medication.

For most patients with thromboembolic stroke, daily aspirin is effective in reducing the risk of repeat ischemic events. Patients with atrial fibrillation or other cardiac sources of emboli may need to remain on oral anticoagulation therapy. Control of hypertension is also critical because this is one of the major risk factors for stroke. Those stroke patients who smoke cigarettes should be encouraged and helped to stop smoking. Patients with high cholesterol or diabetes mellitus must achieve optimal control of these conditions through proper diet and medication when necessary.

III. SEIZURES

A. Clinical Relevance

1. Types of Seizures

A seizure is a sudden alteration of neurological function resulting from abnormal and excessive discharges in cerebral neurons (5). Epilepsy refers to a group of conditions in which recurrent unprovoked seizures occur. The manifestations of the seizure and its presumed mechanism of onset determine its classification, and this has implications for diagnosis and treatment. In a seizure with primary *generalized* onset, all cortical areas apparently discharge simultaneously, resulting in a sudden loss of consciousness. In a seizure with *partial* onset, the discharge initiates in one portion of the brain, resulting in more focal symptoms and signs such as speech arrest or uncontrolled movements of one limb. A *complex partial* seizure may have an experiential aura (sensing a smell or other unusual sensation or having an unusual cognitive experience such as déjà vu) and altered behavior without a complete loss of consciousness. A seizure with partial onset may become secondarily generalized, with loss of consciousness and convulsive movements, and when this occurs rapidly, it may be difficult to differentiate from a generalized onset seizure. Usually a period of unconsciousness or confusion follows a generalized seizure. This postictal period may last from minutes to days and tends to be longer in the elderly.

2. Epidemiology

After the age of 60, the annual incidence of seizures increases exponentially. Between the ages of 20 and 60, the rate is relatively stable at approximately 40/100,000, but between 60 and 80 it rises to 140/100,000 (7). This is the result of increased frequencies in the elderly of neurological diseases associated with seizures and increased vulnerability of the aged brain to those systemic conditions that affect the seizure threshold (5). In older adults, partial onset seizures are more common (7), reflecting the fact they are commonly caused by focal brain disease. The immediate morbidity of a seizure results from the potential for injury during the convulsion, the possibility of airway obstruction during the event, and from sustained seizures (status epilepticus) causing brain injury. Although all new onset seizures require immediate attention, a seizure that is primarily or secondarily generalized represents a life-threatening emergency.

B. Immediate Diagnostic Approach

When a patient is seen in the middle of a generalized motor seizure (rhythmic and symmetric jerking movements of the limbs) or in a postictal stupor, the physician must first ensure that the patient is breathing without impairment and is protected from injury. A rubber, oral airway is usually sufficient, but family observers and medical personnel should not attempt to force any object, including their fingers, past the clenched jaws of a patient in the throes of a convulsion. A pillow or cushion should be placed under the head, and only gentle restraint may be applied to prevent the patient from injuring herself or himself against nearby objects. Forceful restraint to hold a convulsing patient still will most likely cause greater damage to the patient or the observer. Although a generalized seizure is dramatic and frightening, it usually stops spontaneously within 1 or 2 minutes. When generalized seizures are continuous for 30 minutes or recur before the patient regains consciousness, the patient is in status epilepticus. Status epilepticus is more common in the elderly (5) and requires emergency treatment.

The initial diagnostic approach and treatment measures must proceed simultaneously. Emergency medical personnel should start an intravenous (IV) line and draw blood samples for immediate analysis of serum glucose, electrolytes and calcium, complete blood count, toxicology screen, and arterial blood gases. If the patient is continuing to have convulsions, thiamine, 100 mg IV, followed by an IV bolus of dextrose (25–50 g) is administered. Giving thiamine first protects against Wernicke's encephalopathy in a patient who may be having alcohol withdrawal seizures, and the dextrose treats possible hypoglycemia, another common cause of seizures. If the patient is in status epilepticus, the next steps in treatment must be immediate. However, if the patient is not having an active seizure, further diagnostic evaluation can be made first.

The first step is to ascertain that the patient had a seizure and not another type of neurological event. When the patient has had a sudden loss of consciousness associated with sustained tonic-clonic movements and incontinence, it is fairly clear she or he has had a seizure. However, episodic loss of consciousness with brief tonic-clonic movements can also result from syncope from a variety of cardiovascular conditions in the elderly, particularly if the patient is held upright during the fainting spell. An electrocardiogram with rhythm tracings, postural blood pressure readings, and chest x-ray films may provide the clue to syncope. Transient ischemic attacks do not typically cause a loss of consciousness. However, it may be difficult to differentiate a TIA from a partial seizure. It is rare to have uncontrolled movements in a TIA; this is more characteristic of a partial seizure. Residual weakness after a partial onset seizure is called Todd's paralysis and is difficult to distinguish from a stroke without a good history. An electroencephalogram (EEG) will help if it shows characteristic abnormalities such as focal or generalized discharges (spikes).

The next phase in evaluation is to determine whether the seizure resulted from a pathological condition of the brain or whether it was provoked by a systemic condition. In the latter case, treatment will be directed at the underlying condition, and the prognosis for no further seizures is good (5). Acute metabolic abnormalities such as hypoglycemia, hyponatremia, or hypocalcemia that can precipitate a seizure will be apparent from the serum chemistries. Central nervous system (CNS) infection, such as meningitis or encephalitis, may be suggested by history of a prodromal illness, fever, stiff neck on physical examination, and elevated white blood cell count. An accurate history is necessary to diagnose an alcohol or drug withdrawal seizure, although toxicological studies of blood or urine may help. These provoked seizures tend to be generalized in onset and they may be single or multiple. Once the underlying cause is identified and treated, long-term management with antiepilepsy drugs is not necessary.

In the elderly, a variety of brain disorders can cause seizures. Unlike in children and young adults, the onset of idiopathic epilepsy is unusual in the elderly. Seizures with partial onset, such as complex partial seizures, are common whether they proceed to become generalized seizures or not (7) because they so often result from focal brain pathology, including stroke, mass lesions, and head injury. Approximately, 30% to 40% of new-onset seizures in the elderly result from stroke (5). A high percentage of patients with a cerebral neoplasm will initially be seen with a seizure. Among patients with Alzheimer's disease, perhaps 20% will have seizures as the disease progresses (8). Because chronic conditions are the cause for so many cases of seizures in the elderly, long-term treatment is necessary when these occur.

To help identify these conditions, a brain imaging study is a necessary part of the evaluation. If persistent loss of consciousness, a history or evidence of head trauma, or acute stroke has occurred, an emergency CT or MRI scan must be obtained. It helps to obtain an EEG as soon as possible after the event to help differentiate a seizure from other causes of episodic loss of consciousness. Obviously, if a CNS infection such as meningitis is suspected, CSF evaluation is critical.

C. Therapeutic Intervention

The most critical intervention is for status epilepticus. The morbidity and mortality of status epilepticus is greater in older patients in part because of the severity of the underlying diseases causing the seizures. The approach to the older patient is not different, however. To treat status epilepticus properly, the patient must be well ventilated, with intubation and ventilator assistance if necessary; must have vital signs and electrocardiographic monitoring; and must have an IV line. After thiamine and glucose have been given, lorazepam (0.1 mg/kg IV at 2 mg/min up to 4 mg) or diazepam (0.2 mg/kg IV at 5 mg/min up to 20 mg) should be given. Both are effective and both may cause respiratory depression and hypotension. Lorazepam will control seizures for a longer duration than diazepam, but its side effects will also persist longer.

As an alternative to benzodiazepines or after their use, longer acting antiepilepsy drugs are available. Either phenytoin (20 mg/kg IV at 50 mg/min) or fosphenytoin (at 20 phenytoin equivalents/kg IV at 150/min) can be given. The advantage of fosphenytoin is that it can be administered at a faster rate without cardiovascular complications. If seizures continue after these interventions, the patient must be managed in an intensive care unit by a neurologist, intensivist, and anesthesiologist. They will induce barbiturate coma or general anesthesia with intensive monitoring including continuous EEG.

D. Follow-up Management

If the patient had a first seizure but is not having continuous seizures, the physician must decide whether the patient needs long-term antiepilepsy drugs (AEDs).

This depends on the underlying cause of the seizure. Patients with provoked seizures but no intrinsic brain disorder usually do not need AEDs long term. Because many older patients experience first-time seizures as a result of underlying brain pathological conditions, the risk for recurrence is high in this group (9).

Many AEDs are now available for the treatment of generalized seizures. The older AEDs such as phenytoin, carbamazepine, and valproate are generally effective and well tolerated in the elderly. Phenobarbital tends to be too sedating and causes confusion in older patients. The standard AEDs have many drug-drug interactions, which is especially problematic in a population characterized by multiple chronic illnesses and the use of many medications. Newer agents such as gabapentin and lamotrigine appear to be effective, have a favorable side-effect profile, and have few drug interactions (9). However, studies on the specific use of these agents in the elderly have not yet been published. Although patients with seizures from brain disorders usually require therapy for life, the response to medication is usually good. Patients taking any AED need to be monitored for side effects and toxicity specific to each agent.

IV. SPINAL CORD COMPRESSION

A. Clinical Relevance

The acute or subacute onset of weakness in both legs (paraplegia) or in all limbs (quadriplegia) indicates a high probability of spinal cord injury and constitutes a true medical emergency. The syndrome may be accompanied by pain in the neck or back and may have varying degrees of sensory loss, incontinence, and autonomic dysfunction. In young adults, acute trauma is the most common cause of spinal cord injury. Neoplasms, infarction, and trauma superimposed on degenerative disease of the vertebral bodies are more likely causes in the older adult. Spinal cord compression from extradural metastases affects 5% to 10% of patients with cancer (10).

B. Clinical Manifestations

In case of acute injury to the spine, usually a combination of acute pain, loss of muscle strength, and a sensory level on the trunk below the level (within two vertebral bodies) of the spinal cord lesion are present. Spinal injury may be unilateral (Brown-Séquard syndrome) with ipsilateral loss of power and proprioception and contralateral loss of pain and temperature. Whenever serious head injury is present, an associated neck injury may be present. High cervical lesions (above C5) may cause respiratory failure. When acute paraplegia develops over hours in the absence of trauma, ischemic damage from occlusion of the vascular supply to the spinal cord may have occurred. This usually is at the midthoracic level and affects the anterior spinal cord, sparing some of the sensory fibers in the posterior cord.

Patients who have a known cancer and complain of back pain should be evaluated for possible metastases to the vertebrae as soon as possible to prevent irreversible cord damage. Other signs of spinal cord injury depend on the level of the lesion. Gait difficulties or unsteadiness may proceed to noticeable weakness of the legs with thoracic or lumbar spine lesions. Clumsiness of the hands or arm weakness indicates a cervical lesion, but the symptoms can progress to cause paralysis of the legs also. Incontinence of urine or feces occurs late in the course of an extrinsic compressive lesion.

C. Immediate Diagnostic Approach

Although plain radiographs of the spine may reveal a fracture or dislocation in cases of trauma or erosion of the vertebral bodies or pedicles in metastatic cancer, they are insufficiently sensitive to exclude spinal cord injury (11). Therefore, a MRI examination is necessary to determine whether a spinal lesion with compression exists. When the syndrome is acute, this should be done as an emergency because treatment within hours may preserve neurological function (11).

D. Therapeutic Intervention

The first step in case of fracture-dislocation of vertebral bodies is to stabilize the lesion. The patient should be moved carefully by use of a board and bracing the patient to prevent lateral and flexion-extension movements. If a high cervical lesion and respiratory failure are present, the patient may need to be intubated by use of a blind nasotracheal technique without extension of the neck. The neurosurgeon will determine whether traction reduction and immobilization are sufficient or whether decompression laminectomy is necessary (11).

When cord compression results from a neoplasm, high-dose glucocorticosteroids reduce interstitial edema. Dexamethasone, 24 mg/day in divided doses, should be used initially. Radiation therapy should then be started as soon as possible. This usually prevents new neurological symptoms and may allow some recovery of affected motor function (10).

E. Follow-up Management

The glucocorticosteroids should be continued until the completion of the radiotherapy and then tapered. The patient with quadriplegia or paraplegia will need bladder and bowel care, frequent turning and attention to the prevention of skin breakdown, and pain control. Many patients will benefit from psychological counseling to deal with the loss of neurological function.

In situations in which the primary neoplasm was not known before the discovery of the metastasis to the spine, an evaluation for common primary cancers should include chest x-ray film, mammogram or prostate-specific antigen, and abdominal CT scan (10).

REFERENCES

1. Ropper AH, Martin JB. Acute confusional states and coma. In: Braunwald E, Fauci AS, Isselbacher KS, Kasper DL, Hauser SL, Longo DL, Jameson JL, eds. Harrison's On-Line. New York: McGraw-Hill, 1999, Chap. 24.
2. Mahler ME. Confusion and delirium. In: Yoshikawa TT, Cobbs EL, Brummel-Smith K, eds. Ambulatory Geriatric Care. St. Louis: Mosby, 1993, pp 324–332.
3. Babikian VL, Kase CS, Wolf PA. Cerebrovascular disease in the elderly. In: Albert ML, Knoefel JE, eds. Clinical Neurology of Aging. 2nd ed. New York: Oxford University Press, 1994, pp 548–568.
4. Vuadens P, Bogousslavsky J. Diagnosis as a guide to stroke therapy. Lancet 1998; 352(suppl III):5–9.
5. Hauser WA. Seizures and epilepsy in the elderly. In: Albert ML, Knoefel JE, eds. Clinical Neurology of Aging. 2nd ed. New York: Oxford University Press, 1994, pp 595–610.
6. Fisher M, Bogousslavsky J. Further evolution toward effective therapy for ischemic stroke. JAMA 1998;279:1298–1303.
7. Rowan AJ. Reflections on the treatment of seizures in the elderly population. Neurology 1998;51 (suppl 4):S28–S33.
8. Romanelli MF, Morris JC, Askin K, Coben LA. Advanced Alzheimer's disease is a risk factor for late onset seizures. Arch Neurol 1990;47:847–850.
9. Consensus statements. Medical management of epilepsy: consensus conference on current clinical practice. Neurology 1998;51(suppl 4):S39–S43.
10. Gucalp R, Dutcher JP. Oncologic emergencies. In: Braunwald E, Fauci AS, Isselbacher KS, Kasper DL, Hauser SL, Longo DL, Jameson JL, eds. Harrison's On-Line. New York: McGraw-Hill, 1999, chap. 104.
11. Hauser SL. Diseases of the spinal cord. In: Braunwald E, Fauci AS, Isselbacher KS, Kasper DL, Hauser SL, Longo DL, Jameson JL, eds. Harrison's On-Line. New York: McGraw-Hill, 1999, chap. 373.

21
Psychiatric Emergencies

Indumathi Raghavan and L. Jaime Fitten
UCLA School of Medicine, Los Angeles, and Department of Veterans Affairs Medical Center, Sepulveda, California

I. CLINICAL RELEVANCE

Although other authors in this textbook have stated the demographics of aging, it is worthwhile to underscore that in 2030, one in five Americans will be 65 years and older (1). However, the population 85 years and older has been growing at a rate almost three times that of all persons age 65 and older. It has been estimated that by the turn of the century this segment of the population will be about 5.4 million, and by the year 2020 it will number 7.6 million (2).

Approximately 12% to 15% of persons 65 years and older have psychiatric problems that warrant professional psychiatric intervention (3,4). However, this percentage may dramatically increase in certain subpopulations such as those in nursing facilities. Psychiatric emergencies in the elderly constitute 10% to 15% of all emergency department (ED) visits (5–7). In the aging population, health problems become more complex and chronic and result in more physician visits. ED visits, hospitalization, and enduring disability all increase with age. In addition, growing social isolation, financial difficulties, multiple medical problems, increased somatization of psychiatric illness, and failure to recognize psychiatric problems in the ED, as well as failure to make appropriate referrals to psychiatrists, increase the psychiatric morbidity in the elderly.

Despite the evidence for increased psychopathological conditions, the use of psychiatric services by older persons has not increased proportionately, although ED visits are definitely higher in this population. Elderly patients with psychiatric problems are more likely to be referred to the ED by friends, family, police, or caregivers than by self-referral.

The principal psychiatric emergencies seen in the elderly involve anxiety and mood disorders, which include suicide attempts and acute psychoses; delusional disorders, dementia, and delirium; alcohol and substance abuse; and medication reactions and side effects that often manifest as delirium and other ''organic'' presentations.

Elderly persons tend to somatize their emotional problems more than younger persons and are afraid to reveal social, family, financial, and personal problems that they experience, which often leads to distress and visits to the ED. Individuals aged 75 and older have the highest rates of ED visits—55.8/100 persons, which is 56% greater than the national average of 35.7/100 persons (6). Women between the ages of 65 and 75 years make emergency visits more often than men do. However, this difference between sexes disappears after the age of 75. The elderly (those 65 years and older) visit the ED more frequently than their younger counterparts who are between the ages 25 and 44 (i.e., 1.7 more visits per person per year compared with the young) (8). About 5% of all ED visits by the elderly are for psychiatric problems (9,10). Several studies have examined ED psychiatric presentations in the elderly. Approximately half of ED visits by older patients result in admission to a psychiatric unit in contrast to one-third of ED visits by younger patients (11,12).

Perez and Blown, in their study on psychiatric emergency consultation in the elderly (13), found that 30% of older patients had no prior psychiatric history or treatment, and 70% were currently receiving no treatment at the time of presentation to the ED. Most studies have found that the elderly receive a diagnosis of ''organic brain syndrome'' (OBS) on presentation (9,10,14). Acute mental confusion or delirium is often a harbinger of an underlying physical illness and is a common presentation to clinicians. Studies by Lipowski (15) and Erkinjuntti et al. (16) have found that 40% of patients with dementia age 55 and older were delirious on admission, and 25% of those who were delirious were also demented.

Baker and Scholhamer (17) reported OBS, alcohol abuse, and psychotic illness as the predominant diagnostic groupings in men and psychotic illness, OBS, and adjustment disorder in women, in declining order.

As noted by Wragg and Jeste (18), the eastern Baltimore site of the Epidemiological Catchment Area (ECA) study on the care of the elderly revealed that 1% of patients aged 65 to 74 years saw a mental health specialist, but none older than the age of 75 saw such a specialist. However, 18% of those 65 to 74 years old and 10% of those 75 years and older with mental disorders reported discussing emotional problems when they visited physicians for their general medical care.

Herst (19) reported that depression, confusional states, and paranoid disorders are the most common geriatric psychiatric emergencies. Perez and Blown (13) noted that the common diagnoses seen in psychiatric emergency consultation patients were depression, side effects from psychotropic medication, and psychotic symptoms (i.e., delusions and hallucinations).

In another study on geriatric psychiatric emergencies by Thienhaus and Rowe (14), the most common diagnoses found were major affective disorders and organic mental syndromes other than dementia. In their study, one-third of patients were sent home compared with one-half sent home in a younger population. One-half of the elderly were admitted in contrast to only one-third of the younger population.

Few studies have examined the problem of suicide specifically in the elderly. This seems to be an understudied area. Approximately one in five of all suicides are by older adults (20), with white men older than 75 years of age having the highest rate in any group.

Alcohol consumption is also a serious problem. Studies have shown that 10% to 15% of all elders who seek help have an alcohol-related problem (21). One-year prevalence rates for alcoholism in patients aged 65 years and older was greater than 3%, making it the third most common psychiatric disorder in the aged population (22).

In summary, as reported by several studies, the most common psychiatric problems seen in EDs involve patients with symptoms of confusion or agitation, mood perturbations, and psychoses of varying causes. Alcohol-related problems are also still prevalent.

II. IMMEDIATE DIAGNOSTIC APPROACHES

A. General Principles

The goals of an initial ED psychiatric evaluation are to rapidly assess the patient, provide emergency treatment, and arrange for an appropriate disposition. Nonpsychiatrists, such as nurses and ED physicians, usually conduct these initial evaluations. They must, thus, be knowledgeable and sensitive to psychiatric problems in the elderly and be able to assess the urgency of a problem to request a psychiatric consultation.

It is imperative that a thorough physical examination be done to identify underlying medical and neurological conditions before obtaining psychiatric consultation because medical conditions often mimic, cause, or exacerbate psychiatric symptoms, such as depression, anxiety, agitation, delusions, and hallucinations. Furthermore, a medication history should accompany the physical examination to identify whether medications or substances are contributory to the presenting problem.

Because it is often not possible to obtain detailed information on the patient's symptoms from the patient (i.e., chronology and progression of present psychiatric symptoms, past psychiatric history and treatment, prior hospitalizations), an attempt should be made to get collateral information from family members, friends, or other caregivers or witnesses. Physicians prescribing medication to the patient should be contacted to obtain supplemental information.

A thorough mental status examination of the patient is necessary in making a diagnosis, planning treatment, and providing disposition. Eliciting information about past medical and psychiatric history through *open-ended* questions will help determine the organization of a patient's thinking processes.

The patient's ability to cooperate with the interview and relate to the interviewer, as well as his or her dress and appearance, grooming, mood, psychomotor activity, and speech, all help to reveal the patient's psychiatric status. During the course of the interview, suspiciousness, delusions, hallucinations, and suicidal and homicidal ideations may be elicited and should be thoroughly and actively explored.

The content, nature, complexity, and organization of the delusions and hallucinations should be assessed, and the interviewer should determine whether the patient has the potential to act on these delusions and hallucinations or whether he or she has specific plans to hurt himself or anyone else. Hallucinations and the sensory modality in which the patient experiences them can be a useful aid to diagnosis. In schizophrenia, they are usually auditory, whereas visual or tactile hallucinations usually suggest that an underlying medical or neurological condition as the cause.

In depressed patients, it is critical to assess their suicide potential (i.e., whether passive or active suicidal ideation is present and whether an intent or a definite plan to carry it out exists). It is important to obtain additional information about prior suicide attempts and other risk factors such as substance abuse, agitation, anxiety, hopelessness, psychotic symptoms, or alcohol abuse. These factors increase the risk of an actual attempt. Other factors are a family history of suicide or a poor support system. The depressed, potentially suicidal patient should be examined for cuts, scars, and possession of a weapon. Younger depressed patients who actually attempt suicide have often visited their physicians a short time before the attempt is made. Not much, however, is known about the activity of older patients in terms of physician visits before suicide attempts.

Cognitive functioning must also be assessed in the context of the mental status evaluation. A useful rapid screening instrument beyond tests of orientation is the popular Folstein Mini-mental State Examination. Scores of 25 or less are suggestive of a dementing process in patients with essentially normal attention capacity. Continuous performance tasks such as the ''A'' test (patient raises finger every time he hears the examiner say the letter ''A'' as the latter utters a string of about 20 consecutive letters including 6 or 7 interspersed A's) will help screen out attentionally disordered patients, such as those with delirium, who have many errors of omission and commission on this test. ED physicians should be familiar with the administration and interpretation of tests that help screen for delirium and dementia.

B. Confusion/Agitation

Cognitive problems in association with behavioral disorders are fairly common in older persons. Delirium accounts for most acute confusional states seen in the ED when patients are 65 years of age and older and will be discussed in more detail in another chapter in this book. (See Chapter 20.) Dementia is often associated with delirium.

Elderly patients are often brought to the ED from nursing homes and other institutional settings in an agitated or aggressive state. These patients produce an excessive amount of purposeless activity, motoric or vocal or both, and may threaten or strike out at their entourage. About 80% to 90% of nursing home patients have a physical or psychiatric illness. Of these, 50% have dementia and 20% to 30% have a diagnosis of depression (23). These conditions are believed to play an important causal role in the behavioral disruptions that bring them to the attention of the ED.

A common cause of agitation is delirium. Agitation can also be a result of dementia, particularly when patients have psychotic symptoms, such as delusions or hallucinations, or when environmental or caregiver stressors make excessive demands on these demented patients and overwhelm them. This is referred to as a ''catastrophic reaction.''

Importantly, agitation can also result from a serious underlying physical illness and can be associated with aggressive or assaultive behavior that may disrupt family life and result in earlier institutional placement.

C. Mood Disorders

Common mood disorders with criteria as described in the *Diagnostic and Statistical Manual of Mental Disorders*, fourth edition (DSM IV), generally have a lower prevalence in patients older then 65 years. The ECA study showed that 1% to 2% of the elder population had DSM III major depressive disorder. This is in contrast to the 4% prevalence rate reported in that study for younger individuals. Other studies, however, have shown that 10% of elders living in the community experienced depressive symptoms that do not meet criteria for a DSM IV major depressive disorder but nonetheless may be clinically significant. Furthermore, the prevalence of depression is about 50% in patients living in institutions providing long-term or short-term care, whereas the prevalence of depression in the medically ill is about 12% to 36% (24).

Depression in elderly patients frequently can have an atypical or masked presentation. A despondent mood is not as common a presenting symptom as it is in younger patients. The older person may minimize or even deny being depressed when asked about the state of his or her mood by the physician. Depressive symptoms and signs can be masked by concomitant medical or neurological illness, or depressed patients can have amplified somatic complaints or minimize or deny their depressive symptoms, which then often go undiagnosed. For example, an increase in chronic pain in a patient with degenerative joint disease without any new, objective findings may lead to increased doctor-seeking or medication-seeking behavior. If depression is not suspected and excluded, an important treatment opportunity will be missed, and unnecessary interventions may ensue. Depression reaches psychotic proportions about 5% of the time. Delusions (false beliefs) may be more common than hallucinations (false perceptions), although both can be present. Delusions often are mood congruent as they are in younger patients, but they may not be. Catatonia (manneristic, stereotypic, or akinetic behaviors) or paranoia may also be present. Refusal to get out of bed, lack of self-care for basic needs, or even eating behavior changes can raise concerns in family members and result in an ED visit. Depression can also occur as a result of losses—death of a spouse, financial reverses, and physical illness.

Depression is highly correlated with suicide attempts. However, a few studies have examined this relationship in the aged. Elderly patients who attempt suicide often succeed. They account for 25% of all suicides (20). Major risk factors include age 75 years and older, white, male, widowed, presence of hypochondriacal symptoms, recent significant losses, and agitation. It is important for the ED physician to be aware of the various risk factors that might increase the chances of an elderly patient attempting suicide and to probe for their presence in older individuals presenting to the ED without an obvious acute medical illness.

Bipolar disorder (manic-depression) has a prevalence of 0.1% in the general population and is largely an understudied area in the elderly. Most commonly, bipolar illness is chronic and lifelong after an onset in early adulthood. However, the illness can also begin in later years. A large proportion of these late-onset manic patients have underlying brain pathosis (e.g., small strokes) and may come to the ED in the hypomanic state (e.g., irritability, poor sleep, racing thoughts) rather than a full manic episode (severe hyperactivity, grandiosity, insomnia, flight of ideas, psychosis, hypersexuality, etc,).

D. Anxiety Disorders

Anxiety disorders have a high prevalence in the elderly just as they do in the younger patient population. These disorders are the least studied group of psychiatric problems in the elderly. In the aged, anxiety is often comorbid with other psychiatric and medical conditions and often occurs concomitantly with a serious physical illness. Comorbidity with depressive disorder is particularly high in the aged. When anxiety accompanies depression, the risk of suicide increases in this already-at-risk population.

The rates of anxiety and depression combined are greater than 80% in institutionalized patients (25). These combined conditions are particularly difficult to differentiate in the frail elderly who may be referred or sent to the ED. Alcohol-dependent patients have a higher prevalence of anxiety disorder and often use alcohol to self-medicate the disorder. Anxiety is also highly correlated with cognitive decline and is often accompanied by early dementia.

Although *de novo* panic disorder is uncommon in older patients, those with a lifelong disorder do age and can remain symptomatic. Patients with panic attacks visit the ED frequently. These patients often believe they are having real cardiac events (i.e., angina or myocardial infarction) when they experience palpitations, shortness of breath, chest pain, or discomfort. They experience fear of dying or total loss of control sometimes leading to air hunger and hyperventilation, which can mimic acute pulmonary syndromes. Other phobic disorders (e.g., agoraphobia) or generalized anxiety disorder may occasionally be seen in the ED. Underlying medical conditions such as endocrine abnormalities, cardiac diseases, and pulmonary disorders should be excluded because they may produce similar symptoms as anxiety. A medication history for both prescribed and over-the-counter drugs should be reviewed because in older patients multiple medications can produce symptoms of anxiety as either a side effect or a drug-drug interaction.

E. Acute Psychosis

Older patients seen in the ED with psychoses need to be evaluated carefully for underlying medical or neurological problems. Medical or neurological causes of psychoses in the elderly include delirium and dementia, although depression, when severe, can also be seen with psychosis as noted earlier. Approximately 50% of elderly patients with delirium have psychotic symptoms. Delusions, when present, are persecutory in tone and not well systematized, and hallucinations, if present, are usually visual or tactile rather than auditory. It is also important to exclude sensory deficits as contributors to the development of psychotic symptoms in this population because sensory deprivation over time can be complicated by psychosis.

Psychotic patients can be anxious and agitated. Demented patients frequently experience psychosis that can be accompanied by agitation, particularly in the later stages of the illness. Wragg and Jeste (18) reported delusions (usually persecutory) in 30% of patients with Alzheimer's disease. Hallucinations (visual slightly more common than auditory) are reported in 21% to 49% of patients with Alzheimer's disease.

Mood disorders (depression or mania) may be seen with psychotic features and accompany agitation. A good history and mental status examination will determine whether mood symptoms preceded the onset of psychotic symptoms. Psychotic depression occurs more frequently in older patients than in younger patients.

Patients with a diagnosis of delusional disorder (DSM-IV) can be seen in the ED. Their delusions are usually chronic, well systemized, and more focused on a particular theme or person, unlike those seen in patients with dementia or delirium. Hallucinations, if present, are not prominent. In contrast to the schizophrenic, demented, or delirious patient, these patients are well preserved in other areas of cognitive and daily functioning.

Elderly patients diagnosed with late-onset schizophrenia can be seen in the ED with bizarre delusions, often persecutory in nature, and hallucinations that are usually auditory in nature. An acute exacerbation of chronic schizophrenia may also be seen with delusions or hallucinations in the elderly. This is less frequent, however, compared with younger patients.

Alcohol abuse or dependence or abuse of other substances can lead to delusions or hallucinations. It is important to remember that the older alcoholic individual is more susceptible to the toxic effects of alcohol at lower blood alcohol levels, even though the person is accustomed to alcohol, and that the symptoms of medical illness that bring him or her to the ED may mask a dependence or withdrawal. Abuse of over-the-counter medications (such as those containing anticholinergics or antihistaminics) or of prescribed medications can result in acute psychotic symptoms. Hallucinations tend to be visual or tactile rather than auditory. Delusions, when present, are not well systemized, are fleeting, and often occur on a background of delirium. These older patients may be brought to the ED by family or law enforcement authorities when they become a danger to themselves or to those around them or when they act out on their delusions or hallucinations and become disruptive.

In summary, it is important for the ED physician to attend to underlying medical, neurological, or substance abuse problems in these older patients before seeking psychiatric consultation. In contrast to younger patients, medical and neurological conditions rather than schizophrenia, mania, or depression are more often the cause of psychotic symptoms in the elderly. The *incidence* of traditional psychiatric disorders (as noted earlier) presenting as acute psychoses is more common in younger than older patients.

F. Dementia and Delirium

Delirium is a common ED presentation and often is superimposed on dementia. Older patients, most commonly the cognitively impaired, are sensitive to the effects of underlying medical, neurological conditions, and concurrent multiple medications and thus need to be thoroughly evaluated. Common infections, such as urinary tract infections or pneumonia, can produce sensorium changes and delirium early on as can a worsening congestive heart failure, lung disease, or small strokes. Because this population is such a high consumer of medications, it is important to exclude drug-drug interactions, drug side effects, or abuse of over-the-counter preparations, all of which can lead to delirium. A more detailed account of the causes of delirium is presented elsewhere in this book. (See also Chapter 20.)

Alzheimer's disease, vascular dementia, and diffuse Lewy body disease account for 75% of all dementias in patients 65 years and older. These patients often come to the ED with agitation, confusion, psychotic symptoms (either delusions or hallucinations), or aggressive behavior. The caregiver typically brings the patient in when ''wandering'' or aggressiveness or uncooperativeness can no longer be managed. ''Sundowning'' at home or in the nursing facility may also result in an ED visit. Patients with dementia typically become more confused, disoriented, and even agitated when natural light and other stimuli are gradually withdrawn from their environment, which usually happens in the early evening and night (hence, the term ''sundowning''). In addition, a ''catastrophic'' reaction may result in an ED visit. This can occur when excessive demands are placed on demented patients. They may react with agitation or aggression because they are unable to process and withstand added environmental, psychological, or caregiver-induced stress placed on them.

It is important in these presentations to exclude remediable causes of dementia. Approximately 10% of all dementias are potentially reversible. Assessment of the acuteness of the condition and identification of rapid worsening of cognitive functioning, as well as proper assessment of the potential for normal pressure hydrocephalus, hypothyroidism, electrolyte imbalance, the dementia syndrome of depression, or substance abuse, will lead to the correct diagnosis and the appropriate corrective intervention.

G. Elder Abuse

Elder abuse is discussed in Chapter 24.

III. THERAPEUTIC INTERVENTION

A. Agitation and Confusion

After acute medical and neurological problems are excluded, the differential diagnosis should include other causes such as dementia, agitated depression, hypomania, medication side effects, and drug interactions. This might require admitting the patient to a medical or psychiatric ward, as appropriate, for further evaluation and management.

A low dose of a short-acting benzodiazepine such as lorazepam (0.5–1 mg 4–6h) or a low dose of a neuroleptic may be used to contain the agitation. In the elderly, the newer atypical agents such as risperidone and olanzapine are useful in low oral doses such as 1.0 to 2.0 mg of risperidone or 2.5 to 5.0 mg of olanzapine, particularly if psychosis is present and agitation is not severe. Haloperidol has been used extensively in doses as low as 0.5 mg orally every 6 hours and has been effective, although its potent extrapyramidal side effects are not well tolerated by the frail and by the very old. However, in more severe agitation, when the patient may become a danger to self or others, haloperidol, 1.0 to 3.0 mg (dose depending on age), may be the treatment of choice because it can be administered parenterally and has a rapid onset of action. It is important to remember that because of diminished organ reserve, altered pharmacokinetics, and increased disease burden that are characteristic of elderly patients, it is essential to start with low psychotropic doses (one-third to one-half normal) and increase doses gradually and cautiously only if clearly indicated.

B. Mood Disorders

Once underlying medical conditions that could mimic or cause depression, such as hypercalcemia or hypothyroidism, have been excluded, it is imperative to evaluate suicide risk in the patient. The degree of suicide risk determines the patient care plan and need for hospitalization. Patients who have significant depression accompanied by identifiable suicide risk factors should be evaluated by a psychiatrist, as should patients who are evasive or noncommittal about their suicidal thoughts.

Evaluation of the severity of the depression forms an important part of the treatment plan. Among the conditions to be evaluated are whether the patient has lost a significant amount of weight or whether the depression is so severe that the patient is refusing or unable to feed himself or herself. Marked psychomotor retardation may also dramatically incapacitate a patient. In severe cases, in which patients are unable to feed or care for themselves, a course of electroconvulsive therapy (ECT) will help improve vegetative and motor functions much faster than antidepressants. ECT would, however, require admission to the psychiatric unit. Psychotic depressions, which are more common in aged patients, also respond well to ECT. When psychosis is present, psychiatric consultation should be sought. In milder forms, psychotic depression can be treated with well-tolerated antidepressants such as one of the selective serotonin reuptake inhibitors (e.g., paroxetine, sertraline, citalopram) starting with one-half the normal adult initial dose and titrating up gradually until response is observed and a maintenance dose is established. Adding a low-dose neuroleptic such as risperidone, 0.25 to 1.0 mg/day, from the beginning helps to control psychotic symptoms.

C. Acute Psychoses

In the ED acute psychosis is often accompanied by substantial agitation and may require immediate symptomatic treatment regardless of cause. Once the diagnosis of psychosis and agitation is made, palliative treatment may be initiated while the cause is investigated. A low-dose antipsychotic that can be given intravenously or intramuscularly should be used. Low-dose haloperidol, as described earlier, or a short-acting, parenteral benzodiazepine is an effective treatment for this condition in the ED.

D. Dementia and Delirium

The detailed management of delirium is addressed elsewhere in this book. (See Chapter 20.) Usually the patient with cognitive deterioration caused purely by a dementing process does not initially come to the ED unless an acute medical, environmental, or interpersonal stressor has caused decompensation leading to worsened cognition and behavior. In some instances, the modest stress that leads to cognitive or behavioral decompensation may serve to reveal the new diagnosis of dementia, which was not obvious earlier. In other cases, a known demented patient is brought in with a recent history of rapid cognitive or behavioral deterioration. In either case, the task of the ED physician is to identify the factors involved in the decompensation, particularly those of medical and neurological origin, that can be treated. It is, therefore, important to obtain as accurate a history from collaterals as possible and to perform a complete physical and neurological examination of the patient with cognitive and behavioral impairment, whether dementia has been previously established or is only currently suspected.

Laboratory tests intended to identify medical causes of decompensation, such as complete blood count, electrolytes, blood urea nitrogen, urinalysis, and thyroid function tests, should be obtained. If new, focal, or lateralizing neurological signs are present, neuroimaging of the head should be performed. Patients with dementia complicated by other acute medical comorbidities may require hospitalization. These patients often have a delirium superimposed on their dementia, and it is important to remember that the demented patient recovers slowly from delirium. If dementia is detected for the first time and decompensating factors are satisfactorily addressed, an appropriate referral (e.g., geriatric psychiatrist or neurologist) should be made to ensure that the correct diagnosis of dementia type is eventually reached. This has treatment and management implications for such conditions as Alzheimer's disease, vascular dementia, and the dementia syndrome of depression. The ED physician can always manage the acute psychiatric and behavioral manifestations of the demented patient with sedative or neuroleptic medications in the manner suggested previously.

IV. FOLLOW-UP MANAGEMENT

Once the evaluation of the acute phase has been completed, a disposition must be made. If the patient with psychiatric symptoms is sufficiently medically ill, he or she may require hospitalization and, in some cases, eventual institutional placement for variable lengths of time. If psychiatric consultation was obtained, it is important for the consulting psychiatrist to take appropriate steps to establish follow-up care for the patient. This may occur as an inpatient in a psychiatric unit if behavioral and psychiatric symptoms are severe enough and if functional capacity is greatly reduced. In milder cases, follow-up care can be provided as an outpatient after the patient is discharged from the ED. Outpatient options for treatment include pharmacotherapy with psychotropic or cognitive enhancers, interpersonal therapies such as individual or group psychotherapy, and supportive day treatment centers for the cognitively impaired. In the case of cognitively compromised patients, the patient's family or caregiver should be informed and instructed with regard to the treatment options and recommendations. These patients, once medically and psychiatrically clear, need to be released only under the care of a significant other. Adult protective services may be needed in the case of the potentially abused patient.

REFERENCES

1. United States Bureau of the Census, Washington DC, 1985.
2. Gustafson DH, Sainfort F, Johnson SW, Sateia M. Measuring quality of care in psychiatric emergencies: construction and evaluation of a bayesian index. Health Serv Res 1993;28:131–158.
3. McCraig LF. National Hospital Ambulatory Medical Care Survey. 1992 Emergency Department Summary Advance Data from Vital and Health Statistics, No. 245, Hyattsville, MD: National Center for Health Statistics, 1994.
4. Colenda C, Greenwald BS, Crossett JH, Husain MM, Kennedy GJ. Barriers to effective psychiatric emergency services for elderly persons. Psych Serv 1997;4(3):321–325.
5. Beland F, Lemay A, Philibert L, Maheux B, Gravel G. Elderly patients' user of hospital-based emergency services. Med Care 1991;29(5):408–416.
6. Tueth MJ. Diagnosing psychiatric emergencies in the elderly diagnostics. Am J Emerg Med 1994;12(3):364–369.
7. Ettinger WH, Cusani JA, Coon PJ, Muller DC, Piazza-Arpel K. Patterns of use of the emergency department in elderly patients. J Gerontol 1987;42:638–642.
8. Johnson RE, Mullooly JP, Greenlick MR. Morbidity and medical care utilization of old and very old persons. Health Serv Res 1990;25(4):549–665.
9. Waxman H, Dubin W, Klein M, Weiss KJ, Carner EA. Geriatric psychiatry in the ED, II: Evaluation and treatment of geriatric and non-geriatric admissions. J Am Geriatr Soc 1984;32(5):343–349.
10. Waxman H, Carner E, Dubin W, Klein M. Geriatric psychiatry in the ED: Characteristics of geriatric and non-geriatric admissions. J Am Geriatr Soc 1982;30:427–432.
11. Blixen CE. Differences in the use of hospital based outpatient mental health services by the elderly. IMAGE: J Nurs Scholarship 1994(Fall);26(3):195–200.

12. Burns B, Taube C. Mental health services in general medical care and in nursing homes. In: Fogel B, Furino A, Gottlieb G, eds. Mental Health Policy for Older Americans. Protecting Minds at Risk. Washington DC: American Psychiatric Press, 1990, pp 63–84.
13. Perez EL, Blown J. Psychiatric emergency consultations to elderly patients in a Canadian general hospital. J Am Geriatr Soc 1986;34:91–94.
14. Thienhaus O, Rowe C. Geropsychiatric emergency services utilization and outcome predictors. Hosp Commun Psych 1989;39(12):1301–1305.
15. Lipowski ZJ. Delirium in the elderly patient. N Engl J Med 1989;320:578–582.
16. Erkenjuntti T, Wikstron J, Palo J, Autio L. Dementia among medical inpatients: evaluation of 2000 consecutive admissions. Arch Intern Med 1986;146:1923–1926.
17. Baker FM, Scholhamer N. The evaluation of elderly patients by a psychiatric emergency services. J Natl Med Assoc 1988;80(2):793–799.
18. Wragg RE, Jeste DV. Overview of depression and psychosis in Alzheimer's disease. Am J Psychiatry 1989;146:577–587.
19. Herst LD. Emergency psychiatry for the elderly. Psychiatr Clin North Am 1983;6: 27–280.
20. Conwell Y. Suicide in elderly patients. In: Schneider LS, Reynolds CF, Lebowitz BD, eds. Diagnosis and Treatment of Depression in Late Life. Washington DC: American Psychiatric Press, Inc., 1994:397–418.
21. National Institute Study on Alcohol and Alcohol Abuse Amongst the Elderly. A study of legal drug use by elder Americans. Washington DC: US Department of Health Education and Welfare, 1979.
22. Kaplan HI, Sadock BJ. Comprehensive Textbook of Psychiatry. 6th ed. 1995; Vol 2. Anxiety disorders, Section 49.6, Lippincott Williams & Wilkins, Philadelphia, PA, 1995, pp 2572–2573.
23. Blazer D. Depression in the elderly. N Engl J Med 1989;320:164–166.
24. Sadavoy J, Smith I. Depression in geriatric patients and chronic medical illness. Int J Geriatr Psychiatry 1990;5:187–192.
25. Rovner BW, Kafonek S, Filipp L, Lucas MJ, Folstein MF. Prevalence of mental illness in a community nursing home. Am J Psychiatry 1986;143:1446–1449.

22
Acute Vision Impairment or Loss

Charles Wesley Flowers, Jr., and Glenville A. March, Jr.
Charles R. Drew University of Medicine and Science, Martin Luther King, Jr.–Charles R. Drew Medical Center, and Jules Stein Eye Institute, UCLA School of Medicine, Los Angeles, California

I. APPROACH TO EYE EXAMINATION

Acute visual loss is an ophthalmic emergency that requires prompt diagnosis and treatment. In the elderly, visual loss is nothing less than catastrophic, considering that many of these individuals have pre-existing physical disabilities, mental disabilities, or both. Consequently, the loss of sight in one or both eyes can significantly compromise their ability to function in society and diminish their quality of life. Age is the single most important predictor of blindness and visual impairment, with visual impairment being the second most prevalent physical disability observed among the elderly population (1).

Because much of the elderly's ongoing medical care is provided in a primary care setting, the primary care physician is often the first to encounter these patients during an episode of acute visual loss. Thus, it becomes imperative that primary care physicians possess the requisite knowledge to perform an adequate preliminary assessment and initiate the appropriate therapy before referral. Early diagnosis and treatment can often avert permanent visual loss in these patients.

A. Medical History

The approach to any patient with acute visual loss begins with a thorough medical history and a detailed history of the present illness describing the nature and extent of the visual loss. On initial examination, the examiner must determine

Table 1 Clinical Parameters Used to Assess Acute Visual Loss in the Elderly

1. The immediate circumstances surrounding the visual loss (e.g., was the patient involved in strenuous activity or subject to physical trauma?).
2. Time of visual loss versus the time of presentation.
3. Previous occurrences of visual loss.
4. Rate of visual loss (sudden versus gradual).
5. Binocular versus monocular involvement. If monocular, how and when was the visual loss detected?
6. Transient versus sustained?
7. The presence or absence of pain or headache. If pain is present, what is the temporal sequence of the pain in relation to the visual loss?
8. Is visual loss confined to a particular portion of the visual space (central versus peripheral vision or both)?
9. The presence of pre-existing ocular disease or previous ocular surgery or trauma.

the nature and extent of the visual loss with respect to nine important clinical parameters (Table 1). Eliciting information with respect to these parameters provides an effective way of narrowing the differential diagnosis and rapidly identifying the cause of the patient's visual loss (Table 2). Ascertaining the immediate circumstances surrounding the visual loss is important in any patient with a systemic condition that may have direct or indirect ocular manifestations (i.e., diabetes mellitus, hypertension, coronary artery disease, and cerebrovascular disease). Patients with advanced cardiovascular or cerebrovascular disease are prone to losing vision during physical exertion either from vertebrobasilar or carotid artery insufficiency or hypotension from a cardiac dysrhythmia. These patients may also experience acute visual loss during strenuous bowel movements or straining to urinate resulting from a vasomotor response. Moreover, elderly patients who sustain head or periorbital trauma from falls or other forms of incidental trauma may experience visual loss from direct trauma to ocular structures or damage to intracranial structures of the visual pathway.

B. Establishing Differential Diagnosis

Table 2 illuminates how establishing monocular versus binocular involvement is a critical differentiating feature in determining the cause of acute visual loss. In general, bilateral processes tend to localize the pathological insult to the central nervous system, whereas unilateral processes tend to localize the pathological insult to the eye. Visual loss can often be the initial sign of an impending stroke

Table 2 Clinical Features Differentiating the Predominant Causes of Visual Loss in the Elderly

	Clinical feature			
Differential diagnosis	Unilateral vs bilateral	Transient vs prolonged	Painful vs painless	Central vs peripheral vision loss
Central retinal artery occlusion	Unilateral	Prolonged	Painless	Both
Branch retinal artery occlusion	Unilateral	Prolonged	Painless	Peripheral
Central retinal vein occlusion	Unilateral	Prolonged	Painless	Both
Branch retinal vein occlusion	Unilateral	Prolonged	Painless	Both
Anterior ischemic optic neuropathy (arteritic/nonarteritic)	Unilateral	Prolonged	Painless	Both
Vitreous hemorrhage	Unilateral	Prolonged	Painless	Both
Acute angle-closure glaucoma	Unilateral	Prolonged	Painful	Both
Amaurosis fugax	Unilateral	Transient	Painless	Both
Chiasmal ischemic syndrome	Bilateral	Prolonged	Painless	Peripheral
Pituitary apoplexy	Bilateral	Prolonged	Painful	Peripheral
Papilledema	Bilateral	Transient	Painful	Both
Vertebrobasilar artery insufficiency	Bilateral	Transient	Painless	Both
Orthostatic hypotension	Bilateral	Transient	Painless	Both

or ruptured cranial aneurysm. Moreover, poorly controlled systemic diseases, such as hypertension or cardiac dysrhythmias can manifest through transient acute bilateral visual loss.

Establishing the temporal nature of the visual loss also provides insight into the underlying cause. Transient visual loss is defined as visual loss varying from slight dimming or blurring of vision to no light perception lasting seconds to hours and returning to normal or baseline within 24 hours. Most often it lasts seconds to minutes. Transient visual loss usually signals a central nervous system or systemic abnormality in much the same way as an acute bilateral decrease in vision. An acute loss of vision that persists beyond 1 hour requires emergency evaluation and treatment. It is important to note that a sustained acute bilateral loss of vision is an uncommon occurrence and is usually due to a cerebrovascular accident. In most cases of acute bilateral visual loss, further questioning reveals that visual loss occurred in one eye first, and the sudden loss reported by the patient was noted when the fellow eye became involved. This situation commonly arises among the elderly, who have a reduced sensory awareness as a result of aging or dementia.

Pain in association with acute visual loss is an extremely helpful clinical sign. First, a limited number of clinical entities produce pain in association with visual loss, and thus pain substantially narrows the differential diagnosis.

Pain in and around the eye typically localizes the disease process to the eye (i.e., infectious keratitis, acute angle-closure glaucoma, optic neuritis), whereas headache localizes the disease process to the central nervous system (i.e., pituitary apoplexy, intracranial aneurysm). Pain in the setting of acute visual loss is an ominous clinical sign because many of the associated clinical entities have dire consequences for life or vision if therapy is not instituted in a timely manner. Therefore, the presence of pain should heighten the urgency with which a patient is evaluated and treated.

C. Essential Components of Eye Examination

In the setting of acute visual loss, the ophthalmic examination performed by the primary care physician should consist of the following five elements.

Visual acuity
External examination
Confrontational visual fields
Pupillary examination
Ophthalmoscopic examination

Ideally, visual acuity testing should be performed at distance with a Snellen chart and at near with a Rosenbaum card. If a distance Snellen chart is not available, near vision testing will suffice. If neither measurement device is available, visual acuity can simply be assessed by having the patient attempt to read an office magazine or educational brochure. Newspaper and magazine print roughly equates to a near visual acuity of 20/40. The patient should be wearing the eyeglasses or contact lenses normally used for distance or near viewing. The main focus of attention is the visual deficit that cannot be restored with corrective lenses. If the patient is unable to see the largest Snellen letter, the visual acuity should be measured according to the following protocol.

Counting fingers: Ask the patient to count the number of fingers you hold up at a distance of 1 to 5 feet. It is important to measure the vision in the eyes separately and to record the distance that the fingers were counted correctly (e.g., count fingers at 3 feet).

Hand motion: If the patient cannot see well enough to count fingers, ask the patient to distinguish between your horizontal and vertical hand movements at 1 foot. This maneuver should also be performed on each eye separately.

Light perception: If the patient is unable to see hand movements, illuminate each eye separately with a bright light and ask whether the patient sees the light.

The external examination need only entail inspecting for ocular redness (conjunctival injection) and corneal opacification with a penlight. The presence of either of these signs immediately localizes the disease process to the eye and warrants immediate ophthalmic referral. Conjunctival injection is a nonspecific sign that is seen anytime the eye is inflamed. Corneal opacification, on the other hand, is a much more specific sign and often has dire implications. The presence of corneal opacification or haze should alert one to the possibility of an infectious keratitis, which if not treated in a timely manner could lead to corneal perforation within 24 hours. Corneal opacification or haze in the setting of acute visual loss should also alert one to the possibility of acute angle-closure glaucoma.

Confrontational visual field testing provides a quick way of screening for gross visual pathway abnormalities. This test lacks the sensitivity to detect small visual field defects, and thus visual field deficits detected during this examination often indicate that the field defects are large and the damage to the visual pathway is substantial.

The pupillary examination provides a sensitive means of assessing optic nerve function. The direct light response and the swinging light test are used to evaluate patients with acute visual loss. The direct light response assesses both the efferent (pupillary constriction) and afferent (retina and optic nerve function) limb of the pupillary light reflex arc (Figure 1). Thus, incomplete or absent pupillary constriction on the direct light response indicates a defect is present in either the efferent or afferent limb of the pupillary light reflex.

The swinging light test is then used to determine whether the defect involves the afferent limb. This test is usually performed after the direct light response and is performed by swinging a penlight between the two eyes (Figure 2). By comparing the direct and consensual pupillary responses in each eye individually, the swinging light test is used to detect the presence of a relative afferent pupillary defect (rAPD) or Marcus Gunn pupil. A rAPD signifies a disturbance in the afferent limb of the pupillary light reflex, which typically localizes the lesion to the optic nerve or retina. It is important to note, however, that damage to greater than 90% of the retina is required to produce a rAPD, whereas relatively subtle damage to the optic nerve can produce this clinical sign. Thus, the presence of a rAPD usually indicates optic nerve compromise.

Ophthalmoscopic evaluation with a direct ophthalmoscope is specifically used to check for the presence of normal red reflexes in each eye, the presence of retinal hemorrhages or exudates, and the presence of optic nerve pathology. Normal red reflexes indicate that the optical media of the eye (i.e., cornea, anterior chamber, lens, and vitreous) are free of disease. Assessment of the optic nerve

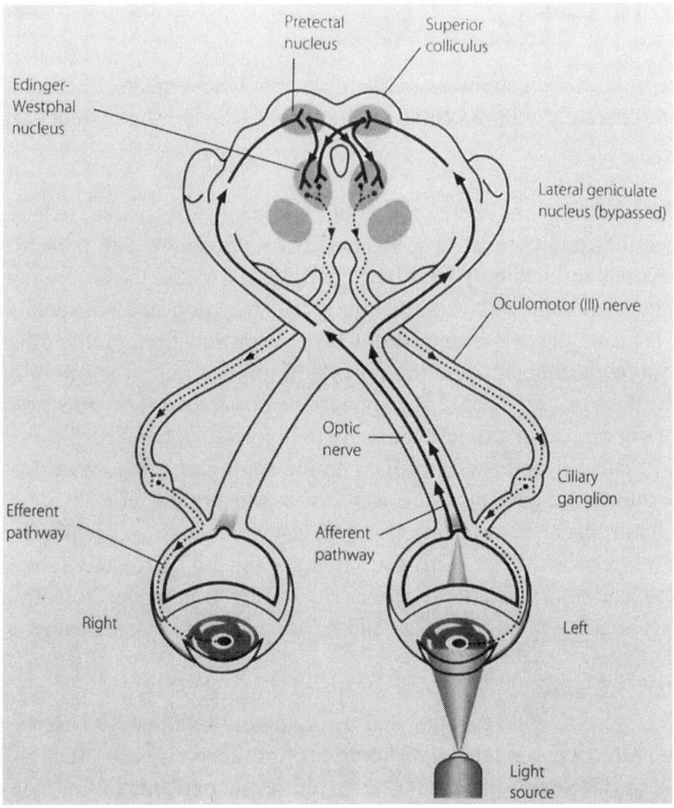

Figure 1 Pupillary light reflex pathway. In this schematic, the solid line represents the afferent pathway and the dotted line represents the efferent pathway. Light falling on the left retina will generate pupillary impulses that travel up the left optic nerve to the chiasm, where some of the impulses cross and travel up the right optic tract and some of the impulses continue on up the left optic tract. From the optic tracts the pupillary impulses bypass the lateral geniculate body to synapse in the pretectal nuclei. From the pretectal nuclei pupillary impulses pass to the Edinger-Westphal nuclei, which form part of the third cranial nerve nuclear complex. In traveling from the pretectal nuclei to the Edinger-Westphal nuclei, pupillary impulses are distributed to the nuclei on both the right and left side. The afferent pupillary impulses that reach the left and right Edinger-Westphal nuclei stimulate the cells that initiate the efferent pupillary light reflex pathway by triggering the pupillary constrictor response. From the Edinger-Westphal nuclei, pupillary constrictor impulses travel through the pupillary motor fibers within the third cranial nerves on both sides to each iris sphincter, causing both pupils to constrict. Thus, light stimulation in one eye leads to bilateral innervation of the Edinger-Westphal nuclei because of the crossing of fibers at the chiasm and the pretectal nuclei, which in turn produces bilateral pupil constriction (direct and consensual pupillary response). (From Gurland JE, Hamed LM, Johns KJ, Wilhelmus KR, Wilson II FM. Pupillary examination. In: Wilson II FM, ed. Practical Ophthalmology: A Manual for Beginning Residents. San Francisco: American Academy of Ophthalmology, 1996, p 127.)

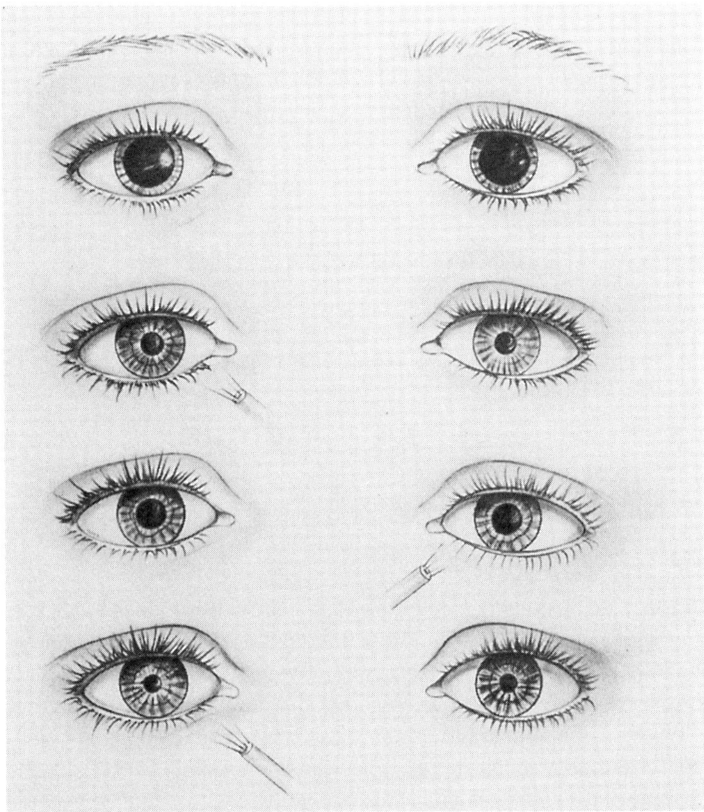

Figure 2 Swinging-light test. The swinging light test entails placing the patient in a dimly lit room and having him or her fixate on a distant target. The examiner then shines a penlight into one eye of the patient. (By convention, the test begins in the right eye.) The penlight is then swung rapidly over the bridge of the nose to directly illuminate the opposite eye. Normally because of the consensual light reflex, illumination of one eye causes the pupil to constrict equally in the illuminated and nonilluminated eye. As the light passes over the bridge of the nose, there is a momentary period when neither eye is illuminated and thus both pupils begin to dilate slightly. Once the light falls on the previously nonilluminated eye, the pupils in each eye should constrict. If the pupils dilate, this is an abnormal response and indicates optic nerve dysfunction or a rAPD. (From Liesegang TJ, McPhee TJ. Neuro-ophthalmology. In: Bartley GB, Liesegang TJ, eds. Essentials of Ophthalmology. Philadelphia: J.B. Lippincott, 1992, p 173).

should entail evaluation of the nerve color (pink, normal; white, abnormal), cup size (less than half disc radius, normal), presence of spontaneous venous pulsations (which are not present in 20% of the normal population), and margin contour (flat and distinct, normal; raised and indistinct, abnormal).

II. SUSTAINED ACUTE UNILATERAL VISUAL LOSS

The leading causes of sustained unilateral acute visual loss arise primarily from vascular insults, with retinal arteriole and venous occlusions being the most common among the elderly (Table 2).

A. Central Retinal Artery Occlusion

1. Clinical Relevance

Central retinal artery occlusions (CRAOs) primarily arise from atherosclerosis-related thrombosis. However, embolization of the central retinal artery appears to be the cause in approximately 20% of cases (2). Systemic associations include atherosclerotic disease of the carotid arteries, cardiac valvular disease, cardiac dysrhythmias, hypertension, diabetes mellitus, giant cell arteritis, collagen vascular disease, hypercoagulable states, sickle cell disease (including trait), and oral contraceptive use. Ipsilateral carotid artery disease is the most common systemic association in the elderly, with about one-third of patients having this condition (2). Approximately 10% of CRAOs in this group are due to giant cell arteritis, and consequently, giant cell arteritis must be excluded in any patient older than 50 years of age manifesting a CRAO (2). Collagen vascular disease, sickle cell disease, and oral contraceptives are frequent causes of CRAO in young adults.

2. Clinical Manifestations and Immediate Diagnostic Approach

Visual loss from a CRAO manifests as a sudden painless loss of vision in one eye. The visual loss is profound, with patients typically presenting with vision of counting fingers to light perception and the presence of a rAPD. On external examination,the eye will appear normal, and confrontational visual field testing will reveal deficits in all four quadrants. On funduscopic examination, the retina will appear pale white as a result of retinal edema produced by ischemia. All the edema occurs in the inner retinal layers, which are absent in the fovea, thus the fovea maintains its reddish orange hue and stands out as a cherry-red spot among the surrounding white retina (Figure 3).

3. Therapeutic Intervention

CRAO is considered an ophthalmic emergency, and therapy must be instituted promptly. Experimental studies have demonstrated that irreversible damage to the retina will occur after a CRAO if blood flow is not re-established within 97 minutes (3). Clinical reports have documented visual recovery in patients seen up to 2 days after the onset of symptoms (4–6). The mainstay of therapy for this condition includes ocular massage or compression coupled with inhalation therapy with a 95% oxygen and 5% carbon dioxide mixture administered by mask for 10 minutes every hour during the waking hours and every 4 hours at night. In addition to these two measures, the lowering of intraocular pressure with intravenous or oral acetazolamide (Diamox), 500 mg, and the administration of aspirin are believed to be useful therapeutic adjuvants. All these measures are targeted at dislodging the thrombus/embolus that led to the artery occlusion. After the

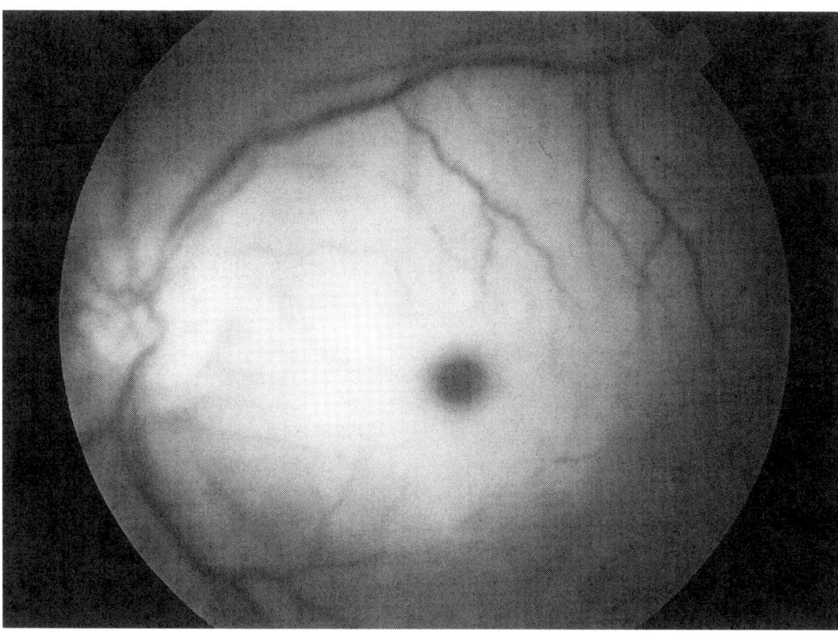

Figure 3 Central retinal artery occlusion. Note how well the fovea stands out compared with the other retinal structures. (Courtesy of K. Sparks, MD, Los Angeles, California.)

institution of the measures stated previously, the patient should be promptly referred for more in-depth ophthalmic evaluation.

4. Follow-up Management

Patients with CRAO require aggressive treatment of the underlying systemic disease. The elderly patient with a CRAO is at an increased risk for cerebrovascular and cardiac ischemic events. In a study of patients with CRAO and branch retinal artery occlusion (BRAO), Savino and colleagues (7) found that the annual stroke mortality in these patients was four times the rate expected. In addition, they found that ischemic heart disease was the most common cause of death among this patient cohort. Therefore, evaluation for carotid artery occlusive disease and ischemic heart disease is warranted in these patients, and some have advocated prophylactically placing these patients on aspirin (8).

B. Central Retinal Vein Occlusion

1. Clinical Relevance

Central retinal vein occlusions (CRVOs) arise from thrombosis of the central retinal vein. Ninety percent of patients with a CRVO are older than 50 years of age, and it is therefore primarily a disease of the elderly. The systemic risk factors most commonly associated with CRVO include atherosclerosis, systemic hypertension, diabetes mellitus, and hyperviscosity states (multiple myeloma, leukemia, Waldenström's macroglobulinemia). In the hyperviscosity disorders, it is important to point out that hyperviscosity retinopathy is a known entity that can mimic a typical CRVO; however, unlike a CRVO, hyperviscosity retinopathy is seen bilaterally and can be reversed by plasmapheresis (9). Patients with preexisting glaucoma are also at risk for a CRVO developing.

2. Clinical Manifestations and Immediate Diagnostic Approach

A CRVO manifests in a similar fashion to a CRAO, with an abrupt unilateral painless loss of vision. Visual loss is usually profound, with patients manifesting visual acuities of 20/200 or worse and a rAPD. Visual field testing will reveal complete visual field loss in the affected eye. Funduscopic examination classically reveals extensive intraretinal hemorrhaging and dilated tortuous retinal veins (blood and thunder fundus) (Figure 4). Patients may also manifest disc edema, cotton wool spots, and macular edema.

3. Therapeutic Intervention

Prompt ophthalmic referral is indicated in any patient suspected of having a CRVO. At present, no therapeutic intervention reverses the visual deficits; thus, therapy is aimed at preserving the vision that remains.

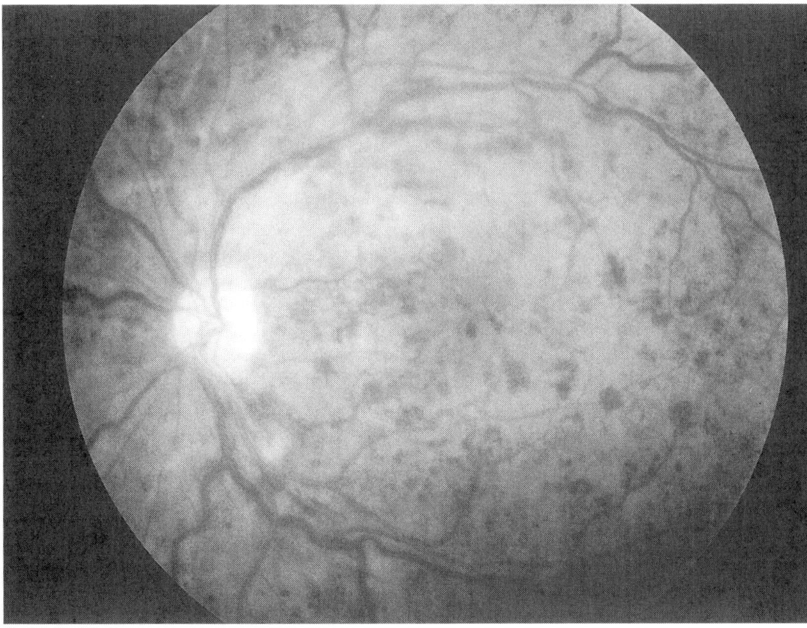

Figure 4 Central retinal vein occlusion. (Courtesy of K. Sparks, MD, Los Angeles, California.)

4. Follow-up Management

Patients who have CRVO's develop are at high risk for neovascularization of the retina, optic nerve, and iris developing, which can lead to spontaneous vitreous hemorrhages, intractable glaucoma, and retinal detachments.

These complications typically arise within 6 months of the onset of a CRVO, and, therefore, these patients require close ophthalmic follow-up. Treatment of the underlying systemic condition is essential in preventing the other eye from becoming affected.

C. Branch Retinal Vein/Artery Occlusion

1. Clinical Relevance

Branch retinal vein and artery occlusion share the same demographic and systemic risk factors as CRVO and CRAO. They differ, however, in their clinical presentation and prognosis for useful vision.

2. Clinical Manifestations and Immediate Diagnostic Approach

A branch retinal vein occlusion (BRVO) manifests in the exact same manner as a CRVO or CRAO, except that the amount of visual loss is much less and the prognosis for visual recovery is much better. The vision on presentation varies but is usually 20/50 or worse. Patients may complain of a blind spot in their field of vision. External ocular findings are absent, and no associated rAPD is present. Funduscopic examination classically shows scattered intraretinal hemorrhages, cotton wool spots, and retinal edema involving a single sector of the retina, with the superotemporal quadrant being the most common site (Figure 5). The acute decrease in vision is primarily due to changes in the macula, which can take the form of either edema, hemorrhage, or ischemia. In general, 50% to 60% of patients with BRVO maintain a visual acuity of 20/40 or better at 1 year (10).

Branch retinal artery occlusions like BRVOs only involve the sector of the retina supplied by the compromised arteriole. In contrast to BRVO, the predominant clinical finding is retinal edema and opacification (Figure 6). In general, the temporal retina is more commonly affected, and emboli are the primary cause

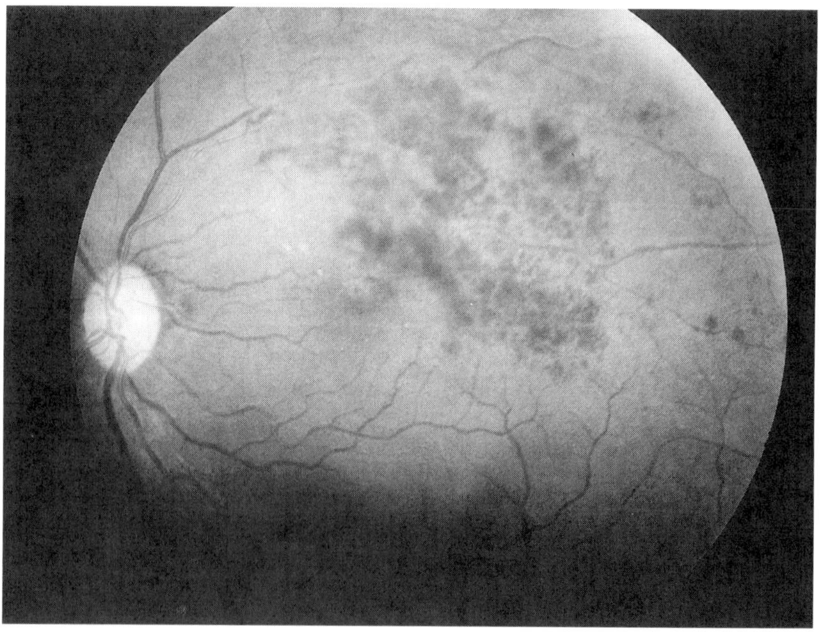

Figure 5 Branch retinal vein occlusion: note sectoral distribution of the hemorrhage. (Courtesy of K. Sparks, MD, Los Angeles, California.)

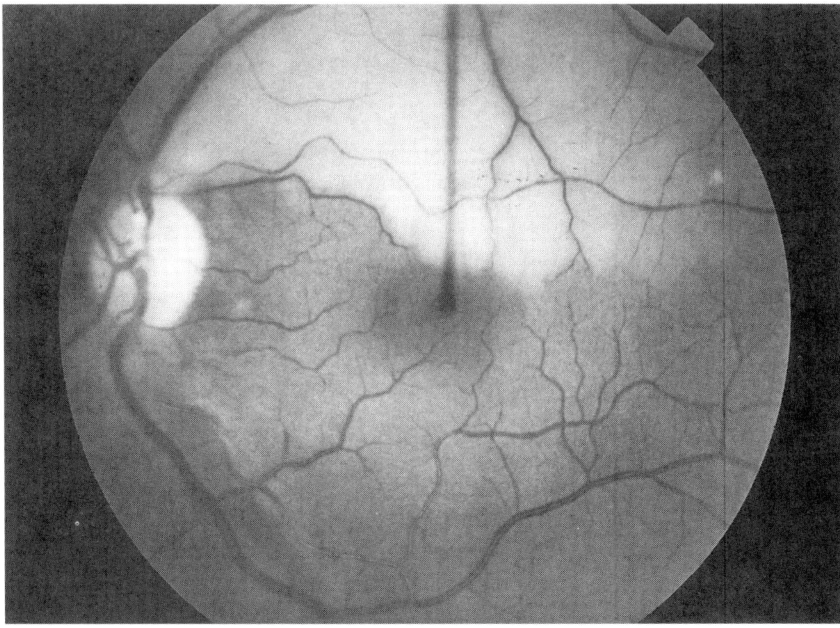

Figure 6 Branch retinal artery occlusion.

of vascular occlusion. Cholesterol, calcium, fibrin, and platelet emboli have all been implicated. The ipsilateral carotid artery is the most common source of emboli in the elderly, and the emboli are typically composed of cholesterol. In younger patients, the most common source of emboli is a defective cardiac valve. Central vision is often maintained, so patients typically complain of peripheral field deficits. As with the other vascular occlusions, the onset is abrupt and painless. Pupillary responses and external examination are normal, and on rare occasion the funduscopic examination may reveal an atheromatous embolus lodged in a retinal arteriole. In most instances, the visual loss is not severe and will completely resolve once the emboli have dissolved or pass on through the vascular system.

3. Therapeutic Intervention

Observation and documentation is the principal ophthalmic intervention. Thus, patients should be referred to an ophthalmologist in a timely manner. The mainstay of therapy for these conditions is treatment of the underlying systemic disease.

4. Follow-up Management

Patients with BRVO are similarly at risk for ocular neovascularization as patients with CRVO and, therefore, require the same level of close ophthalmic follow-up.

D. Anterior Ischemic Optic Neuropathy

Anterior ischemic optic neuropathy (AION) is the most common cause of visual loss associated with optic disc swelling in patients older than 55 years of age (11). The underlying pathophysiological mechanism is vascular occlusion of the blood supply to the optic disc. Clinically, AION manifests in two forms: arteritic and nonarteritic (Table 3). Giant cell arteritis (GCA) or temporal arteritis represents the arteritic form of the disease, which is more severe and has a significantly poorer visual prognosis. Nonarteritic anterior ischemic optic neuropathy (NAION) is considered the less severe form of the disease because the visual loss tends to be less profound and the incidence of bilateral optic nerve involvement is significantly less (Table 3). The hallmark presentation of AION is acute painless unilateral visual loss in an elderly patient associated with optic disc swelling. The presence of optic disc swelling is considered a requisite for making the diagnosis. The absence of this finding in an elderly patient who has abrupt unilateral visual loss essentially excludes AION as a diagnostic possibility. A normal ap-

Table 3 Anterior Ischemic Optic Neuropathy

	Arteritic (giant cell/temporal arteritis)	Nonarteritic
Peak incidence (yr)	70–80	60–65
Visual loss	Severe	Minimal to severe
Pupillary response	rAPD	rAPD
Field defect	Altitudinal, central scotoma	Altitudinal, central scotoma
Optic nerve	Disc swelling, CRAO Flame hemorrhages	Disc swelling, often segmental Flame hemorrhages
Systemic associations	Headache, jaw claudication Scalp tenderness, polymyalgia Malaise, weight loss, fever	Hypertension, diabetes
ESR (Westergren)	Markedly elevated	Normal
Fellow eye involvement (%)[a]	75	30–40
Corticosteroid response	Very responsive	None

RAPD, Relative afferent pupillary defect; CRAO, central retinal artery occlusion; ESR, erythrocyte sedimentation rate.

Source: Modified with permission from Glaser JS. Neuro-ophthalmology. Philadelphia: JB Lippincott, 1990, p 138.

[a] If inadequately treated with systemic corticosteroids.

pearing disc in this clinical situation places carcinomatous infiltration of the optic nerve sheath and a rapidly expanding basal tumor at the top of the differential diagnosis.

1. Giant Cell Arteritis (Arteritic Anterior Ischemic Optic Neuropathy)

Clinical Relevance. Giant cell arteritis constitutes an ophthalmic emergency. If left untreated, this condition will lead to bilateral blindness or a bilateral loss of functional vision. Giant cell arteritis is a systemic vasculitis affecting medium to large-sized arteries. The arteries most commonly involved include the superficial temporal, vertebral, ophthalmic, and posterior ciliary. The incidence has been reported to be as high as 25/100,000 patients, with the disease rarely affecting individuals less than 50 years of age, and the peak incidence occurring between 70 and 80 years (12,13).

Women are affected at a rate twice that of men (14), whites are affected in significantly higher proportions than African Americans (15), and the incidence increases with age (16).

Clinical Manifestations and Immediate Diagnostic Approach. Patients generally have an acute, nonprogressive, painless unilateral loss of vision. Visual loss is abrupt and profound, with patients typically demonstrating vision of count fingers or worse. Because of the systemic nature of the disease, patients may also have one or more of the following associated constitutional symptoms: antecedent or simultaneous headache, jaw claudication (pain with chewing), scalp tenderness (tenderness with hair combing), proximal muscle (shoulder, neck, thigh, and buttock) and joint aches (polymyalgia rheumatica), anorexia, weight loss, or low-grade fever. External examination may reveal firm, tender, and nonpulsatile temporal arteries. Visual field testing classically reveals a superior or inferior hemifield defect respecting the horizontal meridian (altitudinal field defect). Pupillary examination demonstrates a rAPD, and funduscopic examination is remarkable for optic disc swelling with associated flame-shaped hemorrhages (Figure 7).

Ophthalmic consultation/evaluation should be obtained promptly and laboratory testing initiated to assess the erythrocyte sedimentation rate (ESR), C-reactive protein, serological testing for syphilis and various collagen vascular diseases, complete blood count (CBC), lipid profile, and fasting blood glucose. The Westergren method is the most reliable for measuring the ESR.

Therapeutic Intervention. If the ESR confirms the diagnosis of GCA or the clinical constellation of symptoms and signs are highly suggestive of GCA, the patient should be admitted and started on systemic corticosteroids immediately. In addition, a temporal artery biopsy should be performed within 1 week of initiating systemic corticosteroid therapy to establish a definitive diagnosis. Corticoste-

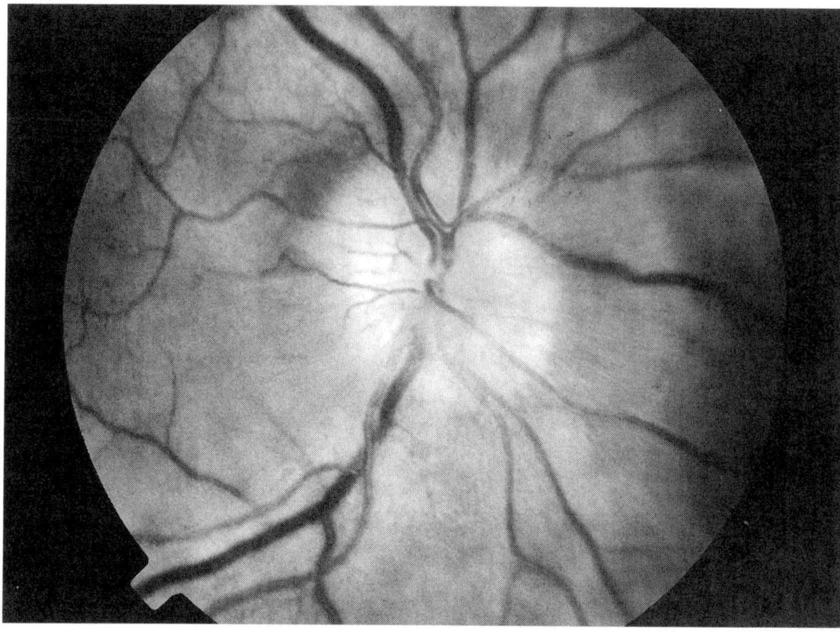

Figure 7 Anterior ischemic optic neuropathy. Note the blurring of disc margin produced by the disc swelling and the disc elevation at the superior left margin.

roid therapy is aimed primarily at preserving the vision of the fellow eye, because the visual loss sustained at the time of presentation is often irreversible. Without treatment, a greater than 75% chance exists that the contralateral eye will be affected. In the absence of adequate systemic corticosteroid therapy, fellow eye involvement generally occurs within days to weeks but can occur within 24 hours. The generally recommended dosing regimen for systemic corticosteroids is 250 mg of methylprednisolone administered intravenously every 6 hours for 12 doses, followed by 80 to 100 mg of oral prednisone taken daily for 2 to 4 weeks until the symptoms reverse and the ESR normalizes.

Follow-up Management. The ESR and symptom constellation are used to monitor disease activity and guide the rate of tapering corticosteriods. Corticosteroid treatment is usually maintained for at least 3 to 6 months but may extend up to 1 year or more, depending on the disease activity. Given the extended period of corticosteroid use, patients also require close monitoring for cortiosteroid-related complications.

2. Nonarteritic Anterior Ischemic Optic Neuropathy

Clinical Relevance. Nonarteritic anterior ischemic optic neuropathy (NAION) is the most common cause of AION accounting for greater than 75% of the cases reported in the literature (17). The clinical presentation of NAION is identical to arteritic anterior ischemic optic neuropathy, except that NAION occurs in a slightly younger cohort, with the peak incidence occurring between 60 and 65 years of age (18).

Clinical Manifestations and Immediate Diagnostic Approach. Clinical examination findings are indistinguishable from those of arteritic AION. Therefore, the recommendations for ophthalmic referral and laboratory testing for arteritic AION apply to NAION. Patients with NAION have a normal ESR, fail to manifest any of the constitutional symptoms seen with GCA, and often have less severe visual loss. Systemic hypertension and diabetes mellitus are strongly associated with NAION, with studies showing a significantly higher prevalence of these conditions in patients with NAION compared with age-matched controls (17–21). Approximately, one-third of fellow eyes ultimately succumbs to the disease.

Therapeutic Intervention. At present, no effective medical or surgical therapy exists for treating NAION; however, spontaneous visual recovery has been documented to occur in approximately 20% of cases (22).

Follow-up Management. Given the strong association with hypertension and diabetes mellitus, patients with NAION deserve close monitoring and aggressive treatment of these conditions in an effort to prevent the fellow eye from becoming affected.

E. Vitreous Hemorrhage

1. Clinical Relevance

Spontaneous vitreous hemorrhage constitutes another major cause of acute monocular visual loss in the elderly. The reported incidence of spontaneous vitreous hemorrhage is 7/100,000 per year, with proliferative diabetic retinopathy, retinal tear, proliferative retinopathy after retinal vein occlusion, posterior vitreous detachment, retinal arterial macroaneurysm, age-related macular degeneration (ARMD), and proliferative sickle cell retinopathy accounting for approximately 87% of all cases (23). In the elderly, the predominant causes of spontaneous vitreous hemorrhage are proliferative diabetic retinopathy, proliferative retinopathy after retinal vein occlusion, posterior vitreous detachment, retinal arterial macroaneurysm, and ARMD. Proliferative retinopathy after retinal vein occlusion accounts for most of the cases in this age group (23,24). Proliferative retinopathy associated with retinal vein occlusion and diabetic retinopathy causes spontaneous vitreous hemorrhages as result of retinal neovascularization. Both conditions produce retinal ischemia, which leads to neovascularization as the retina tries to compensate for the oxygen deficit. The new blood vessels lack the integrity of normal blood vessels and are predisposed to leakage. Spontaneous leakage from these weak blood vessels results in vitreous and intraretinal hemorrhaging.

Posterior vitreous detachment leads to spontaneous vitreous hemorrhaging as a result of age-related degenerative changes in the vitreous. The vitreous is a transparent gel-like tissue that fills the vitreous cavity of the eye and has firm attachments to the retina and retinal blood vessels. With age, the vitreous undergoes a process of liquefaction, which can cause the vitreous to contract. If the vitreous contracts with sufficient force, it will detach from the retina and the retinal blood vessels. Because of its firm attachments to these structures, the vitreous may create tears in the retina or retinal blood vessels as it separates. If a tear in a retinal blood vessel occurs, it will then lead to a vitreous hemorrhage. The peak incidence of posterior vitreous detachments is between the ages of 55 and 65 years, and there appears to be a female predominanance (25).

Retinal arterial macroaneurysms and ARMD are relatively uncommon causes of spontaneous vitreous hemorrhage in the elderly, accounting for approximately 4% of the cases. A retinal arterial macroaneurysm is an acquired retinal vascular lesion closely associated with systemic hypertension and arteriosclerotic vascular disease (26). In most cases, the macroaneurysm will spontaneous involute and require no therapy. In approximately 10% of cases, the macroaneurysm will rupture leading to vitreous hemorrhage (26).

Age-related macular degeneration is the leading cause of legal blindness in adults older than 50 and accounts for 2.2% of monocular blindness in individuals age 65 and older (27). Age-related macular degeneration is generally a slowly progressive, bilateral loss of central vision, developing as a result of the deterioration of the retinal pigment epithelial layer in the central retina (macula). The retinal pigment epithelium (RPE) is the cell layer beneath the retina that provides the retina with vital nutrients. In approximately 10% of patients with ARMD, a neovascular membrane develops in the vascular plexus (choroid) beneath the RPE that provides its blood supply and the blood supply to the outer retina. Because of the fragile nature of neovascular blood vessels, bleeding from these vessels can lead to an abrupt loss of vision in ARMD because of either acute hemorrhaging directly into the central retina or in the vitreous. A central retinal hemorrhage (macular hemorrhage) leading to acute visual loss in ARMD is far more common than a spontaneous vitreous hemorrhage.

It is important to point out, however, that several reports have shown that systemic anticoagulation therapy appears to be a significant risk factor for the development of massive vitreous hemorrhage in patients with neovascular ARMD (28–30).

2. Clinical Manifestations and Immediate Diagnostic Approach

The clinical presentation of a spontaneous vitreous hemorrhage is the same for each of the conditions listed previously. Patients will generally complain of an acute, unilateral painless loss of vision. Patients with proliferative diabetic retinopathy, however, have a higher incidence of bilateral visual loss caused by vitreous hemorrhage (24). The visual symptoms and extent of visual loss will vary, depending on the density and location of the hemorrhage. Visual symptoms can range from mild visual haze to light perception vision. Common visual complaints include visual haze or fog, smoke signals, showers of floaters or black spots with associated flashing lights, and the perception of moving shadows and cobwebs. The eye will appear noninflamed, and the pupil reactions will usually be normal, although very dense vitreous hemorrhages have been shown to produce a rAPD (23).

The blood will obscure examination of part or all of the retina, and thus, it is oftentimes difficult to precisely identify the cause of the vitreous hemorrhage initially. The medical history provides important clinical clues in these situations.

3. Therapeutic Intervention

Immediate referral to an ophthalmologist is warranted in any patient suspected of having a vitreous hemorrhage. Use of all anticoagulant agents including nonsteroidal anti-inflammatory drugs should be eliminated unless they are medically necessary. The general approach to vitreous hemorrhage is to allow sufficient time for the vitreous hemorrhage to clear spontaneously. Clearance of blood from the vitreous is a slow process; current guidelines dictate that a period of at least 3 months, but no more than 6 months, be allowed to pass for spontaneous clearance of a vitreous hemorrhage, unless occupational or personal needs demand early intervention. Intervening before 3 months is also recommended in patients with extensive untreated proliferative diabetic retinopathy or proliferative retinopathy after a retinal vein occlusion and in patients who have uncontrollable glaucoma develop as a result of the vitreous hemorrhage. The established treatment option for a nonclearing vitreous hemorrhage is surgical removal by vitrectomy. Patients with proliferative neovascular retinopathy from diabetes and retinal vein occlusion will also require extensive laser photocoagulation therapy. In patients with posterior vitreous detachments, extensive retinal evaluation is required once the hemorrhage clears to exclude an associated retinal tear. If a retinal tear is found, laser photocoagulation is used to seal the tear. Vitreous hemorrhage resulting from retinal macroaneurysms generally clears without visual sequelae. The natural history of vitreous hemorrhage resulting from ARMD is poor, with the vitreous hemorrhage being slow to clear and patients never recovering vision to prehemorrhage levels.

4. Follow-up Management

Patients with vitreous hemorrhage require close ophthalmic follow-up and aggressive treatment of underlying systemic conditions.

F. Acute Angle-Closure Glaucoma

1. Clinical Relevance

Acute angle-closure glaucoma is an ophthalmic emergency and requires immediate therapy to avoid permanent visual loss. Fortunately, it is a rare condition. The peak incidence occurs between the ages of 55 and 65 years (31). A distinct racial predilection exists, with Eskimos and Asians showing the highest incidence (31). Far-sighted individuals also appear to carry a higher risk of this condition developing. Most acute angle-closure glaucoma cases occur spontaneously. Very few cases are actually precipitated by the instillation of pupil-dilating drops.

2. Clinical Manifestations and Immediate Diagnostic Approach

Acute angle-closure glaucoma arises from a blockage in the outflow of aqueous humor leading to an accumulation inside the eye, which results in a precipitous rise in the intraocular pressure. Patients often have intraocular pressures in excess of 45 mm Hg (normal range, 10–22 mm Hg). The clinical presentation is characterized by an acute painful unilateral loss of vision. The pain is severe, localized to the periocular region, and typically described as a deep-seated boring pain. During the acute episode, the visual loss is due to corneal edema produced by the acute rise in intraocular pressure. Patients report their vision as being blurred, foggy, or hazy and perceive halos around lights. Autonomic stimulation produced by the periocular pain often leads to nausea and vomiting, which can be so severe that the patient's symptoms are erroneously attributed to an abdominal source. On examination, the eye manifests marked conjunctival injection and clouding of the cornea as a result of corneal edema. The pupil is in a mid-dilated position and does not react to light, and patients exhibit moderate light sensitivity. The elevation in intraocular pressure can usually be detected by simultaneous digital palpation of both globes. The involved eye will have the consistency of a stone. The retina is often obscured by corneal edema.

3. Therapeutic Intervention

Immediate therapy should be directed toward lowering the intraocular pressure and referring the patient emergently to an ophthalmologist for further diagnosis and treatment. The first-line therapeutic agents consist of topical and systemic inhibitors of aqueous secretion. These agents include topical beta-blockers (Timoptic, 0.5%), topical carbonic anhydrase inhibitors (Trusopt, 2%), topical alpha-$_2$-adrenergic agonist (Iopidine, 0.5% or 1%), and oral or intravenous carbonic anhydrase inhibitors (Diamox, 500 mg). Patients experiencing significant nausea and vomiting will be unable to tolerate oral medication and, therefore, require intravenous administration. Hyperosmotic agents are often used as an adjuvant to the aqueous suppressants and can be helpful in lowering intraocular pressure. Glycerin can be administered orally in a 50% solution in a dosage of 2 to 3 mL/kg. Alternately, oral isosorbide can be given in a dose of 50 to 100 g (1–2 g/kg) over crushed ice. Isosorbide is preferred in diabetics because it is metabolically inactive, as opposed to glycerin, which is contraindicated in diabetics, because it can cause severe hyperglycemia. Intravenous mannitol is the most potent hyperosmotic agent for lowering intraocular pressure and is often used as a last resort because of the increased risk of cardiovascular side effects. Mannitol is administered intravenously in a dose of 1 to 2 g/kg over 45 minutes (a 500-mL bag of 20% mannitol contains 100 g of mannitol). Hyperosmotic agents should be avoided in any patient with congestive heart failure. Topical corticosteroids and systemic analgesics are useful adjuncts to control intraocular inflammation and relieve the patient's pain. The use of miotics should be left to the discretion of the ophthalmologist. If the intraocular pressure is not lowered in a timely manner, patients may have severe permanent visual loss from the development of a CRVO or a CRAO, particularly if the intraocular pressure is elevated greater than the mean diastolic pressure of the central retinal artery.

4. Follow-up Management

Medical lowering of the intraocular pressure in this condition is solely used as a temporizing measure. Once the intraocular pressure has been sufficiently lowered to reduce or eliminate corneal edema, definitive therapy is achieved by performing a laser iridotomy, which provides an outflow passage for the accumulated aqueous humor. A number of ocular diseases can lead to the development of acute angle-closure glaucoma. Consequently, patients with this condition require comprehensive ophthalmic evaluation to identify and treat the underlying disease.

III. SUSTAINED ACUTE BILATERAL VISUAL LOSS

A. General Clinical Problem

1. Clinical Relevance

As noted earlier, a sudden sustained bilateral decrease in vision is an uncommon occurrence. Consequently, very few entities are known to produce this visual complaint. Cerebrovascular accidents are the predominant cause of sustained acute bilateral visual loss in the elderly. Hemorrhagic and ischemic cerebrovascular accidents can produce acute bilateral visual loss and acute neurological motor and/or sensory dysfunction. The nature and extent of the visual loss will depend on the location along the visual pathway the vascular event occurs (Figure 8). Recall that the visual pathway begins at the retina, where representation of the visual space is organized such that the nasal retina provides information on the temporal visual field, the temporal retina provides information on the nasal field, the inferior retina on the superior field, and the superior retina on the inferior field. Axons from the retinal ganglion cells coalesce to form the nerve fibers of the optic nerve. These fibers then course posteriorly through the optic nerve to the optic chiasm, where fibers originating from the nasal retina cross to the contralateral side. Retinal fibers arising from the temporal retina remain uncrossed. These crossing nasal fibers then leave the chiasm to join the uncrossed temporal fibers on the respective side to form the optic tract. The optic tract is then com-

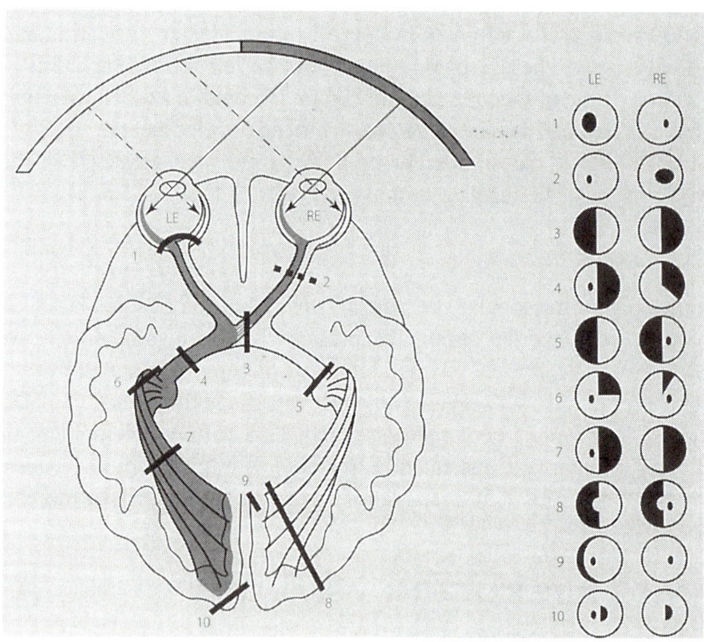

Figure 8 Visual pathway. (From Gurland JE, Hamed LM, Johns KJ, Wilhelmus KR, Wilson II FM. Pupillary examination. In: Wilson II FM, ed. Practical Ophthalmology: A Manual for Beginning Residents. San Francisco: American Academy of Ophthalmology, 1996, p 127.)

posed of temporal retinal nerve fibers from the ipsilateral eye and nasal retinal nerve fibers from the contralateral eye. Within the optic tracts, retinal nerve fibers course laterally and posteriorly to synapse in the lateral geniculate body. Axons leaving the lateral geniculate body then pass posteriorly in the optic radiations to the visual cortex in the occipital lobe. Within the optic radiations, nerve fibers are distributed topographically such that fibers originating from the inferior retinal quadrants course through the temporal lobe en route to the visual cortex, and fibers originating from the superior retinal quadrants course through the parietal lobe en route to the visual cortex. Thus, temporal lobe damage will lead to superior field defects, and parietal lobe lesions will produce inferior field defects. The nerve fibers ultimately reaching the visual cortex in each of the occipital lobe hemispheres will consist of temporal retinal fibers from the ipsilateral eye and nasal retinal fibers from the contralateral eye (Figure 8).

On the basis of the anatomy of the visual pathway, bilateral visual loss will typically arise from damage at or posterior to the optic chiasm (Figure 8). Damage occurring anterior to the chiasm usually results in unilateral visual loss unless the injury occurs bilaterally, which is a rare occurrence. Visual deficits produced by chiasmal and retrochiasmal injury manifest in a fairly consistent pattern. In general, the visual field defects will respect the vertical meridian and, therefore, will either involve the nasal or temporal half of the visual field. A field defect respecting the vertical meridian in this way is referred to as a hemianopic field defect. Field defects involving both eyes are described as homonymous, when the field defect is on the same side in each eye (e.g., the field defect occurs on the left side in both the right and left eyes). The classic visual field defects seen with damage to the various components of the visual pathway are shown in Figure 8. Lesions involving the chiasm will cause visual loss in the temporal portion of the visual field in each eye, a bitemporal hemianopia. Recall that damage to the chiasm will affect the decussating nasal retinal fibers from each eye. Patients will also report a decrease in central vision owing to the high concentration of macular fibers coursing through the chiasm.

Acute bilateral visual loss from chiasmal injury is an uncommon occurrence. Visual loss from disease in this region of the visual pathway generally occurs gradually (32). In the elderly, acute visual loss involving the chiasm is primarily caused by acute ischemia and acute compression (32–41). Acute chiasmal ischemia in this age group is produced by either carotid artery atherosclerosis or GCA (32–34). Acute chiasmal compression, on the other hand, is predominantly produced by pituitary apoplexy (32,35–41).

2. Clinical Manifestations and Immediate Diagnostic Approach

Patients with acute infarction of the chiasm complain of acute bilateral blurring or loss of vision or rapidly progressive bilateral visual field loss. Pupillary responses will typically be normal unless the chiasm is asymmetrically involved. Funduscopic examination will be normal in the acute setting, but patients will eventually have bilateral disc pallor develop. The diagnostic evaluation in any elderly patient with bilateral visual loss should include laboratory studies to exclude GCA (i.e., ESR, C-reactive protein) and an assessment of risk factors for atherosclerosis (i.e., serum cholesterol, triglycerides, and glucose), and neuroimaging to localize the site of injury and identify the underlying cause. Magnetic resonance imaging (MRI) is generally superior to computed tomography (CT) in evaluating the chiasm (35). Ophthalmic evaluation should ideally be performed before sending the patient for neuroimaging studies because the information gleaned from the ophthalmic examination will generally aid the neuroradiologist in determining the region of the brain to focus the study and the best radiologic technique for identifying pathological conditions. Noninvasive carotid artery Doppler ultrasonography studies are also warranted in these patients.

3. Therapeutic Intervention

Therapy will depend on the underlying cause. In the elderly, this will usually entail lowering the patient's atherosclerotic risk factors (i.e., cholesterol lowering medications, better control of hypertension and/or diabetes, elimination of smoking), initiating low-dose aspirin therapy, and referring the patient for evaluation by a vascular surgeon.

In the case of GCA, patients will require the appropriate level of corticosteroid therapy to keep the disease process under control.

4. Follow-up Management

Acute infarction of the chiasm is indicative of advanced atherosclerotic narrowing of the cerebral vasculature. In the cases reported in the literature, the extracranial portions of the carotid arteries were the sites containing the greatest amount of disease (33). Thus, patients require ongoing noninvasive carotid artery evaluation and better control of comorbid atherosclerotic risk factors.

B. Pituitary Apoplexy

1. Clinical Relevance

Pituitary-apoplexy is a rare but potentially life-threatening condition that results from sudden massive enlargement of the pituitary gland, which leads to compression of the optic chiasm. The gland enlargement is usually a result of acute infarction or hemorrhage in a pre-existing pituitary adenoma. Nontumorous apoplexy does occur and is predominantly caused by postpartum pituitary hemorrhaging. The cases of pituitary apoplexy reported in the literature show an even distribution between the ages of 20 and 70 years and a male sex predilection, with a male/female ratio of 2:1 (36). In the elderly, anticoagulant therapy, thrombolytic therapy, and atherosclerosis appear to be significant risk factors for this condition developing (37–41). Several reports have documented pituitary apoplexy developing in elderly patients receiving either anticoagulant or antithrombolytic therapy for the treatment of myocardial infarction (37–40). In addition, Sussman and Parra (41) have reported several cases of pituitary apoplexy arising from atheromatous emboli in a similar patient cohort.

2. Clinical Manifestations and Immediate Diagnostic Approach

Patients generally complain of the sudden onset of a severe headache and visual loss. The headache may be diffuse, retro-orbital, or frontotemporal and is often accompanied by nausea and vomiting. Signs of meningeal irritation and altered consciousness may be present. The visual loss will typically result from compression of the optic chiasm, producing a bitemporal hemianopia and a subjective reduction in visual acuity. In addition, patients may have symptoms of double vision or lid drooping because of cranial nerve involvement if the gland expands laterally to include the cavernous sinus. Cranial nerves III, IV, V, and VI pass through the cavernous sinus and thus potentially could be affected. On the basis of clinical reports, the third cranial nerve is most commonly involved (34). Pupillary responses will often be normal in these patients, and funduscopic examination will usually be negative for signs of optic nerve compromise. The severe headache in association with the other symptoms will generally lead one to pursue neuroimaging studies immediately. MRI is the neuroimaging study of choice and often readily identifies the lesion.

3. Therapeutic Intervention

Pituitary apoplexy is considered a neurosurgical emergency and prompt referral to a neurosurgeon for consideration of surgical decompression should be performed. Surgical decompression is generally indicated in patients with acute severe visual loss or loss of consciousness. In patients who retain consciousness or present in stable condition some time after the onset of symptoms, observation and medical therapy alone is indicated. Medical therapy primarily consists of corticosteroid replacement therapy, which should be instituted immediately after the diagnosis has been established.

4. Follow-up Management

Given the irreversible damage to the pituitary gland, patients will require continued corticosteroid replacement therapy and monitoring for endocrine dysfunction.

C. Retrochiasmal Lesions

Retrochiasmal lesions characteristically do not produce loss of visual acuity unless they are bilateral, which is uncommon. Patients are often unaware of the visual disturbance. It typically comes to their attention when they begin repeatedly colliding into objects in the blind area of their visual field or they are involved in a motor vehicle accident. Given this presentation, retrochiasmal lesions rarely manifest with acute visual loss and, therefore, are not germane to this discussion.

IV. TRANSIENT UNILATERAL ACUTE VISUAL LOSS

A. Clinical Relevance

Transient visual loss is one of the most common visual complaints in the elderly. As defined previously, transient visual loss is an abrupt reversible decrease in vision that lasts less than 24 hours. Typically, the visual loss lasts seconds to minutes, with patients reporting either a complete or partial loss of their visual field in one or both eyes. The major pathophysiological mechanisms underlying transient visual loss include ischemia, neuronal depression after a seizure, and migraine headache. Ischemia is the predominant cause of transient visual loss across all age groups and is the main cause of transient visual loss in the elderly (42). The mechanisms underlying ischemia include thromboembolism, vasospasm, compression, and hypoperfusion, with thromboembolic vascular occlusion being the principal mechanism in the elderly (42,43).

Unilateral transient visual loss is referred to as amaurosis fugax. In the elderly, this condition primarily arises from atherosclerotic disease of the ipsilateral carotid artery or cardiac valvular disease (42,43). A less frequent, but notable, cause of amaurosis fugax in the elderly is extensive atheromatous occlusive disease involving several branches of the aortic arch (44,45). In these patients, visual loss is precipitated by either physical activity (i.e., a change in posture, or exercise) or exposure to bright light. Given the associated systemic factors, many experts believe that amaurosis fugax may be an important marker for generalized atherosclerotic disease and a predictor of future stroke and cardiac death (43,46–48). Poole and Ross Russell (46), for example, found that patients sustaining amaurosis fugax attacks had a four times greater risk of stroke than age-matched controls 6 years after presentation. In addition, these investigators found a four times greater rate of cardiac death in amaurosis fugax patients compared with the general population over the same time period.

B. Clinical Manifestations

Patients with amaurosis fugax typically manifest an abrupt unilateral loss or decrease in vision with or without associated neurological symptoms, lasting between 2 and 10 minutes. Patients may describe the visual loss as a dimming or darkening of their vision, a diffuse blurring of their vision, or a shade or veil being pulled over a portion of their visual field. Patients may also experience a complete loss of vision during the amaurotic episode. Visual loss usually begins in the superior visual field and rarely in the inferior field. Attacks can recur several times throughout the day, and no obvious precipitating factors can usually be identified except in those cases caused by extensive atherosclerotic occlusive disease of aortic arch branch arteries (44,45).

C. Immediate Diagnostic Approach

The ophthalmic examination is often noncontributory to the diagnostic evaluation in these patients except in the rare instance that a retinal arterial embolus is seen during funduscopic examination. These emboli are most commonly associated with atheromatous lesions of the ipsilateral carotid artery, and their presence on retinal examination indicates a greater than 50% chance of high-grade ipsilateral carotid artery stenosis (42,43). Amaurosis fugax in the elderly can precede the development of anterior ischemic optic neuropathy from GCA (13). Consequently, the diagnostic evaluation of any patient older than age 50 who is seen with transient monocular visual loss should begin with a laboratory and clinical investigation to exclude GCA. Clinical history taking should explore concurrent cerebral ischemic symptoms (i.e., dizziness, syncope, extremity weakness or parasthesias, confusion, dysarthria), arteriosclerotic risk factors (i.e., hypertension, diabetes mellitus, familial arteriosclerotic disease, smoking), and heart disease, particularly valvular disease, angina pectoris, and atrial fibrillation. In addition to the laboratory studies directed at diagnosing GCA, laboratory investigation should include a CBC, and serum cholesterol, triglyceride, and glucose testing. Complete ophthalmic examination by an ophthalmologist should be performed to ascertain whether localized ocular pathosis is the source of the visual symptoms. Noninvasive carotid artery studies (carotid Doppler ultrasonography) and evaluation by a vascular surgeon are indicated in every elderly patient with transient visual loss. If carotid artery Doppler ultrasonography studies reveal 70% to 90% reduction in luminal diameter (flow-limiting stenosis), carotid angiography is indicated to determine the patients candidacy for endarterectomy.

Given the increased risk of cardiac death in patients with amaurosis fugax caused by carotid artery disease, a cardiac assessment for ischemic heart disease and sources of cardiac emboli should be performed (47,48).

D. Therapeutic Intervention

Therapy will depend on the underlying cause of the transient visual loss. In the elderly, treatment is usually focused on aggressively controlling arteriosclerotic risk factors in conjunction with low-dose aspirin (300–325 mg/day) therapy. Routine anticoagulation with heparin or warfarin is not recommended because of inconclusive evidence regarding its efficacy in reducing the risk of stroke in patients with amaurosis fugax (42,43). Carotid endarterectomy is indicated in those patients with greater than 75% stenosis located at a surgically accessible site (i.e., extracranial carotid artery). In patients with less than 75% stenosis, endarterectomy may be indicated if amaurosis fugax is associated with cerebral hemispheric transient ischemic attacks, retinal emboli observed on ophthalmoscopy, ulceration of the carotid bulb, or evidence of cerebral infarction on CT scan (43).

E. Follow-up Management

Patients with amaurosis fugax require aggressive long-term monitoring of their cerebrovascular system and cardiac status. In addition, adequate control of comorbid conditions must be achieved to effectively reduce the risk of future stroke or sudden cardiac death in these patients.

V. TRANSIENT BILATERAL VISUAL LOSS

Transient bilateral visual loss is generally a sign of cerebral or systemic disease. The predominant causes include papilledema from any cause, vertebrobasilar artery insufficiency, orthostatic hypotension, cardiac dysrhythmia, severe systemic hypertension, migraine headache, and seizure activity. In the elderly, the conditions most likely to produce transient bilateral visual loss are papilledema, vertebrobasilar artery insufficiency, and orthostatic hypotension (42).

A. Papilledema

1. Clinical Manifestations

The principal visual symptom associated with papilledema is a brief decrease in vision lasting seconds, referred to as a transient obscuration of vision (42,49). Transient visual obscurations are quite specific for papilledema and are not produced by other causes of disc edema. On average, these visual obscurations last between 5 and 15 seconds and recur several times a day. They are often incited by orthostatic or postural changes and because of their fleeting nature, patients will frequently ignore them initially. Amaurosis fugax, by contrast, lasts between 2 and 10 minutes and readily comes to the patient's attention. The visual loss produced by papilledema will be bilateral and may be described as a blurring or dimming of vision or a complete blackout of vision over the entire visual field.

The transient visual obscurations may be accompanied by headaches, nausea, and vomiting.

2. Immediate Diagnostic Approach

On examination, visual acuity, pupillary responses, and confrontational visual fields will usually be normal. The funduscopic examination is the key to the diagnosis. The optic disc in early papilledema will be markedly swollen and elevated and manifest intense hyperemia (Figure 9). Visualization of the disc vessels will be obscured at the disc margin because of swelling of the surrounding retinal nerve fiber layer. Flame-shaped hemorrhages at the disc margin are usually present, as well as venous dilation and the loss of spontaneous venous pulsations. These optic nerve changes will be present bilaterally and often show a high level of symmetry. On the basis of the funduscopic findings, patients should be immediately referred for neuroimaging studies to exclude a mass lesion followed by lumbar puncture if an intracranial mass lesion is not detected.

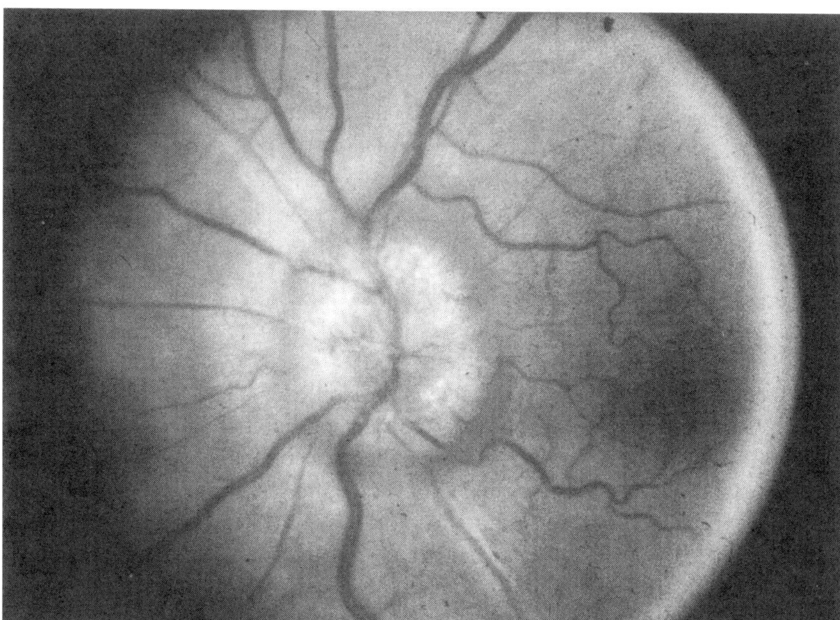

Figure 9 Papilledema: note the elevated and obscured disc margins and associated disc hemorrhages.

3. Therapeutic Intervention

Papilledema is a neurological emergency and, as such, requires immediate referral to a neurologist or neurosurgeon for definitive management.

4. Follow-up Management

Ongoing follow-up will generally be provided by the neurologist and/or neurosurgeon.

B. Vertebrobasilar Insufficiency

1. Clinical Relevance

Vertebrobasilar insufficiency is a term that refers to a heterogeneous group of vascular occlusive disorders affecting the posterior cerebral circulation. These posterior-circulation occlusive disorders generally have been categorized according to the site of the vascular occlusion or posterior circulation vessel involved (50). The vertebrobasilar arterial system consists of the two vertebral arteries that traverse the neck through the transverse foramina of the cervical vertebrae (C6-C2) to enter the cranium where they fuse to form the basilar artery. The basilar artery supplies branches to the brain stem and cerebellum and ultimately bifurcates to give off the two posterior cerebral arteries. The vertebrobasilar arterial system provides blood flow to the brain stem, cerebellum, occipital lobes, and the medial temporal lobe. Patients with vertebrobasilar insufficiency will have neurological deficits that coincide with the site or sites of occlusion (50,51). In the case of transient bilateral visual loss, the site of occlusive disease is the posterior cerebral arteries, which supply the visual cortex in the occipital lobes.

Occlusive disease in this portion of the vertebrobasilar system primarily arises from emboli, with cardiac and proximal vertebrobasilar lesions being the main embolic sources in the elderly (52,53). In addition, intrinsic atherosclerotic narrowing of the posterior cerebral artery has been shown to be an important source of occlusive disease in this age group (54). The predominant causes of posterior cerebral artery occlusion in young adults include migraine headache, hypercoagulable states, collagen vascular diseases (systemic lupus erythematosus, polyarteritis nodosa), and idiopathic sources of embolism (53).

2. Clinical Manifestations

The visual symptoms produced by vertebrobasilar insufficiency in the territory of the posterior cerebral artery typically mimic those of amaurosis fugax except that the visual deficits occur bilaterally and the attacks are of much shorter duration usually lasting less than a minute (42). In a very rare instance, patients with vertebrobasilar insufficiency may complain of transient episodes of vertical inversion of visual images (55). Because embolic and intrinsic atherosclerotic occlusive disease of the posterior cerebral artery generally indicates significant atherosclerotic disease in the more proximal portions of the vertebrobasilar arterial system, the visual symptoms are frequently accompanied by signs of brain stem ischemia (50–54). The brain stem ischemic symptoms commonly reported include facial or limb numbness, ataxia, lethargy, upper and/or lower extremity weakness, diplopia, and dysarthria.

3. Immediate Diagnostic Approach

Given that the risk factors and underlying pathological condition for vertebrobasilar insufficiency mirror those for carotid artery disease, the diagnostic evaluation will be the same as that for amaurosis fugax except that vascular studies will be directed toward the vertebrobasilar arterial system. Ophthalmic examination will generally be noncontributory in this situation as well.

4. Therapeutic Intervention

Treatment considerations for vertebrobasilar insufficiency also mimic those for carotid artery disease.

5. Follow-up Management

The ongoing management issues are no different from those of patients with carotid artery disease.

C. Orthostatic Hypotension

1. Clinical Relevance

Orthostatic hypotension is a common and clinically important disorder among the elderly (56). The major causes of orthostatic hypotension in this age group include impairment of the autonomic orthostatic response, cardiac dysrhythmia, and over aggressive treatment of systemic hypertension. Approximately 20% of the population age 65 and older and 30% to 50% of the population older than age 75 suffer from this condition (57).

The major pathogenic factors leading to the development of orthostatic hypotension in the elderly appear to be the age-related decrease in autonomic nervous system function (baroreceptor reflex), vascular rigidity, and cerebral blood flow autoregulation. Other contributing factors include antihypertensive agents and other medications that lower blood pressure to some degree, diseases that cause autonomic dysfunction, and cerebrovascular disease. Volume depletion from dehydration, anemia, and electrolyte imbalance in the elderly are also important contributory factors (Table 4).

2. Clinical Manifestations

Patients will generally complain of transient dizziness, light-headedness, mental clouding, and bilateral blurring or dimming of vision immediately after a change in posture. Symptoms are most prominent in the morning shortly after arising because baroreceptors are often slow to respond after a period of prolonged recumbency. Patients may also report a worsening of symptoms in association with a hot shower or bath, after exercise, and after heavy meals (57).

3. Immediate Diagnostic Approach

Ophthalmic examination will generally aid in assessing the severity of contributory comorbid conditions, such as diabetes mellitus, hypertension, and atherosclerotic disease. Visual acuity, pupillary responses, and confrontational visual fields will usually be normal. The assessment for orthostatic hypotension entails measuring the patient's blood pressure and heart rate in the supine and upright position. The upright measurements should only be obtained after the patient has rested in the supine position for 15 to 30 minutes and on standing; several measurements should be performed at 1-minute intervals for 3 to 5 minutes (57). In addition, the patient's symptoms should be monitored. A drop in systolic blood pressure greater than 20 mm Hg is considered diagnostic for orthostatic hypoten-

Table 4 Factors Contributing to Orthostatic Hypotension in the Elderly

Multiple medication use
Antihypertensives
Diuretics
Tricyclic antidepressants
Nitrates
Phenothiazines
Diseases affecting autonomic function
Parkinson's disease
Diabetes mellitus
Peripheral neuropathy
Increase in cerebrovascular disease
Intravascular volume depletion
Dehydration
Anemia
Electrolyte imbalance

sion. A basic cardiac evaluation should be performed to assess for dysrhythmias, myocardial ischemia, and valvular disease. The presence of carotid bruits should also be investigated.

4. Therapeutic Intervention

Treatment for this condition usually begins with a thorough assessment of the patient's specific contributory factors. Once these factors are identified, an attempt should be made to modify or eliminate them. Offending medications should be withdrawn or reduced in dosage and contributing medical conditions properly treated. In addition, general supportive measures should be instituted, such as sleeping with the head of the bed elevated, increasing sodium and fluid intake, avoiding prolonged standing, and changing positions slowly. If these therapeutic measures fail to provide symptomatic relief, low-dose mineralocorticoid therapy with fludrocortisone acetate (Florinef) should be initiated at a dose of 0.1 mg/day. Fludrocortisone increases intravascular and extravascular volume, and thus, patients must be monitored closely for the development of congestive heart failure, hypertension, and hypokalemia.

5. Follow-up Management

Behavior modification, close monitoring of fluid and electrolyte status, appropriate treatment of contributing medical disorders, and the judicious use of systemic medications are the therapeutic strategies used to provide effective long-term care for patients with orthostatic hypotension.

REFERENCES

1. Ensrud KE, Newitt MC, Yunis C, Cauley JA, Seeley DC, Fox KM, Cummings SR. Correlates of impaired function in older women. J Am Geriatr Soc 1994;42:481–489.
2. Duker JS, Sivalingham A, Brown GC, Reber R. A prospective study of acute central retinal artery obstruction. Arch Ophthalmol 1991;109:339–342.
3. Hayreh SS, Kolder HE, Weingeist TA. Central retinal artery occlusion and retinal tolerance time. Ophthalmology 1980;87:75–78.
4. Augsburger JJ, Magargal LE. Visual prognosis following treatment of acute central retinal artery obstruction. Br J Ophthalmol 1980;64:913–917.
5. Nielsen NV. Treatment of acute occlusion of the retinal arteries. Acta Ophthalmol 1979;57:1078–1083.
6. Stone R, Zink H, Klingele T, Burde RM. Visual recovery after central artery occlusion: Two cases. Ann Ophthalmol 1977;9:445–450.
7. Savino PJ, Glaser JS, Cassady J. Retinal stroke: Is the patient at risk? Arch Ophthalmol 1977;95:1185–1189.

8. Barton JJS, Corbett JJ. Neuro-ophthalmologic vascular emergencies in the elderly. Clin Geriatr Med 1991;7:525–548.
9. Kearns TP. Differential diagnosis of central retinal vein obstruction. Ophthalmology 1983;90:475–480.
10. The Branch Vein Occlusion Study Group. Argon laser photocoagulation for macular edema in branch vein occlusion. Am J Ophthalmol 1984;98:271–282.
11. Miller NR. Anterior ischemic optic neuropathy: Diagnosis and management. Bull NY Acad Med 1980;56:643–654.
12. Keltner JL. Giant-cell arteritis: signs and symptoms. Ophthalmology 1982;89:1101–1110.
13. Ghanchi FD, Dutton GN. Current concepts in giant cell (temporal) arteritis. Surv Ophthalmol 1997;42:99–123.
14. Beri M, Klugman MR, Kohler JA, Hayrech, SS. Anterior ischemic optic neuropathy VII. Incidence of bilaterality and various influencing factor. Ophthalmology 1987; 94:1020–1027.
15. Smith CA, Fidler WJ, Pinals RS. The epidemiology of giant cell arteritis. Report of a ten-year study in Shelby County, Tennessee. Arthritis Rheum 1983;26:1214–1219.
16. Hauser WA, Ferguson RH, Holley KE, Kurland, LT. Temporal arteritis in Rochester, Minnesota, 1951 to 1967. Mayo Clin Proc 1971;46:597–602.
17. Guyer DR, Miller NR, Auer CL, Fine SL. The risk of cerebrovascular and cardiovascular disease in patients with anterior ischemic optic neuropathy. Arch Ophthalmol 1985;103:1136–1142.
18. Boghen DR, Glaser JS. Ischaemic optic neuropathy: The clinical profile and natural history. Brain 1975;98:689–708.
19. Ellenberger C Jr. Ischemic optic neuropathy as a possible early complication of vascular hypertension. Am J Ophthalmol 1979;88:1045–1051.
20. Hayreh SS. Anterior ischemic optic neuropathy: I. Terminology and pathogenesis. Br J Ophthalmol 1974;58:955–963.
21. Repka MX, Savino PJ, Schatz NJ, Sergolt, RC. Clinical profile and long-term implications of anterior ischemic optic neuropathy. Am J Ophthalmol 1983;96:478–483.
22. Movsas T, Kelman SE, Elman MJ, Miller NR, Dickersin K, Min YI. The natural course of non-arteritic ischemic optic neuropathy (abstr). Invest Ophthalmol Vis Sci 1991;32(suppl):951.
23. Spraul CW, Grossniklaus HE. Vitreous hemorrhage. Surv Ophthalmol 1997;42:3–39.
24. Dana MR, Werner MS, Viana MA, Shapiro MJ. Spontaneous and traumatic vitreous hemorrhage. Ophthalmology 1993;100:1377–1383.
25. Novak MA, Welch RB. Complications of acute symptomatic posterior vitreous detachment. Am J Ophthalmol 1984;97:308–314.
26. Rabb MF, Gagliano DA, Teske MP. Retinal arterial macroaneurysms. Surv Ophthalmol 1988;33:73–96.
27. The International ARM Epidemiology Study Group. An international classification and grading system for age-related maculopathy and age-related macular degeneration. Surv Ophthalmol 1995;39:367–374.

28. Feman SS, Bartlett RE, Roth AM, Foos RY. Intraocular hemorrhage and blindness associated with systemic anticoagulation. JAMA 1972;220:1354–1355.
29. El Baba FE, Jarrett WH, Harbin TS, Fine SL, Michels RG, Schachat AP, Green WR. Massive hemorrhage complicating age-related macular degeneration. Ophthalmology 1986;93:1581–1592.
30. Lewis H, Sloan SH, Foos RY. Massive intraocular hemorrhage associated with anticoagulation and age-related macular degeneration. Graefes Arch Clin Exp Ophthalmol 1988;226:59–64.
31. Stelmack T. Angle closure glaucoma. In: Lewis TL, Fingeret M, eds. Primary Care of the Glaucomas. Norwalk, CT: Appleton & Lange, 1993, pp 347–361.
32. Burde RM, Savino PJ, Trobe JD. Chiasmal visual loss. In: Burde RM, ed. Clinical Decisions in Neuro-Ophthalmology. St. Louis: Mosby–Year Book, 1992, pp 74–103.
33. Lee KF, Schatz NJ. Ischemic chiasmal syndrome. Acta Radiol 1975;347:131–148.
34. Cha JK, Kim HT, Kim MH. Two cases of suspected arteriosclerotic optical chiasmal syndrome. J Korean Med Sci 1990;5:169–172.
35. Hupp SL. Magnetic resonance imaging of the optic chiasm. Surv Ophthalmol 1991; 36:207–216.
36. Reid RL, Quigley ME, Yen SSC. Pituitary apoplexy: A review. Arch Neurol 1985; 2:712–719.
37. Fuchs S, Beeri R, Hasin Y, Weiss AT, Gotsman MS, Zahger D. Pituitary apoplexy as a first manifestation of pituitary adenomas following intensive thrombolytic and antithrombotic therapy. Am J Cardiol 1998;81:110–111.
38. Oo MM, Krishna AY, Bonavita GJ, Rutecki GW. Heparin therapy for myocardial infarction: An unusual trigger for pituitary apoplexy. Am J Med Sci 1997;314:351–353.
39. Hyer SL, Soo SC, Taylor W, Nussey SS. Spontaneous hemorrhage into pituitary tumor after streptokinase therapy. Postgrad Med J 1993;69:244.
40. Nourzaden AR, Pitts FW. Hemorrhage into pituitary adenoma during anticoagulant therapy. JAMA 1965;193:623–625.
41. Sussman EB, Porro RS. Pituitary apoplexy: The role of atheromatous emboli. Stroke 1974;5:318–323.
42. Burde RM, Savino PJ, Trobe JD. Transient visual loss. In: Burde RM, ed. Clinical Decisions in Neuro-Ophthalmology. St. Louis: Mosby–Year Book, 1992, pp 117–144.
43. The Amaurosis Fugax Study Group. Current management of amaurosis fugax. Stroke 1990;21:201–208.
44. Ross Russell RW, Page NGR. Critical perfusion of brain and retina. Brain 1983; 106:419–427.
45. Furlan AJ, Whisnant JP, Kessing JP. Unilateral visual loss in bright light: An unusual symptom of carotid artery occlusive disease. Arch Neurol 1979;36:675–676.
46. Poole CJM, Ross Russell RW. Mortality and stroke after amaurosis fugax. J Neurol Neurosurg Psychiatry 1985;48:902–905.
47. Hurwitz BJ, Heyman A, Wilkinson WE, Haynes CS, Utley CM. Comparison of amaurosis fugax and transient cerebral ischemia: A prospective study. Ann Neurol 1985;18:698–705.

48. Muuronen A, Kaste M. Outcome of 314 patients with transient ischemic attacks. Stroke 1982;13:24–31.
49. Walsh TJ. Blurred vision. In: Walsh TJ, ed. Neuro-Ophthalmology: Clinical Signs and Symptoms. Baltimore: Williams & Wilkins, 1997, pp 387–464.
50. Caplan LR. Large-vessel occlusive disease of the posterior circulation. In: Caplan LR, ed. Stroke: A Clinical Approach. Boston: Butterworth-Heinemann, 1993, pp 237–271.
51. Caplan LR. Vertebrobasilar disease: Time for a new strategy. Stroke 1981;12:111–114.
52. Castaigne P, Lhermitte F, Gautier J, Escouiolle R, Derouesue C, Deragopian P, Popa C. Arterial occlusions in the vertebral-basilar system. Brain 1973;96:133–154.
53. Pessin MS, Lathi ES, Cohen MB, Kwan ES, Hedges TR, Caplan LR. Clinical features and mechanism of occipital infarction. Ann Neurol 1987;21:290–299.
54. Pessin MS, Kwan ES, DeWitt LD, Hedges TR, Gale D, Caplan LR. Posterior cerebral artery stenosis. Ann Neurol 1987;21:85–89.
55. Stracciari A, Guarino M, Ciucci G, Pazzaglia P. Acute upside down reversal of vision in vertebrobasilar ischaemia. J Neurol Neurosurg Psychiatry 1993;56:423.
56. Robbins AS, Rubenstein LZ. Postural hypotension in the elderly. J Am Geriatr Soc 1984;32:769–774.
57. Rubenstein LZ, Josephson KR, Robbins AS. Falls in the nursing home. Ann Intern Med 1994;21:442–451.

23
Hypothermia and Hyperthermia

Arnel M. Joaquin
Charles R. Drew University of Medicine and Science, and Martin Luther King, Jr.–Charles R. Drew Medical Center, Los Angeles, California

One of the earliest problems that confronted man was survival and protection against the extreme ranges of environmental temperatures. Although lower forms of animals, such as the poikilotherms and even some mammals (through mechanisms such as hibernation) are able to tolerate a wide range of environmental temperatures, man is dependent mostly on behavioral modification and autonomic regulation to maintain a narrow range of normal core body temperature. As such, when these two mechanisms are impaired, as in the aging individual and those with chronic illnesses, temperature-related events pose a major threat to survival.

The body normally produces heat, and heat is dissipated to a large extent by radiation, which accounts for up to 50% of heat loss. Heat loss from evaporation from skin and airways constitute 25% and 5%, respectively. Conduction is responsible for 15% of heat loss and convection another 5%. The balance between heat loss and heat production is regulated by the hypothalamus, the dominant thermoregulatory controller in mammals. Thermal input goes to the hypothalamus from other parts of the brain, the spinal cord, deep abdominal and thoracic tissues, and the skin surface, resulting in voluntary behavioral regulation and autonomic regulation. Shivering causes an increase in metabolic rate from a baseline of 40 to 60 kcal/h to as high as 300 kcal/h. Other autonomic effects include vasoconstriction/dilation and sweating. In the geriatric patient, physiological, pathological, and environmental factors combine to disrupt this balance (1,2).

Hypothermia and hyperthermia are significant causes of morbidity and mortality in the geriatric population. Deaths from hypothermia and hyperthermia occur at higher rates in the elderly population. Indeed, aging carries with it multiple risk factors for bad outcomes from thermal disorders, even in optimally treated cases. Table 1 shows some age-associated factors that contribute to in-

Table 1 Age-Related Factors Affecting Temperature-Related Morbidity and Mortality

Intrinsic factors	
Nervous system	Decreased responsiveness and precision of thermoregulatory mechanism
	Deranged ability to detect changes in temperature
	Decreased ability to alter environment (nonambulatory, bed ridden)
Cardiovascular system	Diastolic dysfunction, reduced cardiac output and inotropic response
Pulmonary system	Decreased reserve
Skin	Atrophy of skin layers, decreased sweat production, decreased vasoconstriction
Skeletal muscle	Decreased lean body mass, decreased shivering, decreased strength
Liver	Decreased reserve
Kidneys	Decreased reserve
Extrinsic factors	
Drugs	Beta-blockers, anticholinergics, antipsychotics, anesthetics, opioids, diuretics, alcohol
Social issues	Living alone, low income, poor social support

creased incidence and increased morbidity and mortality in hypothermia and hyperthermia in the geriatric age group. In addition, delay in diagnosis may cause further organ damage because both hyperthermia and hypothermia may be associated with life-threatening conditions, such as sepsis and cerebrovascular accidents.

This chapter will discuss the management of hypothermia and hyperthermia of various causes, whether environmental, drug-induced, or as part of disease/pathological process.

I. HYPOTHERMIA

A. Clinical Relevance

From 1979 to 1995, hypothermia deaths in the United States averaged more than 700 cases per year, and approximately half of the cases are in persons aged 65 years and older (3). In 1979, deaths for persons 75 years and older, representing only 4% of the population, accounted for 28% of total deaths from hypothermia for that year. The geriatric population is at high risk for hypothermia primarily because of inadequate physiological responses related to aging (e.g., lack of vasoconstriction to cold, decreased metabolic rate, impaired shivering mechanism) and underlying diseases (e.g., diabetes mellitus, heart failure, peripheral vascular disease). Malnutrition, decreased mobility, and poor economic conditions are also contributing factors in the elderly. It is not uncommon to find an inappropriately clothed elderly person in an inadequately heated apartment because of the high cost of utilities. Alcoholism, which occurs in the elderly, places a person at high risk for hypothermia.

Core body temperature is normally maintained at 36°C (4). This is affected, however, by environmental conditions and the body's capacity for thermoregulation. When the elderly patient is exposed to adversely low temperatures, appropriate behavioral modifications may be affected, which impairs their ability to adjust accordingly. In addition, with aging physiological responses are compromised as stated earlier. The elderly can be hypothermic even in only moderately cool environments. Their low lean body mass and reduced energy reserves contribute to increased susceptibility.

B. Immediate Diagnostic Approach

Taking an adequate history is important in determining the cause and duration of hypothermia. Family members can also help establish certain historical details such as previous medical conditions, medications, and home environment. Medical conditions that can cause hypothermia should be initially considered and excluded (e.g., hypothyroidism, sepsis, hypoadrenalism). Any history of trauma must be documented. Inquiry on the intake of alcohol should also be done. Early signs of hypothermia may be nonspecific and may be confused with other conditions in the elderly patient. A patient may have mental confusion, disturbance of judgment, and other signs of delirium. During surgery, the only manifestation may be difficulty in achieving hemostasis because of inactivation of clotting factors at low temperatures. Patients with burns are susceptible because of increased loss of heat from vasodilation and increased skin circulation. A delay in diagnosis and immediate corrective measures may adversely affect outcome.

The only reliable method for diagnosis of hypothermia is by measuring the core body temperature. A core body temperature of 35°C (95°F) or less constitutes hypothermia. Several methods and sites are used for measuring temperature. Thermometers that measure temperatures as low as 15°C (59°F) should be used. Thermocouples are bimetal junctions often between copper and constantan that generate tiny temperature-dependent voltage and are precise and accurate in measuring temperature. Thermistors, semiconductors whose resistance decreases as temperature increases, are also reliable instruments. Liquid crystal skin-surface thermometers estimate core temperature from skin temperature by means of a constant offset value near 2°C (assume constant skin to core gradient). Infrared thermometers have become inexpensive and reliable enough for routine use, although their use in cases of hypothermia have not been evaluated in published studies. It is best to remeasure core temperature accurately when a reading of less than 35°C is obtained. The preferred temperature measurement is by a rectal thermocouple probe inserted at least 15 cm.

Monitoring sites for standard core temperatures include the distal esophagus, tympanic membrane, nasopharynx, and pulmonary artery. They are generally accurate to about 0.2°C and precise to about 0.1°C. Intermediate sites are mouth, axilla, bladder, and rectum. Their accuracy and precision is to 0.5°C and 0.2°C, respectively. These intermediate sites can fail for a variety of reasons.

Hypothermia can be classified into mild, moderate, and severe. Mild hypothermia is a temperature between 34°C and 35°C (4). Patients may have poor coordination, muscle shivering, stumbling, slurred speech, amnesia, and hallucinations. Blood pressure may initially be increased, as well as heart and respiratory rates. Peripheral vasoconstriction manifests as cool extremities and acrocyanosis. Cardiac output decreases. Moderate hypothermia is a temperature between 30°C and 34°C (4). The patient becomes more obtunded or comatose, muscle tone is increased, and blood pressure falls. Muscle shivering may be absent. Severe hypothermia is a temperature less than 30°C (4). At this temperature, cardiac arrest is imminent because of spontaneous ventricular fibrillation. Brain stem function and deep tendon reflexes are usually absent, and the patient has agonal breathing.

Hypothermia can also be classified as primary or secondary. Primary hypothermia results directly from an overwhelming cold stress, whereas secondary hypothermia is part of other clinical conditions. The diagnosis of primary hypothermia may be quite obvious, but secondary hypothermia may need a high index of suspicion. A good physical examination may reveal clues as to the cause of hypothermia (e.g., trauma, alcohol breath, needle marks). Sepsis is a common cause of hypothermia and was a cause in up to 40% of hypothermia cases in one urban hospital. Hypothermia is common in severe hypothyroidism because of the reduction of the metabolic rate by as much as 40% below normal. Other conditions such as hypoglycemia, diabetic ketoacidosis, and hyperosmolar coma may cause hypothermia by suppressing the hypothalamic temperature regulation or through inhibition of shivering. Hypothalamic tumors, spinal cord tumors, and first thoracic nerve tumors can also lead to hypothermia. The latter two conditions lead to lower temperatures by blocking shivering and interrupting cold-induced compensatory reflexes mediated by the lateral spinothalamic tracts.

When the patient is first seen, hypothermia has already caused several changes in the bodily functions, and assessment should include trying to determine both the cause of hypothermia and the immediate organ system damages. The patient may have shock caused by intravascular volume depletion from cold diuresis, a condition resulting in reduction of the absorptive capacity of renal tubular cell.

A complete physical examination should be done quickly, noting any evidence of trauma. Doppler ultrasonography may be needed for measuring blood pressure accurately because of the intense peripheral vasoconstriction. The extent of frostbite and tissue necrosis, especially of the ears, nose, and extremities, should be assessed. The neurological examination should focus on finding focal signs that point to an intracranial pathological condition.

Laboratory evaluation should include a complete blood count, serum biochemical profile (electrolytes, blood urea nitrogen [BUN], creatinine, glucose, calcium, magnesium, phosphorous, amylase, liver enzymes), thyroid function, serum cortisol, prothrombin and partial thromboplastin times (PT/PTT), blood cultures, urinalysis, arterial blood gases, electrocardiogram, chest x-ray films, and toxicological and alcohol screening. The electrocardiographic finding in hypothermia (i.e., Osborne J-wave [a positive deflection occurring at the junction of the QRS complex and the ST segment]) is pathognomonic of hypothermia.

C. Therapeutic Intervention

As always, initiating and maintaining cardiopulmonary resuscitation is done to make sure that there is airway patency, adequate breathing, and maintainance of circulation. The hypothermic body is able to tolerate prolonged periods of hypoxia, and this should be taken into account in the management, particularly in cases of accidental hypothermia. Assessment of permanent organ damage is inaccurate until the patient is properly warmed. Electroencephalographic findings during severe hypothermia may be isoelectric, which is not an indication of brain death and may in fact be reversible. Prompt return of normal body temperature is the primary goal. An algorithm for patients with hypothermia is shown in Figure 1. Depending on the severity of hypothermia, interventions may range from simple passive warming to invasive cardiopulmonary bypass.

Geriatric patients with accidental exposure tend to have severe forms of hypothermia because of their decreased threshold for shivering and other factors mentioned previously. In addition, they may have taken drugs that may further aggravate the condition.

Several ways are effective in rewarming the hypothermic geriatric patient. Passive rewarming is the use of the patient's own heat-generating capacity, whereas active rewarming is giving heat from an external source. Active rewarming can be administered either externally or internally (core). Dry blankets are effective in reducing heat loss by 30% to 50%, depending on the number and thickness used. Avoiding exposure to water and wind will also help in conserving heat. If the hypothermic victim is unable to shiver, especially with core temperatures less than 30°F, active external rewarming techniques can be used, including electric heating blanket, body-to-body warming, forced-air heating, hot water bottle, and warm water immersion. External forced-air heating has been shown to attenuate the drop in core temperature during rewarming (''afterdrop'') and

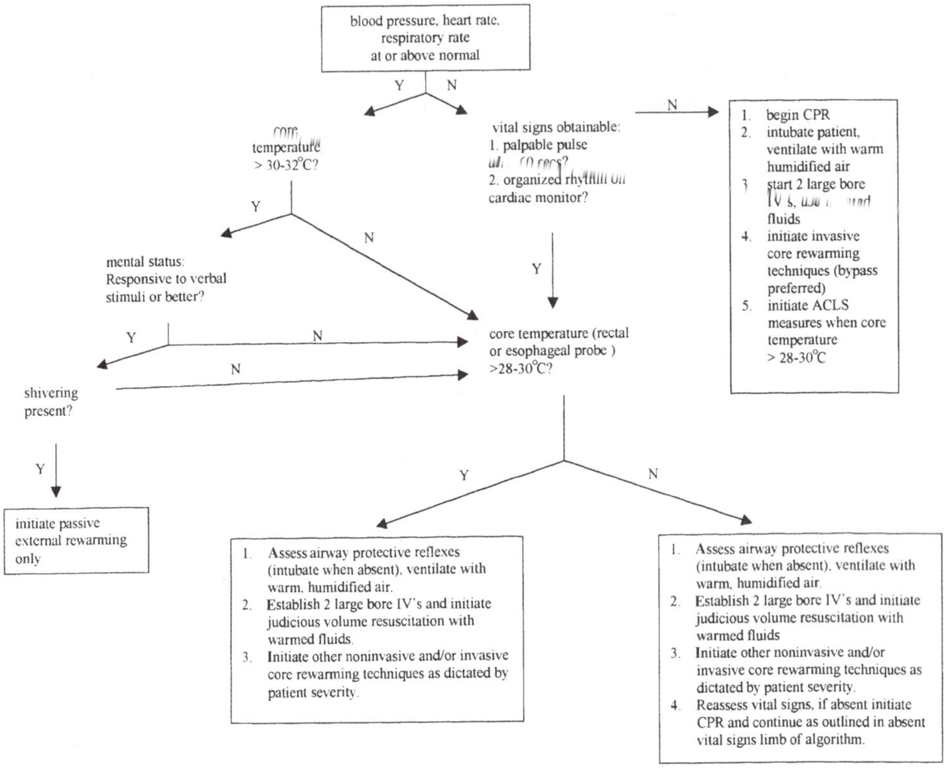

Figure 1 Therapeutic algorithm for patients with hypothermia. Y, yes; N, no; ACLS, advanced cardiac life support; IVs, intravenous lines; CPR, cardiopulmonary resuscitation. (From J. Christopher Farmer, Critical Care, Civetta JM, Taylor RW and Kirby RR, Lippincott-Raven Publishers, Philadelphia, PA, 1997.)

the metabolic stress and shivering in mild hypothermic volunteers with temperatures from 34.5°F to 35.5°F (5). Most radiant heaters may not be effective because they do not have enough surface area to transfer a clinically significant amount of heat to hypothermic patients.

Active internal rewarming interventions include warmed intravenous (IV) fluids. A liter of (IV) fluid at room temperature would decrease the patient's mean body temperature by 0.25°F. In animal studies, IV fluids at 149°F (65°C) were administered safely. In cases in which the patient is extremely dehydrated from cold diuresis and little intake of water, several liters of fluids are used and may delay rewarming if the IV fluids used are not properly warmed. A possibility of ''rewarming shock'' caused by vasodilation exists after return to normal temperature. Intravenous fluid administration should prevent this complication. Theoretically, the use of warm IV fluids should rewarm the heart in parallel to other core and peripheral structures. This would eliminate a discrepancy in the peripheral tissues' increasing metabolic demands and the heart's capacity to deliver oxygen. However, studies have shown no difference in the survival and clinical or histopathological morbidity between active external rewarming and core-rewarming methods (6,7). Little heat is lost by respiration, and the use of active or passive airway heating and humidification adds little to the core temperature. However, airway heating may be beneficial in preventing bronchospasm and decreasing nosocomial pneumonia. Aside from the higher cost, active airway heating and humidification is not shown to be more effective than the least expensive passive method.

Hemodialysis and peritoneal dialysis with warm dialysate are also effective core rewarming techniques. In severe cases of hypothermia complicated by cardiac arrest, cardiopulmonary bypass is the treatment of choice for rewarming, if available.

D. Follow-up Management

After initial stabilization, hypothermic patients need to be in the intensive care unit for close monitoring. Atrial fibrillation with slow ventricular response is common at less than 32°C. The most fatal dysrhythmia is the susceptibility of the cardiac muscle for ventricular tachycardia and fibrillation, especially at core temperatures less than 30°C. Hypothermia triples the incidence of ventricular tachycardia and morbid cardiac events (8). Mild hypothermia also increases sympathetic activity and may induce myocardial ischemia. Bretylium is the treatment of choice to lower ventricular fibrillatory threshold (9–11). The role of transvenous pacemakers is limited, and attempts at placement may cause irritation and initiate a life-threatening ventricular dysrhythmia. Similarly, the placement of a central venous catheter for monitoring is not routinely recommended for the preceding reasons.

Nosocomial infections, particularly pneumonia, may complicate the condition of hypothermia. Obtunded hypothermic patients are prone to aspiration pneumonia. Early intubation for airway protection is recommended if any doubts exist about the patient's own ability to protect his or her airway. Empiric antibiotics, if pneumonia cannot be ruled out convincingly, should include broad-spectrum antibiotics to cover aspiration pneumonia and gram-negative nosocomial pneumonia. The presence of wounds needs special attention. With vasoconstriction compromising oxygen delivery to wounds and the associated decrease in immune function with aging and hypothermia, the elderly patient is at risk for sepsis from infected frostbite and pressure ulcers. Bleeding also occurs as a consequence of coagulation disorders with hypothermia.

Hematologic effects of hypothermia include granulocytopenia, hemoconcentration, thrombocytopenia and platelet dysfunction, and disseminated intravascular coagulation (DIC). Bleeding is not usually responsive to blood component therapy unless rewarming is achieved (12). Laboratory tests for coagulation may be normal with clinical coagulopathy because these tests are performed in heated chambers that warm the blood to normal physiological temperatures.

Education of the elderly and their health care providers, particularly those living in geographic areas with cold temperatures, on the cause, symptoms, and significance of hypothermia should be a primary goal to reduce the risk of hypothermia. Those at highest risk should be targeted, particularly the poverty-stricken, isolated geriatric patient, for close follow-up. Polypharmacy should be avoided, and advice should be given against alcohol use. Adequate food intake and space heating are key preventive measures.

II. HYPERTHERMIA

A. Clinical Relevance

Classic heat stroke typically occurs in elderly individuals as opposed to exertional heat stroke, which is more prevalent in exercising younger individuals. Heat-related death is defined by the National Association of Medical Examiners as exposure to high ambient temperature either causing death or substantially contributing to the death (13). From 1979 to 1995, 62% of deaths from heat exposure caused by weather conditions occurred in persons ≥55 years. During a 1995 heat wave in Chicago, 51% of heat-related deaths were in seniors age ≥75 years. In Dallas county, 15 of 25 heat-related deaths in 1998 were in patients age 65 years and older. Patients living alone, overweight, and taking neuroleptics and tricyclic antidepressants are at highest risk. Alcohol consumption is also a contributing factor. The high prevalence of chronic diseases such as pulmonary and cardiac problems complicate the situation for the geriatric population. In addition, physical or cognitive problems may affect the patient's ability to modify the environment to prevent overexposure to heat.

Two other entities, malignant hyperthermia and neuroleptic malignant syndrome, will also be addressed in this section. Malignant hyperthermia is a rare entity that carries a high morbidity and mortality and most frequently affects the geriatric population and the chronically ill. Neuroleptic malignant syndrome affects the younger population, with a mean age of 40 years (14,15).

Hyperthermia is defined as core body temperature of >38°C. Heat stroke is typically associated with core body temperatures in excess of 105°F (40.6°C). Three different mechanisms exist for hyperthermia: central regulatory failure, inadequate peripheral response, and fever. In a sufficiently warm climate, central thermal regulation is actively maintaining a normal body temperature. When a tumor, stroke, or injury affects hypothalamic function, hyperthermia can result (poikilothermia syndrome) (16). It can also result from intoxication with ethanol, barbiturates, or phenothiazines. Illicit drug use thus markedly increases the risk of heat injury (17,18).

A peripheral response to heat includes behavioral and autonomic thermoregulatory defenses. The most commonly used thermoregulatory defense in humans is behavioral modification. However, this is affected by various factors such as illness, administration of sedatives, strenuous physical activities, and environmental restriction. Under these circumstances, autonomic thermoregulatory defense takes over completely. This may be in the form of dissipation of body heat by conduction, convection, radiation, and evaporation. Only evaporation can dissipate heat when ambient temperature exceeds body temperature. When the humidity approaches 100%, loss by evaporation fails. Hyperthermia can also occur when peripheral thermoregulatory defenses are impaired. Absence of sweating occurs with parasympathetic blockade and dehydration/intravascular depletion. Hyperthermia can also result from excessive heat production as in malignant hyperthermia and neuroleptic malignant syndrome. In malignant hyperthermia, metabolic heat production increases to nearly 10-fold, an amount that usually cannot be dissipated even by intact thermoregulatory defenses. The pathophysiology is unclear for neuroleptic malignant syndrome, but hyperthermia is probably due to increased heat production from muscle contraction, inappropriate vasoconstriction, and altered hypothalamic setpoint.

Fever is different from the other mechanisms of hyperthermia in that it is normal physiological response to pyrogenic cytokines (e.g., interleukin-1, tumor necrosis factor, interleukin-6) and is not due to excessive exposure or inability to dissipate heat. Through a prostaglandin-based pathway, pyrogenic cytokines affect the hypothalamus indirectly to reset thermoregulatory response thresholds to a higher level. The hypothalamus activates a series of behavioral and metabolic responses (vasoconstriction, increased metabolic rate, shivering) to conserve and generate heat, which results in elevation of the temperature. Fever probably enhances the ability to survive infection, but its effects are not favorable to geriatric patients. Fever increases oxygen consumption and is deleterious to the elderly if marginal cardiac and cerebral supply is present. Treatment of fever in the acutely ill patient reduces oxygen consumption and carbon dioxide (CO_2) production (19), as well as gives comfort to the patient. However, it has not been shown to have long-term benefits.

B. Immediate Diagnostic Approach

The occurrence of severe hyperthermia in the setting of fever (response from infection, malignancy, or autoimmune processes), environmental exposure, neuroleptic malignant syndrome, and malignant hyperthermia causes cellular and physiological damages that require immediate response. Identifying hyperthermia is usually not a problem, except in patients with neuroleptic malignant syndrome not yet manifesting a high temperature in whom suspicion always needs to be present. Patients with heat exhaustion may have symptoms of headache, confusion, drowsiness, visual disturbances, fatigue, hyperirritability, and anxiety. On physical examination they have tachycardia, dry mucous membranes, and orthostatic hypotension. In extremely hot conditions, classic heat stroke often affects the elderly, who have limited ability to adapt. These patients have altered mental status and seizures, and a history may not be immediately available. The finding of absence of sweating is usually a late sign and not universal in patients with classic heat stroke. In the elderly patient, hemodynamic instability comes early, especially in those with limited cardiac and vascular reserve.

In malignant hyperthermia, trismus is the first sign that appears after anesthetic administration in 50% of the cases. This is followed by whole body rigidity and a rapid increase in body temperature. Lactic acidosis and CO_2 production also ensue because of depletion of adenosine triphosphate and initation of anaerobic metabolism. Anesthetics implicated usually are succinylcholine and decamethonium and the potent inhalation agents ether, methoxyflurane, cyclopropane, halothane, enflurane, isoflurane, desflurane, and sevoflurane (20). The timing of when symptoms develop is variable, occurring either during induction or thereafter. Other signs of malignant hyperthemia include hypertension, sweating, cyanosis, mottling of the skin, and dysrhythmias. When the temperature starts to rise, the rate could be as fast as 1°C every 5 minutes. Relying on rectal temperature monitoring may not be sufficient because rectal temperature may not change quick enough during malignant hyperthermia (21). The anesthetist or anesthesiologist should measure not only the patient's temperature but also the arterial and venous blood gases, and the end-tidal CO_2 concentration by monitoring the soda lime carbon dioxide absorber for color and heat. These absorbers turn blue and hot when saturated with CO_2 from the patient's respiration.

In neuroleptic malignant syndrome, muscular rigidity, dystonia, unexplained catatonic behavior, and hyperpyrexia occur after administration of a neuroleptic agent or withdrawal of dopaminergic agents. Patients typically have symptoms 5 days after institution of therapy. Hyperpyrexia may not be immediately apparent, and diagnosis of this syndrome may be delayed. Indeed, this syndrome has an insidious onset and its diagnosis is often overlooked by physicians in the early part of its course.

C. Therapeutic Intervention

Attention to the essentials of cardiopulmonary resuscitation is necessary in the initial management of hyperthermic patients. Patients with coma who are unable to protect their airway need to be intubated. Hypotension, when present, is ominous and signifies severe dehydration and possible myocardial dysfunction. Large-bore IV catheters and Foley catheters need to be in place for monitoring fluid input and output. After identifying the proximate cause of the hyperthermia, expedited cooling should be instituted. Survival depends on the intensity and duration of hyperthermia (22,23). Removal of the elderly patient from a hot environment, taking away warm clothing, and discontinuing active warming (as in heating blankets) will usually be effective in treating passive hyperthermia. Sponge baths with ice water or alcohol, immersion in an ice water bath, and cooling fans also hastens heat dissipation. One caveat with body immersion is that it impairs the ability to perform other resuscitative measures (cardiac monitoring, airway protection, etc). In addition, total body immersion in cold water may trigger shivering, which generates more heat, and vasoconstriction, which reduces heat loss. Applying ice packs regionally to the body in rotation may avoid these potential complications. When complicated by dehydration, volume resuscitation with refrigerated normal saline can effectively bring down temperature (0.5°F/L infused) and correct volume depletion (24).

In malignant hyperthermia, removal of the offending agent and hyperventilation up to three times the normal minute ventilation rate with 100% oxygen should be done immediately. Dantrolene is the only specific and effective treatment and should be given as soon as possible. Dosage is 1 to 2.5 mg/kg IV every 5 to 10 minutes, up to the maximum dose of 10 mg/kg, followed by oral dantrolene, 4 to 8 mg/kg/day in four divided doses, 1 to 3 days after the acute event, if necessary. Calcium channel blockers have no role in malignant hyperthermia and may be deleterious to myocardial function. It should be completely avoided. In neuroleptic malignant syndrome, cessation of the offending agent and initiation of dopaminergic agonist like bromocriptine (2.5 to 20 mg orally in 3 divided doses) controls extrapyramidal symptoms within a day. Nondepolarizing agents or dantrolene may also have a role in relaxing the muscles and prevent further excessive heat generation.

Other cooling measures include active internal cooling. If hyperthermia does not respond to external cooling measures, internal cooling can be done. Bladder and gastric lavage and peritoneal lavage with sterile iced saline are effective in malignant hyperthermia and refractory hyperthermia. In extreme circumstances, hemodialysis or cardiopulmonary bypass with cooling of blood may be performed.

It is best to manage hyperthermic patients with temperatures greater than 40°C and with altered mental status in the intensive care unit. Tachycardia is one of the most common consequences of hyperthermia and this could be detrimental to elderly patients, especially those with the most marginal cardiac conditions. Tachycardia can reduce cardiac output in the diastolically impaired heart and increase myocardial oxygen demand, precipitating angina and ultimately myocardial infarction. It is believed that tachycardia results from a direct temperature-dependent effect on the sinoatrial node (25). At extreme levels of hyperthermia, coagulopathy can develop. In cases of hyperthermia caused by exposure to extreme heat and thermoregulatory failure, it should be emphasized that antipyretics are not effective because the mechanism for hyperthermia is not related to prostaglandins.

If hyperthermia is due to fever (≥41°C), nonsteroidal anti-inflammatory drugs and acetaminophen can be administered around the clock. In the elderly, fever often is due to bacterial infection. Although a significant proportion of the elderly population will not mount a febrile response to infection, most (70%–80%) do (26). Fever usually responds well to treatment of underlying infection and only occasionally requires an antipyretic. However, liver and kidney dysfunction and coagulopathy may be present, which makes these antipyretics contraindicated. When fever is due to noninfectious causes such as in extensive tissue necrosis and inflammation, malignancy, allergic reaction, and hypermetabolic states, corticosteroids and diphenhydramine (Benadryl) may be of benefit. Caution is, however, needed with the use of these agents, especially diphenhydramine, which could cause further mental status deterioration and make it difficult to assess the clinical course. As stated earlier, the use of extensive active cooling in high-temperature states has some potential disadvantages. Cutaneous cooling can provoke more vasoconstriction and shivering, which further elevates core body temperature. In addition, these measures are extremely uncomfortable for patients. Meperidine, an opiate agonist, and morphine, as well antipsychotics such as prochlorperazine and chlorpromazine, may be useful in preventing shivering. Among the opiates, morphine is safer to use in the elderly. Combining the two classes of drugs has an additive effect, but care must be given in prescribing these agents singly or in combination to avoid hypotension.

D. Follow-up Management

Electrolyte abnormalities (low sodium, potassium, phosphate, calcium, and magnesium) are frequent findings in the early clinical course of hyperthermia. The magnitude of loss of sodium, potassium, and magnesium may be massive from increased sweating. Replacement of these electrolytes accordingly should be performed for optimal outcome. Hypokalemia impairs sweating ability and decreases skeletal muscle blood flow, further impairing heat dissipation (22). In patients with significant rhabdomyolysis, hyperkalemia, hypocalcemia, and creatine kinase elevation occur. However, hypocalcemia should be corrected only when serious ventricular dysrhythmias supervene because of hyperkalemia. In these cases, glucose, insulin,and calcium solutions should be given emergently. Hemodialysis may be needed in some cases.

Evaluation for sepsis should be done to exclude all possible foci of infection in the elderly. Infections may be present even when hyperthermia is from other causes and may only be a contributing factor. Other disease entities that may be in the differential diagnosis of fever include thyrotoxicosis, pheochromocytoma, and systemic sclerosis.

Acid-base disorders occur in hyperthermia. The most common acid-base disorder is metabolic acidosis and respiratory alkalosis. However, malignant hyperthermia and metabolic and respiratory acidosis occur as a result of an increase in CO_2 production associated with the syndrome. Hyperventilation occurs with hyperthermia, and tissue hypoxia produces lactic acidosis with respiratory compensation. In arterial blood gas determinations, correction for temperatures should be done to avoid an inaccurate assessment (falsely low $Paco_2$ and Pao_2 and elevated pH). Disseminated intravascular coagulation is rare and seen only in severe cases; if present, this is a poor prognostic marker.

Clinical monitoring should focus on the associated complications such as myocardial infarction, congestive heart failure, dysrhythmias, acute renal failure, rhabdomyolysis, seizures, hepatic failure, respiratory failure and adult respiratory distress syndrome, and DIC. Serial cardiac enzymes and electrocardiography need to be performed because the heart may have been affected by hypoperfusion from hypovolemia. Heat can have toxic effects on myocytes, and myocardial infarctions can occur even in the absence of significant coronary artery disease (27). Placement of a central pulmonary artery catheter may help in determining volume and cardiac status. Echocardiography should be done early if hypotension does not improve after hydration of the elderly patient. If myocardial dysfunction exists, dobutamine is an effective choice for inotropic support. In malignant hyperthemia, procainamide should be started because of the likelihood of ventricular fibrillation in this syndrome. Acute renal failure may take 24 to 48 hours to develop and is associated with increased mortality. The central nervous system, particularly the Purkinje cells of the cerebellum, is particularly sensitive to hyperthermia. Some patients may have residual cerebellar dysfunction. If seizure occurs, intravenous diazepam or other benzodiazepines should be given. The liver suffers reversible damage in the face of hyperthermia within 24 to 48 hours. Death from fulminant liver failure is rare. Adult respiratory distress syndrome especially when complicated by DIC, has a mortality rate of 75%.

For most cases of hyperthermia, prevention is important in the face of the preceding consequences. Education of the geriatric patient and health care provider is again of paramount importance. Reduction of physical activity, drinking extra liquids, and increasing time spent in air-conditioned places are proper preventive measures, especially during heat waves. Adequate salt intake is also important, but salt tablets are not recommended and may be harmful for patients with hypertension and heart failure. At very high temperatures (90°F) fans are ineffective for cooling and may increase heat stress and the risk of heat stroke. Thus, programs that distribute fans to senior citizens during summer months may not be effective in reducing the risk for hyperthermia. In reviewing reports on hyperthermia deaths during heat waves, it is noted that a lag of about 2 days exists after the onset of a heat wave and the first cases of death. This may represent a significant window of opportunity to focus efforts and try to decrease the morbidity and mortality associated with hyperthermia in the geriatric population.

In cases of malignant hyperthermia, genetic predisposition is implicated. The gene for malignant hyperthermia is found on chromosome 19 (28,29), although many believe that malignant hyperthermia results from a heterogeneous group of mutations. The ''gold standard'' test for screening for malignant hyperthermia is the in vitro muscle contraction test, although its specificity and sensitivity are also questioned. Individuals susceptible to malignant hyperthermia have sustained contraction develop on biopsied muscle exposed to halothane, caffeine, or ryanodine (30). A clinical grading scale is also available for the prediction of malignant hyperthermia (31). Future testing may involve genetic sequencing and isolation of specific genes in potentially susceptible patients. Agents that may be used safely in susceptible patients include nitrous oxide, opiates, barbiturates, benzodiazepines, and local anesthetics. When encountering susceptible patients, temperature and end tidal volume CO_2 measurements should be performed, and therapy should be instituted if patients show signs of progression of full-blown malignant hyperthermia.

REFERENCES

1. Inouye Y, Nakao M, Araki T, Murakami H. Regional differences in the sweating responses of older and younger men. J Applied Physiol 1991;71:2453–2459.
2. Khan F, Spence VA, Belch JJF. Cutaneous vascular responses and thermoregulation in relation to age. Clin Sci 1992;82:521–528.
3. CDC. Hypothermia-associated deaths—Georgia, January 1996—December 1997, and United States, 1979–1995. MMWR 1998;47:1037–1040.
4. Adam K. Human body temperature is inversely correlated with body mass. Eur J Appl Physiol 1989;58:471–475.
5. Giesbrecht GG, Schroeder M, Bristow GK. Treatment of mild-immersion hypothermia by forced air-warming. Aviat Space Environ Med 1994;65:803–808.
6. Ledingham IM, Mone JG. Treatment of accidental hypothermia: a prospective clinical study. BMJ 1980;280:1102–1105.
7. Moss JF, Haklin M, Southwick HW, Roseman DI. A model for the treatment of accidental severe hypothermia. J Trauma 1986;26:68–74.
8. Frank SM, Fleisher LA, Breslow MJ, Higgins M, Alson KF, Kelly S, Beattie C. Maintenance of normothermia with forced-air warming reduces the incidence of electrocardiographic and morbid cardiac events (abstr). Anesthesiology 1996; 85(3A):A106.

9. Dronen S, Nowak RM, Tomalanovich MC. Bretylium tosylate and hypothermic ventricular fibrillation (letter). Ann Emerg Med 1980;9:335.
10. Kochar G, Kahn SE, Kotler MN. Bretylium tosylate and ventricular fibrillation in hypothermia (letter). Ann Intern Med 1986;105:624.
11. Orts A, Alcaraz C, Delaney KA, Goldfrank LR, Turndorf H, Puig MM. Bretylium tosylate and electrically induced cardiac arrhythmias during hypovolemia in dogs. Am J Emerg Med 1992;10:311–316.
12. Ellis FP. Mortality from heat illness and heat aggravated illness in the United States. Environ Res 1972;5:1–58.
13. Donoghue ER, Graham MA, Jentzen JM, Lifschultz BD, Luke JL, Mirchandani HG. National Association of Medical Examiners Ad Hoc Committee on the Definition of Heat-Related Fatalities. Criteria for the diagnosis of heat-related deaths: National Association of Medical Examiners. Am J Forensic Med Pathol 1997;18(1):11–14.
14. Caroff SN. The neuroleptic malignant syndrome. J Clin Psychiatry 1980;41:79–83.
15. Kurlan R, Hamill R, Shoulson I. Neuroleptic malignant syndrome. Clin Neuropharmacol 1984;7:109–120.
16. Mckenzie MA, Hermus Rmm, Wollersheim H, Pieters GF, Smals AG, Binkhorst RA, Thien T, Kloppenborg PW. Poikilothermia in man: pathophysiology and clinical implications. Medicine 1991;70:257–268.
17. Kalant H, Le AD. Effects of ethanol on thermoregulation. Pharmacol Ther 1984; 23:313–364.
18. Dominguez de Villota E, Mosquera JM, Shubin H, Weil MH. Abnormal temperature control after intoxication with short acting barbiturates. Crit Care Med 1981;9:662–665.
19. Manthous CA, Hall JB, Olson D, Singh M, Chatila W, Pohlman A, Kushner R, Schmidt GA, Wood LDH. Effect of cooling on oxygen consumption in febrile critically ill patients. Am J Respir Crit Care Med 1995;151:10–14.
20. Gronert GA. Malignant hyperthermia. Anesthesiology 1980;53:395–423.
21. Satinoff E. Neural organization and evolution of thermal regulation in mammals—several hierarchally arranged integrating systems may have evolved to achieve precise thermoregulation. Science 1978;201:16–22.
22. Knochel JP. Environmental heat illness: an eclectic review. Arch Intern Med 1974; 133:841–864.
23. Tom PA, Garmel GM, Auerbach PS. Environment-dependent sports emergencies. Med Clin North Am 1994;78:305–325.
24. Sessler DI. Consequences and treatment of perioperative hypothermia. Anesth Clin North Am 1994;12:425–456.
25. Ikeda T, Sessler D. Temperature monitoring. In: Tobin MJ (ed.). Principles and Practice of Intensive Care Monitoring. New York: McGraw Hill, Inc., 1998, pp 1151–1162.
26. Yoshikawa TT, Norman DC. Fever in the elderly. Infect Med 1998;15(10):704–706, 708.
27. Zahger D, Moses A, Weiss AT. Evidence of prolonged myocardial dysfunction in heat stroke. Chest 1989;95:1089–1091.
28. Heffron JJ, McCarthy TV. Current views of the molecular basis of the malignant hyperthermia syndrome. Acta Anaesthesiol Belg 1990;41:73–78.

29. McCarthy TV, Healy JM, Lehane M, Heffron JJ. Recent developments in the molecular genetics of malignant hyperthermia: implications for future diagnosis at the DNA level. Acta Anaesthesiol Belg 1990;41:107–112.
30. Hopkins PM, Ellis FR, Halsall PJ. Ryanodine contracture: a potentially specific in vitro diagnostic test for malignant hyperthermia. Br J Anaesth 1991;66(5):611–613.
31. Larach MG, Localio AR, Allen GC, Denborough MA, Ellis FR, Gronert GA, Kaplan RF, Muldoon SM, Nelson T, Ording H, et al. A clinical grading scale to predict malignant hyperthermia susceptibility. Anesthesiology 1994;80:771–779.

24

Diagnosis and Treatment of Abuse and Neglect in the Emergency Department

Cheryl E. Woodson
Ingalls Health System, Harvey, Illinois

Emergency department (ED) clinicians are in an excellent position to intervene in cases of abuse and neglect of the elderly (ANE) because of the frequency with which these situations are seen in EDs. When this condition is untreated, admissions to the acute hospital through the ED are common. For these reasons, ED evaluation and intervention can be critical to appropriate long-term management of this condition. Compared with primary care physicians who have the luxury of a longitudinal relationship that allows for multiple assessment opportunities and building confidence with all parties, ED personnel may be at a disadvantage when faced with the more subtle manifestations of ANE. Even so, if ED physicians and staff develop confidence in recognizing key signs that activate the assessment process and develop expertise in accessing appropriate referral resources, they can have significant impact.

I. CLINICAL RELEVANCE

The diagnosis of ANE came to light in 1975 with the publication of a British article on ''granny battering'' (1). In the ensuing 23 years, the incidence of this condition has been difficult to assess because investigators differ in both their definitions of ANE and the age at which ''elderly'' begins. When observers fail to report ANE, whether they are health care professionals, social service workers, law enforcement officials, general citizens, or the involved older adult, the accuracy of incidence data may be further decreased. Observers may not recognize that a situation is abusive, or they may not know how to intervene. Observers may believe their intervention would be seen as intrusive or bring unwanted attention to the caregiver or to themselves. The involved older adult may not seek or may refuse help for fear of relocating from their homes. Alternate residence options are few, and nursing home placement may be neither desirable nor appropriate (2).

The cohort of persons aged 65 years and older is the fastest growing portion of the American population, and the rate of growth is increasing. In the 1990 census, older Americans accounted for 13% of the population. It is predicted that this percentage will increase to 18% by 2020 and 25% by 2050. The fastest growing portion of the geriatric population is adults older than age 85; their total population is expected to double between 2020 and 2050 (3). This group is at the greatest risk of frailty and need of care.

Older adults access the emergency medical system at a rate much higher than their representation in the population (4), and they account for approximately 40% of hospital admissions (5). One study reported that of 182 elders with documented physical abuse, approximately 63% had been evaluated in EDs within 5 years. The median rate was three visits, 30% of which generated an inpatient admission. Two-thirds of the patients had a chief complaint corresponding to an ICD-9 diagnosis code specifying an injury, and for approximately 40% of the patients, their ED visit was consistent with the investigators' retrospective criteria for ''high-probability'' ANE (4). Despite this rich opportunity to diagnose and treat ANE, a national survey of ED physicians reported that their level of confidence and expertise in managing this illness was low and that few ED physicians had protocols and referral guides to assist them (6). A great opportunity for improvement exists here.

A. Risk of ANE

As in any other medical syndrome, risk factors are associated with a higher incidence of ANE. Primary prevention is not usually the purview of the ED, but understanding risk factors may heighten the index of suspicion and lead to increased assessment. The ANE literature describes dependency (physical, cognitive, psychological, or financial) as a risk for becoming a victim and psychosocial stress, isolation, substance abuse, and overwhelming responsibility as risk factors for perpetrating abuse (2,7,8,9). We are on the verge of a caregiving crisis in this country because an increasing number of adults survive to older ages and live with chronic disabilities and increasing care requirements. Smaller family size and changes in other societal factors including stepfamilies, increased mobility, and larger geographical distances between family members often result in care responsibility to be assumed by a smaller number of potential caregivers.

These caregivers are increasingly under additional stress from other responsibilities from the workplace and caring for multiple older adults and children simultaneously. Although these factors increase potential caregiver stress, they are no longer believed to be the primary risk in development of ANE. More recent investigations have identified dysfunctional family relationships where a history of family violence or psychological or financial interdependence exists as the primary risk. The additional stresses of substance abuse and psychological syndromes may also impair the caregivers. All these factors increase the risk that care will be inadequate or inappropriate.

B. Categories of ANE and Definitions

Little improvement has been made on the definitions initially outlined by O'Malley et al in 1987 (10), although several previously combined categories are now often made distinct. *Physical abuse* is the easiest to identify because of obvious physical findings, including burns, bruises, fractures, lacerations, or witnessed use of physical force such as hitting, slapping, pinching, pushing, or restraining. This category also includes forced ingestion of street drugs, alcohol, or other substances. *Physical restraint or confinement* is a form of physical abuse that exists when a patient is tied, held, locked in a restricted area, or otherwise forcibly limited in mobility for reasons other than physical safety or, when for physical safety, without supervision or release. *Sexual abuse* is physical abuse occurring when a patient is touched, fondled, instrumented, or forced to engage in intercourse or other sexual acts against his or her will. *Medication abuse* is seen when medications are either withheld or over used. *Psychological abuse* includes threats, yelling, and demeaning and disrespectful interactions, but it also includes coercion and infantalization. *Financial exploitation* is diagnosed when the older adult's financial resources are used for expenses unrelated to their own care without uncoerced permission. The risk is high when the caregiver is financially dependent on the older adult.

Neglect is usually described in two ways: in *passive neglect*, the caregiver allows a need to remain unmet but is unaware of the circumstances or remedies. The terms *active endangerment* or *willful deprivation* are reserved for instances in which the caregiver is fully aware of the need and does not move to intervene appropriately. *Abandonment* is another type of neglect that is evident when the caregiver abrogates full responsibility and provides no care, often removing himself or herself from the care situation. This can be a complicated legal issue because in most states in the absence of a guardianship, no one has either the right or the responsibility to care for another adult. Durable powers of attorney are conferred by the patient before disability, but in most states they are not mandatory for the designee. For example, it may not be clear that an adult child has the legal responsibility to provide care for an aging parent. *Self-neglect* occurs when an adult refuses to alter a high-risk circumstance or to accept assistance. In this case, the adult's own actions present a danger to himself or herself.

In all types of ANE, the decision-making capacity of the involved older adult is critical to any intervention. A person who understands and accepts the consequences of his or her decisions may choose to stay in a situation that is deemed suboptimal or dangerous by others. The incentive for making this decision is often a desire to remain in one's own home rather than to relocate. This is understandable because few good alternate living arrangements exist for dependent older adults. Most assisted living programs are expensive, and nursing home placement may not be desirable.

II. IMMEDIATE DIAGNOSTIC APPROACH

Factors that may indicate elder abuse and neglect are listed in Table 1. The most important identifying factors in the history are implausible explanations for injuries and evidence that medical attention has been delayed or unsought. It is important that someone interview the caregiver and patient together and separately to observe changes in behavior and to have the opportunity to witness any inappropriate behavior. It is also essential to assess caregiver stress, physical and mental illness, other responsibilities, and caregiving resources. In a busy ED, where the physicians are charged with management of potentially critical injuries and illnesses, this important role can be fulfilled by a social worker or nurse who is specially trained in dealing with ANE.

A. Examples of Elder Abuse and Neglect That May Present to the ED

1. Patient Problem 1

A 76-year-old woman was brought to the ED for chest pain. She was 5′9″ tall and had a 6-cm-wide bandlike bruise around her chest and back just under her breasts. The bruise had many acute features but also showed older, yellowed areas. When asked about this, the caregiver said the patient had been walking in the dining room and bumped into the table. ANE should be suspected because (1) the patient was too tall to have sustained a submammary bruise by walking into a table; (2) such a bruise would not have encircled the entire chest; and (3) the differing stages of resolution in the bruised area suggest that this could not have been a one time occurrence. When these points were raised, the caregiver confessed that the patient was usually tied into a dining room chair all day to keep her from wandering. This family was referred to adult day care and a care-

Table 1 Indicators of Possible Elder Abuse and Neglect

Category	History	Physical examination
Physical	Implausible or inconsistent explanations of events Witnessed physical violence Inordinate delay in seeking medicinal assistance	Evidence of physical injury Location or character of injuries inconsistent with history Multiple lesions in different stages of resolution Evidence of inattention to injury (old, nonset fractures)
Sexual	May not be able to elicit	Evidence of perineal, inner thigh, buttock, oral injury, other sexual contact, or sexually transmitted disease in a patient who denies or is incapable of consent (*Use the Rape Kit*)
Medication	Evidence of prescription refills more frequently than prescribed usage dictates Medication not filled or used	Altered mental status (lethargy or agitation) or other signs of medication/substance intoxication Abnormal drug levels Poorly controlled chronic illness despite available medication
Psychological	Observed changes in behavior of patient of caregiver when interviewed together and separately Threats, intimidation, coercion, disrespect infantilization	May be none
Financial exploitation	Untreated illness, malnutrition, inadequate access to services, medicaiton, clothing, etc., despite adequate reported financial resources Caregiver with ''no visible means of support''	See ''Neglect''
Neglect Passive Willful deprivation/active endangerment Self	Medication not filled or used Caregiver unable to demonstrate knowledge of care plan Older adult refuses offered assistance	Malnutrition Dehydration Poorly controlled chronic illness Unkempt/unclean Frequent ED visits or admissions for similar complaints despite appropriate advice and intervention

giver support group. The categories of ANE seen in this case are physical abuse and restraint or confinement.

2. Patient Problem 2

An 80-year-old man with a history of stroke and left hemiparesis was brought in for evaluation of falling and refusing to eat over the past 2 days. He had been previously admitted to a nursing home, but the family had removed him against advice. The patient was alert and weighed 118 pounds at 5′7″ tall. Several bruises of varying stages of resolution were seen on his chest, back, both shoulders, and both elbows. In the ED he demanded food, consumed several cups of juice, and begged a sandwich from the ED staff. The patient was admitted to the hospital, which provided the opportunity to formally assess his mental status and obtain history adequate to initiate an appropriate care plan. Once he was hospitalized, the patient gave information that his family never awoke before early afternoon. When he was hungry and called out for them before they arose, they threw objects at him. He would then slide out of bed and drag himself around the apartment trying to get food on his own. Many of his falls had occurred when he tried to get out of bed or pull up on chairs in the kitchen. His Social Security check was the main source of income for the household. He was placed in a long-term care facility under an order of protection. Here, he gained weight and progressed in a rehabilitation program, making steady improvement in mobility. He is now being assessed for return to an appropriate level of care in the community with continuation of the order of protection. ANE is suspected in this case example because the history is at odds with the patient's demonstrated voracious appetite and obvious ability to eat. The fact that he is severely underweight and without metabolic derangement confirms that this is long-term malnutrition, not a condition that occurred within 2 days. He also had several injuries in different stages of resolution. A social worker could have ascertained that the caregiver was not employed, raising the question of financial dependence on the patient. The categories of ANE demonstrated here are willful deprivation, physical abuse, and financial exploitation because one motivation for keeping this man out of the nursing home was to have continued access to his Social Security check.

B. Screening Questions for ANE

Several standard questions may help ED personnel to recognize and assess the possibility of ANE.

> Do you feel safe at home?
> Is anyone hurting you, touching you, or treating you in ways you don't like?

Is anyone making you do or sign things you don't want to or don't understand?
Is there anything you need or want that you are not able to get?
Are you satisfied with the time it takes to get the things you need or want?
Is your money being spent the way you want it to be?
Are you afraid? Of what? Of whom?

Neither the checklist nor the questions will be useful if the older adult has significant cognitive impairment. Again, evaluation of mental status is critical to the assessment and management process. The involved adult's perception of the timeliness of care can be unrealistic and, in a cognitively impaired person, responses may be inaccurate, but the patient deserves to have beliefs heard and explored.

III. INTERVENTION AND FOLLOW-UP MANAGEMENT

The nature of an ED is a high-volume, fast-paced, critical care capability service. This does not often lend itself to the in-depth psychosocial assessment usually required to identify subtle forms of ANE and to ameliorate the conditions that caused the risk. Although experienced ANE management teams would be ideal, cost constraints and the decimation of hospital social work departments in favor of discharge planning personnel may make hospital-based ANE crisis teams unrealistic. In some areas, community-based ANE specialists are capable of coming into the ED to provide this service. Unfortunately, the same cost and personnel restraints may make immediate availability of a community-based crisis team equally impractical in many communities.

A suggested management approach for ANE in the ED is described in the following and summarized in Tables 2 and 3.

Table 2 Portions of the Assessment Required on ANE Report

In addition to usual identifying information for patient and caregivers (name, address, phone numbers, birth date, social security number, drivers license number, insurance information) include the following:

- Thorough description of injuries, with drawings or photos (with consent) when possible.
- Document any observed inappropriate behavior, discrepancies in the history, or delays in seeking medical assistance.
- Complete description of mental status.
- Preparation of the Rape Kit when appropriate.

Table 3 Summary of Recommendations for ED Protocols

Consult social worker or ANE experts early in evaluation.
Document mental status.
Document injuries (narrative with drawings or photos).
Do not make assumptions about sexual activity—ask.
Admit to physicians with ANE expertise.
Know criteria for admission under Medicare ANE DRG.
Add ANE risk factors to ED ''frequent flier'' logs.
Include hospital and community-based ANE experts.

ANE, Abuse and neglect of the elderly; DRG, diagnostic-related group; ED, emergency department.

An experienced social worker or local Adult Protective Service (APS) professional should be consulted early in the assessment so they can interview family members before information is diffused or family members leave. The social worker can observe and document interactions between the patient and family members and case transitions by facilitating referral to community agencies or admission to the hospital.

It is essential for ED personnel to document a thorough description of the patient's mental status. The ED record should be part of the database used to reach a conclusion about decision-making capacity, but the legal documents should be prepared by a physician who has had more than one opportunity to evaluate the patient's cognition, is experienced with the procedures, and is willing to testify if necessary.

Injuries should be thoroughly documented with detailed written descriptions. Either drawing injuries on a template or taking photos with signed consent of the patient is preferable. The assumption that older adults cannot be sexually active can result in loss of significant information that could compromise legal intervention. ED personnel should inquire about sexual activity (both consensual and forced), perform the appropriate examinations, and, when indicated, prepare the Rape Kit.

If the situation is potentially life threatening or if adequate follow-up is suspect, hospital admission is possible under the Medicare Diagnostic Related Group (DRG) for Abuse and Neglect when acute medical illness is not present. The codes 444 and 445 allow for approximately 3 days and 5–7 days, respectively.

Suspected ANE patients cannot be placed in the general distribution of unassigned admissions to the hospital (i.e., ''ER call''). Members of the medical staff who are willing to assume responsibility for inpatient management should be proactively identified, and these patients admitted to them preferentially. These physicians should be proficient in providing comprehensive medical care to older adults and willing to serve in this capacity. They should be experienced in assessment of mental status and decision-making capacity, comfortable with obtaining appropriate additional diagnostic resources and consultation to assess cognition, well versed in the local legal requirements, and capable of working in concert with the social service and legal professionals.

The ED protocol should also include clear information on how to directly contact the appropriate local agencies and make referrals when admission is not appropriate. It is advisable to invite the local APS workers to participate in ED and hospital in-service programs so that all staff will be familiar with their names, phone numbers, and protocols. This information will vary by locality and can be obtained by the local APS program, Department on Aging, or Area Agency on Aging. In the case of suspected ANE of a nursing home resident by a nursing home worker, the office of the state ombudsman is contacted.

It would be beneficial to add the ANE risk factors to the written or computerized log, which many ED programs use to identify persons who use the ED repeatedly. The logs are used to either facilitate the ED management of these patients, as in the case of persons with sickle cell crises, or by targeting preventive intervention to decrease unnecessary ED use, as in the case of asthma or congestive heart failure. Monitoring ED visits for conditions listed in Table 1 may also be effective in earlier identification and intervention.

IV. DECREASING THE RELUCTANCE OF ED PERSONNEL TO MAKE REFERRALS—KEY POINTS

Most states have ''good Samaritan'' laws that provide for inviolate anonymity for the reporter. They also absolve the reporter of liability when the report is made in good faith without the possibility of personal gain.

Investigating the possibility of ANE is not necessarily an indictment of the caregiver or family but an opportunity to activate the cascade of support and avoid more serious injury.

In the case of neglect, the intent of the caregiver is not relevant to the ED assessment and referral process. Our first responsibility is to advocate for the patient by creating the opportunity for risk to be reduced. We do that by suspecting, making the diagnosis, and referring to the professionals who can have positive impact. The goal of intervention is usually to protect the vulnerable older adult and to stabilize their care system, not

42% in those age 45 to 64 years (2). Repeated visits to emergency departments are also more common for older patients. The emergency department is a common site for referral of nursing home residents, whose most frequent symptoms are respiratory, altered mental status, gastrointestinal symptoms, and falls (3). More than 40% of these nursing home patients are admitted to the hospital.

Recent studies have identified a small portion of older patients who consistently make extensive use of hospital services and can be readily identified. In the Longitudinal Study of Aging, which followed nearly 7500 patients age 70 years and older for 7 years, 42.6% had no hospital admissions and another 24.7% had infrequent hospitalizations. Only 4.8% had consistently high rates of hospitalization, averaging one or more admissions annually (4). A longitudinal cohort study identified eight independent variables that are risk factors for repeated hospital admission among people age 70 years or older: older age, male sex, poor self-rated general health, availability of an informal caregiver, having ever had coronary artery disease, having had during the previous year a hospital admission, more than six doctor visits, or diabetes mellitus (5). On the basis of the presence of these risk factors, the subjects estimated to have a high probability of repeated hospital admission had rates nearly twice as high as low-risk patients and a higher cumulative incidence of repeated admission, a higher cumulative rate of mortality, more hospital days per person-year survived, and higher hospital charges (5).

The cost of acute hospitalization peaks in the 70- to 79-year age group and declines with age thereafter despite the longer length of stay for those older than age 80 (6). Case-mix is an important determinant of hospital costs. Ancillary costs are lower in the oldest patients and highest in those 70 to 79 years. Costs of care are higher for decedents than for survivors.

These national surveys and cohort studies provide convincing evidence that the oldest patients are more likely to be admitted and readmitted to hospitals, to generate high costs of care, and to define the patient in greatest need of hospitalization in the twenty-first century. Recent prospective cohort studies reveal that a change in functional status may be an important determinant of both hospital length of stay and discharge disposition. The oldest patients are at the greatest risk for functional decline with hospitalization.

B. Functional Decline and Hospitalization

Hospitalization is associated with functional decline or physical disability that occurs during the course of treatment for an acute medical illness. In a study of nearly 1300 community-dwelling patients age 70 years and older who were hospitalized for acute medical illnesses, 31% lost independence in one or more of five basic activities of daily living (ADL) compared with their preadmission baseline status (7). Among survivors, 40% reported a loss of independence in one or more instrumental activities of daily living (IADL) 3 months after hospital discharge. Functional decline was most frequent in patients who were older than age 75 years, had some disability in the performance of IADL preadmission, and had lower mental status scores on admission.

An increased risk of disability in elderly patients is related to specific diseases and other nonmedical factors independent of age. One prospective cohort study found that severe disability (disability in three or more ADL) is most frequently associated with discharge diagnoses of stroke, hip fracture, congestive heart failure, pneumonia, coronary heart disease, and cancer. Progressive disability (disability in one or two ADL) is also seen in patients with diabetes mellitus and dehydration (8).

Functional measures are also important predictors of mortality. In prospective studies of hospitalized patients functional measures are strong predictors of mortality subsequent to hospitalization and contribute prognostic ability beyond that obtained with combined measures of disease comorbidity, severity, disease staging, and diagnosis-related groups (9). In a study of elderly patients in a health maintenance organization, urinary incontinence increased both the risk of hospitalization and the subsequent risk of admission to a nursing home (10). Other studies suggest that functional comorbid conditions, including cognitive dysfunction, immobility resulting in generalized weakness or pressure ulcers, depression, and malnutrition, contribute to the risks of functional decline, nursing home admission, and, in some studies, mortality. The concept of the ''dysfunctional syndrome'' explains how the process of hospitalization contributes to the excess functional morbidity of hospitalization for acute illness in elderly patients (11). The vulnerable patient is exposed to the risks of immobility, undernutrition, polypharmacy, and iatrogenesis and may have negative expectations or depressive symptoms that prevent or delay functional recovery (Figure 1).

C. Iatrogenic Illness

Iatrogenic illness during hospitalization is reported more often in elderly patients. In the Harvard Medical Malpractice study, patients age 65 and older had twice the chance of sustaining injury during hospitalization as younger patients, and they were more likely to suffer from the effects of negligence in hospital (12). The risk of iatrogenic illness increases with greater hospital length of stay. In one study, 58% of patients age 65 years and older suffered at least one iatrogenic complication when hospitalized for 15 or more days. Therapeutic interventions accounted for 44% of complications, whereas diagnostic procedures and errors of omission each accounted for approximately 10% of complications (12,13). The most common causes of iatrogenic illness are adverse drug reactions (ADRs), which often result from polypharmacy. Many ADRs are of minor significance, but some such as excessive bleeding because of warfarin, syncope from alpha-adrenoreceptor blockers or vasodilators, and delirium from anticholinergic and

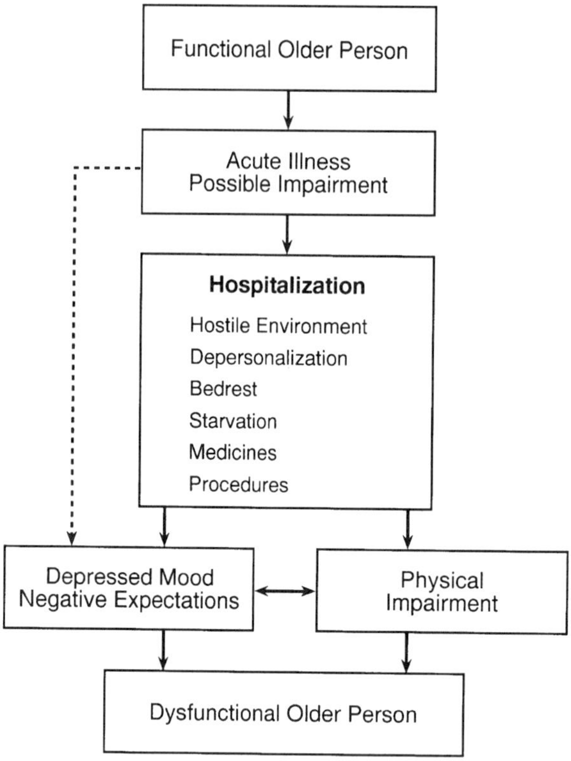

Figure 1 Conceptual model of the dysfunctional syndrome. (From Ref. 11.)

psychotropic medications can have devastating effects on elderly patients. Although nomograms for drug prescribing are useful in specific clinical situations, many elderly patients have multiple comorbid conditions and take several medications that may adversely influence drug binding and drug metabolism and lead to iatrogenic illness (12). In most community hospitals, ADR and drug prescribing errors continue to be problematic. Principles of drug prescribing for elderly hospitalized patients are shown in Table 1. (See also Chapter 3.)

Iatrogenic illness may also result from errors of omission, that is, the failure to evaluate and treat medical conditions in older patients. Recent studies document the underprescribing of potentially life-sustaining treatments in hospitalized patients, including beta-blockers for patients after myocardial infarction and angiotensin-converting enzyme inhibitors for patients with significant systolic dysfunction and heart failure. Although clinical practice guidelines and critical pathways may help lessen the incidence of iatrogenic illness, they may be less useful

Table 1 Principles of Drug Prescribing in Hospitalized Elderly Patients

Review all medications taken by patient before to hospitalization; assess previous compliance.
Avoid unnecessary polypharmacy: use drugs that treat more than one condition (e.g., beta-blockers for both hypertension and angina pectoris) when practical.
When initiating a new medication, choose agents whose pharmacokinetic properties in elderly patients are known.
If patients require multiple medications, avoid, whenever possible, drugs that are inhibitors or inducers of cytochrome P450 hepatic metabolism or are highly bound to albumin. If in doubt, consult a pharmacist, pharmacologist, on-line pharmacology program, or text source.
When the maintenance dose of a medication is not established, ''start low and go slow,'' to titrate the dose against the desired clinical effect.
Use lower than usual maintenance doses of medications that are renally excreted (e.g., aminoglycosides).
Begin with a short-acting agent from a pharmacological class of drugs, but by discharge convert to an agent that is given once or twice daily to enhance patient compliance and reduce caregiver burden at home.
Review all discharge medications with the patient and family and provide written instructions.
Consider an adverse drug effect when patients have new or unexplained medical problems develop: delirium, hypotension, dysrhythmias, renal failure, electrolyte disorders, constipation.

for older patients who have high rates of comorbidity and functional impairments that may contribute to the excess morbidity of an acute illness. Recognition of these common geriatric syndromes is critical to the appropriate assessment and care of the frail patient and the prevention of the dysfunctional syndrome (Table 2).

D. Common Geriatric Syndromes

1. Cognitive Dysfunction (Dementia/Delirium)

Delirium, characterized as an acute disorder of attention and cognition, and dementia most often a result of Alzheimer's disease or vascular diseases, are both common causes of cognitive dysfunction in hospitalized elderly patients. Delirium is especially common in critically ill and postoperative elderly patients, with incidence rates as high as 50% reported in studies (14). (See also Chapter 20.) The incidence of delirium is related to patient predisposing factors, especially baseline cognitive impairment, severe underlying illness, sensory impairment, and dehydration. It may be precipitated by processes of hospital care, including

Table 2 Common Geriatric Problems in Hospitalized Patients

Problem	Clinical features	Management
Delirium	Change in mental status from baseline; inattentive; fluctuating level of alertness; inappropriate behavior or thought processes.	Treat underlying cause; create supportive environment; soft voice, reality orientation; achieve normal sleep-wake cycle; judiciously use psychotropic, drugs, neuroleptics, benzodiazepines.
Malnutrition	Low body mass index; generalized muscle atrophy or weakness; history of unintentional weight loss; anemia, low serum albumin, low serum cholesterol.	Choose enteral over parenteral alimentation; order modified barium swallow when oropharyngeal dysphagia is suspected; add nutritional supplements and calorie-dense foods.
Immobility	Patient unable to transfer from bed to chair, bear weight, or walk without assistance; common causes are physical deconditioning, neurological diseases, medications, and physical restraints.	Prescribe graded aerobic and low-impact resistive exercises: range-of-motion (passive or active), resistance of feet and legs against hands during bedside rounds, assisted ambulation; avoid physical restraints and psychotropic drugs; treat orthostatic hypotension; obtain physical therapy consultation; prescribe assistive devices, walkers, lifts.
Urinary incontinence	Involuntary loss of urine; suspect in patients who are immobile, cognitively impaired, restrained, or are receiving drugs with anticholinergic effects.	Evaluate for overflow incontinence caused by bladder outlet obstruction or an acontractile bladder: suprapubic fullness, large postvoid residual (>200 mL) after urethral catheterization. Use indwelling cather to intermittent straight catheterization for overflow incontinence. Begin toileting schedule, bedside commode, or urinal for stress or urge incontinence.
Pressure ulcers	Patients often immobile, cognitively impaired, malnourished. Pressure ulcer, stage I–IV: nonblanching erythema; blisters or open ulcers to dermis; or through dermis; or through subcutaneous structures.	Reduce pressure on bony prominences, shearing forces, friction, and skin moisture; turn frequently; use air support mattresses, consider skin emollients; skin care nurse consult; surgical consult for stage IV ulcers

Table 2 Continued

Problem	Clinical features	Management
Constipation	Immobile, dehydrated patients; treatment with medications that interfere with colonic motility: narcotics, drugs with antichnolinergic effects; low-fiber diet.	Ensure adequate oral or intravenous hydration; evacuate fecal impactions, then begin water-soluble fiber supplements plus osmolar laxatives; progressive physical activity: up in chair, assisted ambulation, walking.
Depression	Depressive symptoms or history of major affective disorder; failure-to-thrive; uncooperative, poorly motivated; dysphoric mood, anxiety, or impaired concentration.	Supportive environment: encourage family visits, occupational therapies; consultation by nurse specialist or psychiatrist; review of medications (discontinue central nervous system depressants).

immobilization of the patient, use of an indwelling bladder catheter, and use of physical restraints, as well as by dehydration, malnutrition, iatrogenic complications, and environmental and psychosocial factors (14). Delirium is consistently associated with prolonged hospital length of stay, increased costs of care, and greater risk of nursing home placement or death (14). Despite the extreme importance of early detection and the potential to intervene in the management of high-risk or delirious patients, early studies revealed that delirium often goes unrecognized by health professionals; however, both the detection of cognitive impairment and delirium can be enhanced through the use of common and simple bedside screening instruments and scales, such as the Confusion Assessment Method (14).

2. Immobility/Falls

Acutely ill patients are often unable to transfer from hospital bed to chair or to walk. Immobility may be further promoted by orders for bed rest and physical or chemical restraints (15). Falls in hospitals occur more often in older patients and are often associated with physical deconditioning or generalized weakness, the use of psychotropic medications, orthostatic hypotension, and environmental hazards such as unsafe surfaces (15). Patients who fall in the hospital have longer lengths of hospital stay and incur higher charges than nonfallers. Immobility is also a risk factor for incident pressure ulcers, especially in patients with cognitive dysfunction or malnutrition.

3. Malnutrition

Protein-energy malnutrition (PEM), diagnosed by anthropometric and biochemical parameters, is present in approximately one-third of hospitalized medically ill elderly patients. The high prevalence of PEM is associated with age-related factors such as reduced taste and caloric requirements with aging; chronic and acute medical problems, particularly heart failure and chronic obstructive pulmonary disease; and social and lifestyle factors that may adversely effect nutritional consumption, such as alcohol use, social isolation, and functional disabilities (16). Malnutrition is also associated with excess morbidity and mortality. In-hospital starvation or undernutrition is most common in patients with baseline nutritional, functional, and cognitive deficits (17). The diagnosis of PEM is confounded by the effects of acute and chronic inflammation, which increase the incidence of hypoalbuminemia and hypocholesterolemia (e.g., because of the elaboration of various cytokines). Nonetheless, reasonable data support the usefulness of routine protein-energy supplementation in malnourished hospitalized adults (18).

4. Depression

Depressive symptoms are commonly reported by patients at hospital admission but are often left undiagnosed or untreated. Depression may adversely affect hospital outcomes by creating a negative view of clinical treatment, interfering with the patient's decision-making capacity, or creating therapeutic noncompliance. Depressive symptoms are associated with functional decline and an increased risk of mortality even when controlling for severity of illness and comorbid illnesses. Depression is especially difficult to diagnose in patients who are critically ill and whose cognitive function may be impaired or whose verbal abilities may be limited (e.g., intubated patients). Despite the importance of depressive symptoms, screening for depression is not routinely conducted at hospital admission and no studies exist of interventions in elderly hospitalized patients to demonstrate the effects of treatment on functional or other clinical outcomes.

E. Discharge Planning

Until recently, discharge planning for hospitalized elderly patients was the sole responsibility of the attending physician. With growing pressures to decrease hospital length of stay newer systems of discharge planning have evolved and generally use either case managers, individual discharge planners, or interdisciplinary teams (11). Discharge planning, when conducted by nurse specialists for targeted patients (e.g., those with congestive heart failure or pneumonia), reduces the rate of rehospitalization in the time shortly after the patient's discharge.

Despite the intensive effort to improve the rate of completion of advance directives (Living Will or Durable Power of Attorney for Health Care) by older hospitalized patients, especially those who are critically ill, little attention is routinely paid to patient preferences for care, personal comfort, or discussions about end-of-life decision making. Even in the face of terminal illness, many patients, their families, or physicians insist on aggressive interventions for critical illness, suggesting that these decisions need to be decided before the incident of critical illness or at least early in the course of hospitalization (19). (See also Chapter 2.)

The complexity of an elderly patient's illness, the need for rapid assessment of their functional and psychosocial needs, and the pressure facing health professionals to rapidly treat and discharge these patients from the hospital demonstrate the need for a different approach to usual care of acutely and critically ill elderly patients in the medical center of the twenty-first century. Fortunately, a growing body of literature points to opportunities for improving the quality of patient care and outcomes while containing total costs of hospitalization through the development of new systems of hospital care (20).

II. FUTURE DIRECTIONS

A. The Geriatric Medical Center

The current health care system is a complex mixture of separate subsystems of care that have developed rapidly since World War II. Technology has captured the center of attention in the American hospital. In the twenty-first century the challenge to health professionals will be to continue the growth of applied technology while personalizing the hospital environment, maintaining a patient's physical independence and autonomy, and pursuing the most cost-beneficial systems of care. The changes in usual care that occurred in the late twentieth century will be accelerated by financial changes in health care reimbursement to institutions and physicians. The continued growth of Medicare managed care, the alignment of managed care organizations with professional staff organizations, and the continuing pressures to lower hospital length of stay and costs will force the modern medical center to apply the most cost-effective subsystem of care to the patient most likely to benefit from that service. Currently in the United States a panoply of subsystems of care have grown in a patchwork and largely uncoordinated fashion (20). But fresh approaches to coordination of care across subsystems are evolving in integrated health systems and are potentially transportable to most urban communities. A model of the future geriatric medical center, based on subsystems of care that are well established but not usually integrated, is illustrated in Figure 2. In this model, the acute care hospital with its general medical, surgical, and critical care nursing units remains at the center. On the medical center campus is the emergency department, observation unit (clinical decision unit), subacute unit, long-term care unit, and hospital. Contiguous to the

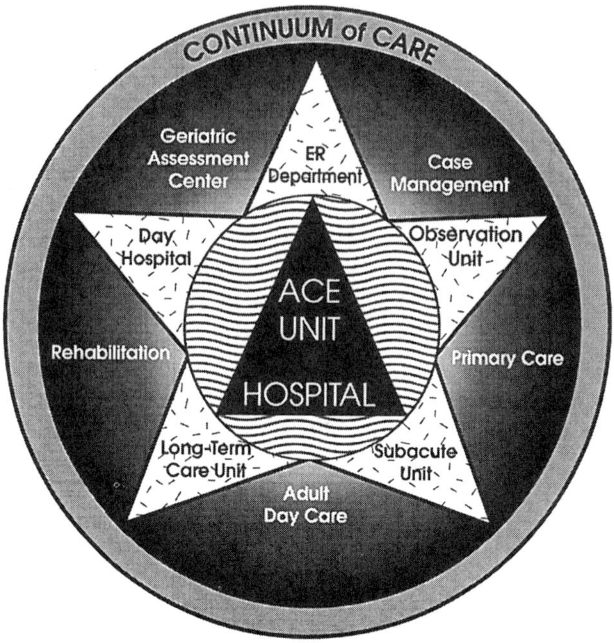

Figure 2 The future geriatric medical center.

geriatric medical center is case management, primary care, adult day care, outpatient rehabilitation, and the geriatric assessment center.

B. The Hospital Environment

The modern urban hospital represents a conglomeration of ''vertically'' developed hospital units, typically designed to meet the needs of health professionals, not patients. Social gerontologists, however, have long recognized the important effects of environmental settings on older people and the need to find congruence of person-environment interaction (11). More recently, clinicians and investigators are coming to understand the biological mechanisms underlying the influence of psychosocial factors on the course of immunologically mediated diseases (21). A positive attitude, a sense of self-efficacy, and a positive perception of healing are potentially helpful to patients as they recover from a serious illness.

In the ideal geriatric medical center, a ''horizontal'' design is preferable and would create a patient-centered environment with a seamless continuum of acute and critical care in the hospital and less intense inpatient services, which are linked to specialty services such as geriatric assessment centers and primary care (Figure 2). The horizontal design combines the promise of more efficient use of professional staff time by concentrating medical services in one area, with less of the stressful burden on patients of transfers from one health care center to another. Unlike vertical hospitals, the horizontal design offers more opportunity for informal ''curbside consultations'' because health care professionals interact with one another to discuss patients in the horizontal corridors (22). Furthermore, this design meets the goal of architects to ''improve personnel productivity while maintaining a greater level of patient comfort and satisfaction'' (23).

1. The Acute Care of Elders Unit

Units for acute care of elders (ACE units) are designed to prevent the dysfunctional syndrome (Figure 3).

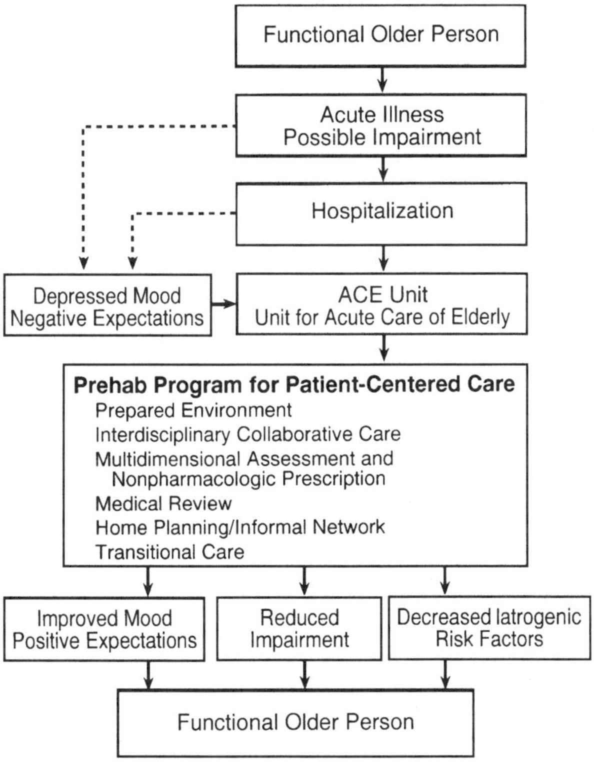

Figure 3 Prevention of the dysfunctional syndrome: Conceptual model. ACE = acute care of elders. (From Ref. 11.)

The ACE unit is a system of care that has four main components: a prepared environment, patient-centered care, interdisciplinary team rounds and discharge planning, and medical care review. The physical environment of the ACE unit is modified to enhance the patient's independent functioning in ADLs and mobility. This is achieved by eliminating clutter in hallway corridors, carpeting hallways and rooms, installing grab bars in bathrooms and rails in hallways, and creating a large common activity room to permit dining outside of rooms, socializing, and light exercise. Patient-centered care begins with a multidimensional assessment performed by the patient's nurse at the time of admission and the use of guidelines to maintain or restore the patient's independent functioning in basic ADLs. Interdisciplinary team rounds and discharge planning are begun on the first hospital day and are fostered by daily brief rounds. Medical care review involves a systematic review of patient's medications, functional status, and planned procedures and assurance that standards of care for treatment of acutely ill patients are maintained throughout the hospitalization. Clinical trials have demonstrated the potential effectiveness of ACE units to improve functional outcomes of hospitalization and to perhaps reduce hospital lengths of stay (24,25). The ideal patient for admission to an ACE unit has not been determined but is likely a community-residing patient age 75 years of age and older who has an acute decline in functional self-care because of physical illness or delirium and who is likely to improve. The principles of ACE can be transported to other settings including the intensive care unit.

2. Emergency Department

Frail elderly patients often are seen in the emergency department with cognitive dysfunction, multiple comorbid illnesses, and significant psychosocial factors that complicate their visit and discharge plans. Elderly patients who are released to home from the emergency department often have considerable loss of functional independence and have subsequently high rates of hospital admission or deaths. A screening or intervention program is needed to identify high-risk patients and refer them to appropriate community services or case management (26). Alternate sites, such as observation units or subacute units, may obviate the need for the emergency department.

3. Observation Units

In the era of managed care, observation units or holding areas in emergency departments have the potential to reduce costs of unnecessary hospitalization of elderly patients. Studies of disease-specific conditions, such as chest pain and asthma, have shown the feasibility of the use of observation or diagnostic units as alternatives to hospitalization (27). Despite their growth in the past 10 years, the role and future of observation units remains controversial. There remains a lack of consensus regarding the indications for admitting and discharging patients from these units and uncertainty regarding the mechanisms of their funding (28).

4. Subacute Unit

Subacute units are skilled nursing facilities that provide short-term, goal-oriented, and intensive restorative and skilled nursing services. Subacute units are ideal alternatives to rehabilitation hospitals or home care for patients who have categorical illnesses, such as hip fracture, and who require extensive interdisciplinary care before their return home. In one study, about half of patients admitted for heart failure to an acute care facility were considered at low risk and could have been managed in a subacute setting, resulting in significant cost savings (29). Subacute care is also ideal for patients who have catastrophic illnesses in the hospital and are severely deconditioned or too ill to return home. The future of subacute care was destabilized by the passage of the Balanced Budget Act of 1997 and the introduction of the Prospective Payment System in 1999. Despite the uncertainties of its future, subacute care will likely grow in importance as an alternative to continued hospitalization for frail elderly patients. In an integrated health system, functionally impaired patients can flow from the ACE unit through the subacute unit and the day hospital.

5. Day Hospital

The geriatric day hospital emerged as a model of care in Great Britain in recognition that many older patients have complex medical problems that cannot be adequately managed in the outpatient clinic but do not require hospitalization (30). The geriatric day hospital is an outpatient facility where frail older patients can receive subacute or acute medical, nursing, social, and/or rehabilitative services over any portion of a full day with return visits as necessary (31). Despite the absence of evidence of their superiority to usual care or of their cost-effectiveness, geriatric day hospitals will likely evolve as alternatives to hospitalization or subacute care because they offer an array of nursing and specialty services in one setting that is not available with usual outpatient care.

6. Long-Term Care Unit

Long-term care is reserved for patients who have severe functional impairments, commonly caused by dementia, and lack adequate social supports at home. Because these patients require "custodial" services, they are not eligible for subacute care under Medicare reimbursement and are too impaired to benefit from the day hospital. In a managed care practice, a small unit attached to the hospital helps case managers and physicians to identify strategies to enable long-term care patients to return home within a reasonable time frame with lower costs.

7. Ambulatory Services Based on Medical Center Campus

Case management generally performed by an nurse specialist or social worker is targeted at high-risk patients (those with functional impairment, chronic progressive diseases, high probability of readmission, or marginal home supports). In managed care organizations an incentive to use case managers to contain the costs of care related to repeated hospitalization or use of the emergency department is present. The need for case management could be identified in any one of the sites in the continuum of care on the geriatric medical center. Screening instruments such as that described by Boult et al (5) can be used to identify patients at risk for hospitalization. Another index identifies hospitalized patients at risk for functional decline during hospitalization, who might improve with aggressive case management (9). The case manager serves as an advocate for the patient and family and helps to coordinate services in the continuum of care.

The geriatric assessment center team performs comprehensive assessments of frail and complex elderly patients. Previous studies have demonstrated that comprehensive geriatric assessment programs that link geriatric evaluation with long-term management are effective in improving survival and function in older persons (32). In some cases, primary care is provided by physicians who have hospital-based office practices. The linking of primary care and consultative geriatric assessment with case management may enable frail elderly patients to retain independent physical functioning, thereby avoiding hospitalization or nursing home placement. Outpatient rehabilitation services are available to patients who do not require an inpatient or subacute admission. Rehabilitative services are offered in both morning and afternoon sessions by an interdisciplinary team, thereby allowing the patient to return home at night. Rehabilitation is also a transitional service for patients who return home after hospital or subacute care for neurological or musculoskeletal illnesses. The day hospital and rehabilitation areas can be combined into a single unit and expanded to include any patients who need intensive interdisciplinary services without an overnight admission.

The geriatric medical center forms linkages with community-based and home care programs. Home care is most often directed to patients who require limited but skilled nursing services (e.g., home intravenous infusion therapy), but choose home care over subacute care, and whose medical condition is stable enough to permit discharge from hospital-based services. Home health care was originally designed to provide transitional care from the hospital to facilitate earlier hospital discharge (33). However, before the Balanced Budget Act of 1997, home health care visits were used primarily to provide long-term care, and no evidence existed that services provided at home replaced hospital services. Home health care services after hospitalization are most often used by patients with the following characteristics: educational level $\leq$12 years, less accessible social support, impairment in at least one instrumental ADL, and prior home health care use (34). Home-based interventions after hospitalization can reduce the rate of unplanned hospital readmission (11). Studies show that patients with congestive heart failure in particular are likely to benefit from home care interventions (35).

Adult day care centers are either attached to the geriatric medical center or are free-standing facilities in the community. Day care centers are ideal sites for frail, usually cognitively impaired, elderly patients who are medically stable but can participate during the day in social and recreational activities or a congregate meal. Adult day care centers offer respite services to caregivers to allow them time away from the dependent elder patient.

An assisted living facility is often indicated for patients who are medically stable but require a low level of informal supervision because of physical or cognitive impairments. Typically the patients live in their own apartment but attend congregate meals and have nursing care services available to them in the facility as required.

C. Medical Information Systems

Perhaps the most striking change in acute hospital care will be in the expanded use of medical information systems. Although hospitals have been slow to adopt computer technology, evidence exists that computerized medical information systems can improve the quality of patient care. A computerized decision-support program linked to computer-based patient records assists physicians in the use of antimicrobial agents and improves the quality of care. In one program a computerized program recommends antimicrobial regimens and courses of therapy for particular patients and provides immediate feedback to the prescribing physician. Significant reductions in orders for drugs to which the patients have reported allergies, excess drug dosages, and antibiotic susceptibility mismatches have been reported after implementation of this computerized program (36). In addition, the total cost of antimicrobial agents and total hospital costs were statistically significantly reduced after implementation of this program. Computerized programs may also reduce the rate of adverse drug events. In a study conducted at a tertiary care hospital, physician computer order entry decreased the rate of serious medication errors by more than half (37). Preventable adverse drug events declined 17%, whereas nonintercepted potential events declined by 84%. As user-friendly computer technology becomes more widely available (e.g., voice activated transcription), computerized order entry will become universal in hospitals. Systems of order entry will lessen the risk of physician error and undesirable variance in the quality of medical care. Computer technology also offers the promise of improving efficiency and documentation of patient care. Palm-held computers allow nurses and physicians to enter data about each patient at the bedside. Computerized databases enable health professionals to access relevant laboratory results, diagnostic studies, and consultation notes without dependence on a paper record. This information can be accessed by physicians off campus, leading to more rapid clinical decision making. Access to medical information is growing easier with the wide availability of CD-ROM programs, on-line texts, and access to MEDLINE and other databases on personal computers.

Another information technology that offers great promise for hospitalized care of elderly patients is telemedicine (38). Although the term ''*telemedicine*'' encompasses a wide range of telecommunications and information technologies, its most attractive application is the medium of interactive video communication. As the technology becomes refined, resolution increases, and costs decrease, telemedicine will become an increasingly important component of both inpatient and outpatient medical practice. Telemedicine permits physicians to view a patient, interpret an electrocardiogram, or analyze the results of simple bedside laboratory tests (e.g., pulse oximetry) from office or home. In rural communities, telemedicine offers the opportunity for primary physicians to obtain consultation from specialists in other communities by way of interactive video transmission. Although many issues remain to be resolved including reimbursement for telemedicine services, liability and malpractice concerns, and issues of confidentiality, the potential of telemedicine to improve the care of hospitalized patients remains enticing.

D. Emerging Models of Care

Most of the recent clinical intervention trials of hospitalized elderly patients have focused on identifying and managing patients at risk for functional decline or on comprehensive discharge planning. With continued aging of the average adult hospitalized patient and the wider availability of newer technologies and palliative therapies (e.g., transplantation of organs), greater emphasis will be placed on functional status and outcomes related to quality of life. Consequently, it becomes increasingly important to detect functional impairments early in the patient's hospitalization and to institute restorative measures promptly. Discharge planning needs to be undertaken early in hospitalization because the patient's ultimate disposition site will be determined largely by his or her ability to perform basic ADLs and the availability of social supports at home. Diagnostic and prognostic precision is key to the process of discharge planning. A variety of models of care that address functional, clinical, and prognostic aspects of the elderly hospitalized patient have evolved in recent years (20). The effectiveness of specialty units such as Geriatric Evaluation and Management Units, ACE units, or stroke units is well documented (11). Multidisciplinary teams, usually nurse-directed, have proven especially effective in the process of discharge planning. Geriatricians have generally served as medical consultants or directors of units. An emerging concept with great potential for the future practice of geriatric medicine is the employment of physician "hospitalists."

1. Hospitalists

Hospitalists are physicians who specialize in inpatient medicine (39). Both hospitals and medical group practices have embraced this inpatient specialist. The hospitalist is viewed positively as an individual who can provide efficient and valuable care and can be an avid member of the interdisciplinary team involved in discharge planning and education of professional trainees. In the geriatric medical center, hospitalists should be either trained geriatricians or internists with additional residency training in geriatric medicine. As geriatricians, they may serve as the medical director of the acute care unit, the geriatric consultant to the hospital medical center, or the primary care physician for hospitalized elderly patients. Emerging data suggest that compared with usual care, hospitalists may provide more cost-effective care to hospitalized adult patients. However, definitive trials of the care of frail elderly patients are lacking. Hospitalists may obviate the need for expensive subspecialty consultation, especially in a group practice, when telemedicine and medical information systems are available to specialists outside of the hospital. Medicare managed care costs can be potentially reduced, and the specialist's time used most efficiently.

2. Nurse-Directed Interventions

Nurses play a pivotal role in the early detection of functional impairments and the psychosocial factors in older patients that may contribute to functional decline. (See also Chapter 4.) Many models of gerontological advance practice nurses have been described. Among these one of the most generalizable is the Yale Geriatric Care Program, which is designed to prevent functional decline in hospitalized elderly patients (40). The program involves an integrated model of primary care nurses, specially trained unit-based resource nurses, gerontological clinical nurse specialists, and geriatric physicians. Nurses routinely assess patients for markers of functional outcomes of hospitalization: skin impairment (pressure ulcers), poor nutrition, incontinence, confusion (delirium or dementia), evidence of falls, or functional impairment. The gerontological clinical nurse specialist makes daily rounds with the geriatric resource nurse, who is a staff nurse with a special interest in geriatrics. The nurses makes rounds with the patient's primary nurse and the geriatric physician to review complicated cases. This model of care appears to be effective in decreasing functional decline in highly targeted elderly hospitalized medical patients (11). Similar models of interdisciplinary teams are used in acute care units and are currently under investigation as an intervention to reduce the rate of physical restraint in patients hospitalized on medical/surgical and critical care units.

Advance practice nurses also play pivotal roles in the process of comprehensive discharge planning. The advance practice nurses coordinate the patient's discharge plans early in hospitalization. Discharge planning directed by nurses has resulted in decreased rates of hospital readmission of patients with targeted medical conditions such as congestive heart failure (11).

3. Geriatric Consultation

Geriatric consultation is usually performed by a geriatrician working with an interdisciplinary team composed of at least a social worker and a nurse. Early studies of geriatric consultations suggested potential benefits, especially on hospital length of stay. However, no studies have demonstrated significant effects on functional status of elderly patients or on total costs of care (11). In one study, for example, inpatient geriatric consultation in a large group practice health maintenance organization did not improve the health or survival of hospitalized patients selected on the basis of screening criteria (41). Geriatric consultation in general appears to have modest effects on functional outcomes of hospitalization for older patients. Consultation, however, may be most effective when performed by geriatricians on specific surgical units such as orthopedics or stroke units or when geriatricians manage the patient's during and immediately after hospitalization. (11,32)

4. ACE Units

Early experiences with acute care geriatric units led to the development of a systematic intervention designed to prevent the dysfunctional syndrome (Figure 3). In this conceptual model of functional decline, the functional older person is admitted to the hospital with an acute illness and possible physiological impairment. The environment is modified to foster independent patient functioning and to promote interdisciplinary collaborative care, multidimensional assessment linked to functional interventions, medical care review, and discharge planning. A randomized clinical trial of one ACE unit, which consisted of 15 beds on a medical/surgical nursing unit, demonstrated modest benefits on functional status of patients who received the ACE intervention compared with usual care. Among 603 patients discharged alive from the hospital, ADL function was better at discharge than on admission in more patients receiving the ACE intervention compared with the usual care, and risk of nursing home placement was significantly reduced. Overall hospital charges and costs were somewhat lower for patients receiving the ACE intervention (24,25). The ACE unit can be either a ''virtual unit'' or a designated free-standing unit. ACE units represent excellent sites for training health professionals in assessment and management of complex elderly patients and can serve as clinical ''research laboratories'' to evaluate the effectiveness of new approaches to patient care. The lessons learned on an ACE unit can then be transported to other areas of the hospital. ACE units also can reduce inefficiency inherent in multidisciplinary care by targeting the services of health professionals at patients who are most likely to benefit from their care.

5. Stroke Units

Stroke units have been carefully evaluated in European trials. Several trials have shown better outcomes for patients treated in stroke units compared with stroke patients treated in general medical wards. Meta-analyses show that the care of stroke patients in stroke units reduces mortality, institutionalization, and functional dependency (11). Stroke units typically use a team including the patient's physician, social worker, physical and occupational therapist, speech therapist, and neurologist. A systematic approach is used to enhance patient recovery after admission and to begin diagnostic and rehabilitative services. Clinical trials have reported improved functional status for patients treated in stroke units and a trend toward increased survival early after stroke (42). The overall effectiveness of stroke units is not restricted to a particular subgroup of patients, and no systematic increase exists in lengths of stay in the hospital or other institutions.

E. Interdisciplinary Care

Interdisciplinary care is a critical component of all clinical trials that have demonstrated improved functional and clinical outcomes of hospitalization of elderly patients. The productivity and efficiency of team members are enhanced through interdisciplinary collaboration in which their services are appropriately targeted to patients and where lengthy individual progress notes are replaced by templates and interdisciplinary team plans. Interdisciplinary health professionals also help to create, define, and refine practice guidelines and clinical pathways. For example, in developing ACE units, focus groups composed of representative members of different health professions (nurses, social workers, dietitians, physical and occupational therapists, speech therapists, discharge planners) created the clinical interventions.

1. Clinical Pathways

Clinical pathways or practice guidelines are useful benchmarks for assessment and management of patients with disease-specific conditions such as stroke or congestive heart failure. However, their application is limited in the care of patients with multiple medical problems and related functional impairments. Because functional status is an independent predictor of functional and prognostic outcomes, functional status needs to be incorporated into clinical pathways related to the care of frail hospitalized patients.

2. The Functional Trajectory

A clinical pathway to describe the functional trajectory (Fig. 4) was used by the interdisciplinary team on the ACE unit (24,25). The functional trajectory pathway begins on the patient's admission when a brief functional assessment is completed by the primary nurse and attending physician. The assessment includes the patient's current ability to perform ADLs (bathing, dressing, transferring, toileting, eating), mobility, cognition, affect, and nutrition. The patient's current status is contrasted to his or her baseline functional status of 1 to 2 weeks before the acute illness. This includes a review of the patient's ability to perform basic and IADLs (medication use, shopping, handling finances, using public transportation, preparing meals, using a telephone); mobility status, including the use of assistive devices; living situation (living alone and in what type of environment); and the patient's informal and formal support network. The baseline functional status serves as the benchmark to predict the patient's discharge functional status, especially in regard to basic ADLs, mobility, and clinical stability. This information is used to determine whether the patient should be discharged to home or to an alternate site by the time their acute medical problems have stabilized and they are ready for hospital discharge. In creating the trajectory of baseline to discharge functional status, patient-centered interventions are implemented as required, including physical therapy to help patients maintain mobility independence, occupational therapy to assess and improve self-care and home safety, medication review by the geriatrician, and nutritional services to prevent undernutrition and to restore nutritional health. The functional trajectory is reviewed daily, and interventions are augmented to achieve the anticipated hospital length of stay and discharge disposition. As an example, consider an 85-year-old woman admitted

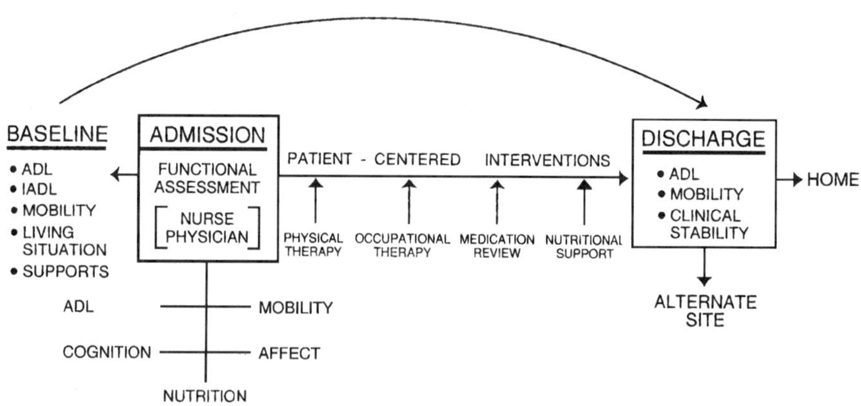

Figure 4 Clinical pathway: the functional trajectory.

from home where she lived alone with a diagnosis of community-acquired pneumonia. At admission the patient is mildly dehydrated and delirious. Her mobility is impaired and she is unable to walk or transfer without assistance. Her mood and affect are normal. At baseline she was independent in her performance of basic ADLs and had a mild gait impairment because of osteoarthritis of the knees but was able to carry out IADLs and enjoyed good informal support from family members. Her primary physician estimates a hospital length of stay of 4 days to adequately evaluate and treat the acute pneumonia, to improve oxygenation, and to prevent relapse of pneumonia. The interdisciplinary team reviews her physical functioning and nutritional status daily, and the geriatrician recommends modifications in the dosing of her medications. Because of delirium and undernutrition intravenous fluids are needed to maintain hydration and oral supplements are added to her diet. By the second day of hospitalization her fever has resolved and her mental status has begun to improve. Physical therapy is intensified: she receives both active and passive range of motion exercises and by the second day of hospitalization assisted ambulation with the use of a walker. By day 3 of the hospitalization, the patient is eating a pureed diet and is walking the hallway corridor using a walker, and her mental status has returned to baseline. At the time of planned hospital discharge she is clinically stable and able to carry out basic activities independently and has adequate mobility to permit safe discharge to her apartment. Because she lives alone, however, home care evaluation is indicated to determine home safety and the ability to comply with nutritional and medical recommendations and continue short-term physical therapy. If, however, the patient had continued to be delirious or physically impaired, discharge to home would be unsafe and the team would have intensified the patient-centered interventions, or plans for an alternate site transfer such as the subacute unit would be undertaken to continue the patient's active inpatient rehabilitation before her return home. In the functional trajectory, any barrier to achieving the desired outcome at the time of discharge is identified and acted on promptly by members of the team.

Although the functional trajectory was not specifically evaluated in the randomized clinical trial of ACE unit, it was the major clinical pathway used by the interdisciplinary team (24,25). Unlike disease-specific clinical pathways, the functional trajectory incorporates a biopsychosocial model of care. It has the potential to reduce hospital length of stay for elderly patients and to improve functional outcomes. The functional trajectory can be a quality indicator in the process of continuous quality improvement.

3. Patient Values and Comfort

Interdisciplinary collaboration can help foster patient comfort and expression of the patient's personal values. (See also Chapter 2.) Health plans are required to ascertain whether patients have advance directives, either a living will or a durable power of attorney for health care, and to include copies of them in the medical record. (See also Chapter 5.) The patient's wishes should be sought for end-of-life care, including cardiopulmonary resuscitation, intensive care, or nutritional support in the event of acute or end-stage illness. Advance directives should be addressed and discussed with patients early in the course of their hospitalization. When advance directives are not available and patients lack medical decision-making capacity, family meetings should be held to review the patient's diagnosis, prognosis, and plans for therapeutic interventions. The need for a review of the patient's values is most evident when potentially futile but life-extending interventions such as intubation of patients with end-stage respiratory failure, or hemodialysis for patients with irreversible uremia are being entertained.

The process of informing and educating patients and their families is enhanced by the use of computer technologies: copies of their diagnostic evaluation, laboratory studies, discharge medications, and information sheets should be provided to them at discharge. From the hospital patients can be linked to any of the services included in the continuum of care offered at the medical center, and high-risk patients can be tracked by case managers. Personal comfort should be addressed. Privacy and quiet at night are important. Family members should be allowed to visit patients even during the nonvisiting hours, and patients should be allowed to dress in their clothes and to bring cherished objects from home. A normal bowel and bladder regimen is maintained with a toileting schedule, a bedside commode, or a urinal for men. Often, fiber supplements or hyperosmolar laxatives (e.g., lactulose) are needed to prevent fecal impaction in patients who are immobile or taking drugs with anticholinergic properties. Prophylactic anticoagulation with unfractionated heparin may prevent deep venous thrombosis in patients with immobility, cancer, recent surgery, heart failure, or a past history of deep vein thrombosis.

F. Alternatives to Hospitalization

The continuum of care of the geriatric medical center creates the opportunity to avoid hospitalization except for patients who need invasive therapies or are unable to be treated at home. In some instances the patient may be initially evaluated in the emergency department or observation unit and briefly hospitalized for an intervention before being discharged to home hospital care. A model of home hospitalization developed in Israel includes therapies directed at the optimization of medical and pharmacological care, treatment of pressure ulcers and wounds, intravenous therapy, enteral feeding by gastrostomy or nasogastric tube, and rehabilitation and supportive therapy for patients with stroke or terminal illnesses (43). Significant cost savings have been identified in clinical studies of patients who have received home hospitalization versus usual care.

In the United States a different version of the home hospital is being developed (44). In this model older persons who face possible acute hospital admission with selected acute medical conditions are identified and brought directly home to receive their medical care. The patient may be initially seen in the emergency department or at home by a physician. The physician makes daily home visits and works closely with nurses who provide direct supervision for the initial part of the home hospital treatment. Although definitive trials of the American model have not been completed, home hospitalization provides an intriguing alternative to inpatient hospitalization for patients who prefer home care and have adequate support services.

III. SUMMARY

The American population is aging, and the proportion of elderly patients in nonfederal hospitals continues to increase even though overall hospital admission rates have declined since the introduction of the Medicare Prospective Payment System. As disease acuity increases and a greater array of technologies and palliative interventions become available to older patients, the importance of efficient and cost-effective treatments becomes magnified. The continuum of care provided at geriatric medical centers will emphasize early detection of patients at risk for functional decline, repeated use of hospital emergency departments, and unplanned hospital readmissions and will link high-risk patients to hospital-based and affiliated medical services, including, when appropriate, subacute units, day hospitals, day care centers, and geriatric assessment centers. Patients will likely move horizontally across hospital-based services. The intensity of patient interventions will be based on the patient's expressed wishes or advance directives and will be monitored through clinical pathways such as the functional trajectory. Health professionals confront the challenge of optimizing the patient's quality of life while constantly striving to reduce the hospital length of stay and costs of care. The challenge will be met through interdisciplinary care, the expansion of computerized information systems, and the efficient access to the subsystems in the continuum of care.

REFERENCES

1. Graves EJ, Gillum BS. National Hospital Discharge Survey: Annual Summary, 1994. National Center for Health Statistics. Vital Health Stat 1997;13:128.
2. Schappert SM. National Hospital Ambulatory Medical Care Survey: 1992 emergency department summary. National Center for Health Statistics. Vital Health Stat 1997;13:125.

3. Ackermann RJ, Kemle KA, Vogel RL, Griffin RC. Emergency department use by nursing home residents. Ann Emerg Med 1998;31:749–757.
4. Wolinsky FD, Stump TE, Johnson RJ. Hospital utilization profiles among older adults over time: consistency and volume among survivors and decedents. J Gerontol (Soc Sci) 1995;50B:S88–S100.
5. Boult C, Dowd B, McCaffrey D, Boult L, Hernadez R, Krulewitch H. Screening elders for risk of hospital admission. J Am Geriatr Soc 1993;41:811–817.
6. Perls TT, Wood ER. Acute care costs of the oldest old: they cost less, their care intensity is less, and they go to non-teaching hospitals. Arch Intern Med 1996;156: 754–760.
7. Sagar MA, Franke T, Inouye SK, Landefeld CS, Morgan TM, Rudberg MA, Siebens H, Winograd CH. Functional outcomes of acute medical illness and hospitalization in older persons. Arch Intern Med 1996;156:645–652.
8. Ferucci L, Guralnik JM, Pahor M, Corti MC, Havlik RJ. Hospital diagnosis, medical charges, and nursing home admissions in the year when older persons become severely disabled. JAMA 1997;277:728–734.
9. Inouye SK, Peduzzi PN, Robinson JT, Hughes JS, Horwitz RI, Concato J. Importance of functional measures in predicting mortality among older hospitalized patients. JAMA 1998;279:1187–1193.
10. Thom DH, Haan MN, Van Den Eeden SK. Medically recognized urinary incontinence and risks of hospitalization, nursing home admission and mortality. Age Ageing 1997;26:367–374.
11. Palmer RM, Counsell S, Landefeld CS. Clinical intervention trials: the ACE unit. Clin Geriatr Med 1998;14:831–849.
12. Riedinger JL, Robbins LJ. Prevention of iatrogenic illness: adverse drug reactions and nosocomial infections in hospitalized older adults. Clin Geriatr Med 1998;14: 681–698.
13. Lefevre F, Feinglass J, Potts S, Souglin L, Yarnold P, Mratin GJ, Webster JR. Iatrogenic complications in high-risk, elderly patients. Arch Intern Med 1992;152:2074–2080.
14. Inouye SK. Delirium in hospitalized older patients. Clin Geriatr Med 1998;14:745–764.
15. Mahoney JE. Immobility and falls. Clin Geriatr Med 1998;14:699–726.
16. Whitehead C, Finucane P. Malnutrition in elderly people. Aust NZ J Med 1997;27: 68–74.
17. Incaldi RA, Jemma A, Capparella O, Cipriani L, Ladi F, Carbonin PU. Energy intake and in-hospital starvation: A clinically relevant relationship. Arch Intern Med 1996; 156:425–429.
18. Potter J, Langhorne P, Roberts M. Routine protein energy supplementation in adults: systematic review. BMJ 1998;317:495–501.
19. Miller DL, Bolla LR. Patient values: the guide to medical decision making. Clin Geriatr Med 1998;14:813–829.
20. Boult C, Boult L, Pacala JT. Systems for care of older populations of the future. J Am Geriatr Soc 1998;46:499–505.
21. Solomon GF. Physiological responses to environmental design: understanding psychoneuroimmunology (PNI) and its application for health care. J Health Care Design 1996;8:79–83.

22. Stoller JK. A physicians view of hospital design: the impact of verticality on interaction. Architecture 1988;12:121–122.
23. Lazzaro PP. Health care system changes and their effect on design and construction. Health Care Facilities Management Series 1995;11:1–9.
24. Palmer RM, Landefeld CS, Kresevic D, Kowal J. A medical unit for acute care of the elderly. J Am Geriatr Soc 1994;42:545–552.
25. Landefeld CS, Palmer RM, Kresevic D. A randomized trial of care in a hospital medical unit especially designed to improve the functional outcomes of acutely ill older patients. N Engl J Med 1995;332:1338–1344.
26. McCusker J, Bellavance F, Cardin S, Trepanier S. Screening for geriatric problems in the emergency department: reliability and validity. Identification of Seniors at Risk (ISAR) Steering Committee. Acad Emerg Med 1998;5:883–893.
27. Roberts RR, Zalenski RJ, Mensah EK, Rydman RJ, Ciavarella G, Gussow L, Das K, Kampe LM, Dickover B, McDermott MF, Hart A, Straus HE, Murphy DG, Rao R. Costs of an emergency department-based accelerated diagnostic protocol vs. hospitalization in patients with chest pain: a randomized controlled trial. JAMA 1997; 278:1670–1676.
28. Brillman J, Mathers-Dunbar L, Graff L, Joseph T, Leikin JB, Schultz C, Severance HW, Werne C. Management of observations units. Ann Emerg Med 1995;25:823–830.
29. Butler J, Hanumanthu S, Chomsky B, Wilson JR. Frequency of low-risk hospital admissions for heart failure. Am J Cardiol 1998;81:41–44.
30. Morishita L, Siu AL, Wang RT, Oken C, Cadogan MP, Schwartzman L. Comprehensive geriatric care in a day hospital: a demonstration of the British model in the United States. Gerontologist 1989;29:336–340.
31. Siu AL, Morishita L, Blaustein J. Comprehensive geriatric assessment in a day hospital. J Am Geriatr Soc 1994;42:1094–1099.
32. Stuck AE, Siu AL, Wieland GD, Adams J, Rubenstein LZ. Comprehensive geriatric assessment: a meta-analysis of controlled trials. Lancet 1993;342:1032–1036.
33. Welch HG, Wennberg DE, Welch WP. The use of Medicare home health care services. N Engl J Med 1996;335:324–329.
34. Solomon DH, Wagner DR, Marenberg ME, Acampora D, Cooney LM, Inouye SK. Predictors of formal home health care use in elderly patients after hospitalization. J Am Geriatr Soc 1993;481:961–966.
35. Stewart S, Pearson S, Horowitz JD. Effects of a home based intervention among patients with congestive heart failure discharged from acute hospital care. Arch Intern Med 1998;158:1067–1072.
36. Evans RS, Pestotnik SL, Classen DC, Clemmer TP, Weaver LK, Orme JF, Lloyd JF, Burke JP. A computer-assisted management program for antibiotics and other anti-infective agents. N Engl J Med 1998;338:232–238.
37. Bates DW, Leape LL, Cullen DJ, Laird N, Petersen LA, Teich JM, Burdick E. Hickey M, Kleefield S, Seha V, Vander Bleit M, Seger DL. Effect of computerized physician order entry and a team intervention on prevention of serious medication errors. JAMA 1998;280:1311–1316.
38. Grigsby J, Sanders JH. Telemedicine: where it is and where it's going. Ann Intern Med 1998;129:123–127.

39. Wachter RM, Goldman L. The emerging role of ''hospitalists'' in the American health care system. N Engl J Med 1996;335:514–517.
40. Inouye SK, Acampora D, Miller RL, Fulmer T, Hurst LD, Cooney LM. The Yale geriatric care program: a model of care to prevent functional decline in hospitalized elderly patients. J Am Geriatr Soc 1993;481:1345–1352.
41. Reuben DB, Borok GM, Wolde-Tsadik G, Ershoff DH, Fishman LK, Ambrosini BL, Liu Y, Rubenstein LZ, Beck JC. A randomized trial of comprehensive geriatric assessment in the care of hospitalized patients. N Engl J Med 1995;332:1345–1350.
42. Ronning OM, Guldvog B. Stroke units versus general medical wards, I: 12- and 18-month survival. A randomized, controlled trial. Stroke 1998;29:58–62.
43. Stessman J, Ginsberg G, Hammerman-Rozenberg R, Friedman R, Ronen D, Israeli A, Cohen A. Decreased hospital utilization by older adults attributable to a home hospitalization program. J Am Geriatr Soc 1996;44:591–598.
44. Leff B, Burton JR. Future directions: alternative approaches to traditional hospital care—home hospital. Clin Geriatr Med 1998;14:851–861.

Index

About the Editors

THOMAS T. YOSHIKAWA is Professor of Medicine at Charles R. Drew University of Medicine and Science, and Martin Luther King, Jr.–Charles R. Drew Medical Center, Los Angeles, California. The coauthor or coeditor of several books, including *Antimicrobial Therapy in the Elderly Patient* (Marcel Dekker, Inc.), he is a Fellow of the Infectious Diseases Society of America, the Gerontological Society of America, and the American College of Physicians, and a member of the American Geriatrics Society, the American Federation for Medical Research, and the American Society for Microbiology. Dr. Yoshikawa received the M.D. degree (1966) from the University of Michigan, Ann Arbor.

DEAN C. NORMAN is Chief of Staff at the Department of Veterans Affairs (VA) Greater Los Angeles Healthcare System, California, and Adjunct Professor of Medicine at the University of California, Los Angeles, School of Medicine. He is a member of the Gerontological Society of America, the Infectious Diseases Society of America, the American Geriatrics Society, and the American Federation for Medical Research, among other organizations. He is the coeditor of *Antimicrobial Therapy in the Elderly Patient* (Marcel Dekker, Inc.) and the author or coauthor of over 120 professional papers, book chapters, and abstracts. Dr. Norman received the M.D. degree (1976) from the University of California at Los Angeles.